SEXUAL ABUSE – BREAKING THE SILENCE

Edited by **Ersi Abacı Kalfoğlu**
and **Rehat Faikoğlu**

Sexual Abuse – Breaking the Silence
Edited by Ersi Abacı Kalfoğlu and Rehat Faikoğlu

Published by InTech

Janeza Trdine 9, 51000 Rijeka, Croatia

Publishing Process Manager Dejan Grgur

Technical Editor Teodora Smiljanic

Cover Designer InTech Design Team

Additional hard copies can be obtained from orders@intechopen.com

Sexual Abuse – Breaking the Silence, Edited by Ersi Abacı Kalfoğlu and Rehat Faikoğlu
p. cm.
ISBN 978-953-51-0425-4

For EU product safety concerns:
IN TECH d.o.o., Prolaz Marije Krucifikse Kozulić 3, 51000 Rijeka, Croatia,
info@intechopen.com or visit our website at intechopen.com.

Meet the editors

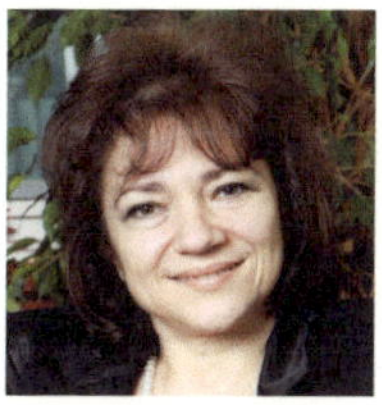

Professor Ersi Abacı Kalfoğlu got her PhD in forensic sciences, following a graduate degree in medical biochemistry. She taught at the Institute of Legal Medicine and Forensic Sciences, Istanbul University, and was the primary investigator of the Forensic Haemogenetics Department for 20 years. Professor Kalfoğlu has spent the last years of her career specializing in sexual abuse and its consequences. She is the author of numerous articles on the subject, published in English and Turkish Scientific Journals. Being aware of the difficulties that sexual assault victims and survivors are facing, she founded a centre for sexual assault victims in Turkey, which now operates in Istanbul, under Yeni Yüzyil University where she is the Dean of the Faculty of Health Sciences.

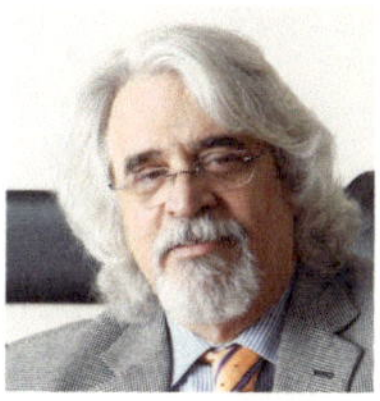

Assoc. Professor Rehat Faikoğlu received his medical degree from the Cerrahpasa Medical Faculty and specialized in Obstetrics and Gynaecology in Istanbul. His experience in examining cases of sexual assault and his awareness of the current situation on that issue directed his research area to this specific topic. He has various publications both in English and Turkish and organizes meetings on this topic in Turkey. He is currently the director of the Sexual Assault Crisis Center at Yeni Yüzyil University and the Director of the Department of Nursing at the same University.

Contents

Preface

Sexual assault can be considered as expression of aggression through sex. This in turn can have serious negative effects on a survivor's social and occupational functioning. Unfortunately, it has been experienced in all cultures for centuries. The accumulation of scientific data about this fact, though, is quite new. We started learning about the ways that women, men, and children are victimized and our methods of disclosing this victimization only started since 1970. In reality, we have very limited knowledge of the actual issue.

Although the number of published research papers has been very high over the last years and the scientific methodology is quite reliable, the results are far from reflecting the truth, because the actual number of cases is enormous compared to what is reported. Victims do not disclose the assault, and they prefer silence.

There are numerous reasons for this kind of refusal, which differ based on the cultural and social environment of the assaulted. It seems that the rhetoric of 'what we know is only the tip of the iceberg' seems to reflect reality. Shame and embarrassment, self blame, fear of exposure, fear of the legal system and the court procedures are some of the international reasons that prevent thousands of sexual assault survivors from reporting the assault.

That is certainly a very serious multidimensional problem, the solution of which is complicated. Various parties have to help in facilitating the solution by approaching the issue from their specific angle.

The institutional approach should involve all those establishments that are involved in a sexual assault case identification and victim rehabilitation. The victims generally complain about re-victimization following the disclosure of an assault. This notion has to be completely erased. How can we achieve that? The answer is in a correct and effective coordination of the various parties. Coping with sexual assault is a truly multidisciplinary process. Lawyers, judges, doctors, nurses, psychologists, psychiatrists and pediatricians are involved and they all have to be educated on the issue of dealing with sexual assault. Besides, the law enforcement has to be aware of that interdisciplinary need. In any case, an organized, well informed group of people must deal with the victims in a way that will ensure that they will not be hurt anymore.

Secondly, the victims themselves, the vulnerable people but also the general public should be aware of the possibility of sexual assault. Awareness-raising activities should be developed according to various age groups and specific policies should be applied. A real success of such an awareness-raising activity can be the empowerment of the survivors. Their fear may be changed to an accomplishment because following their disclosure, others in the community may be protected from becoming victims.

It is known that if the trauma of sexual assault is left unrecognized and unaddressed, a cycle of re-traumatization will always be a high possibility. Therefore, once the case is disclosed or found out, a rehabilitation strategy has to be systematized and psychologists have to be seriously involved.

It is also known that there is a risk of developing a perpetrator from a sexual assault victim if not treated properly.

We can only have progress in this issue in the light of correctly processed and analyzed scientific data.

This book has been organized on that specific approach, by compiling the scientific work of very well-known scientists from all over the world. Three different sections included three different aspects of the issue.

The first part examined the psychological victimization of sexual assault. Sexual assault can be considered as an articulation of aggression through sex which can impair. Sexual assault has been associated with post traumatic stress disorder that may be characterized by mood disorders, anxiety disorders, conduct disorders, substance abuse, and suicidal behaviors, chronic headaches, maladaptive sexual behaviors, dissociative behaviors, depression, alcoholism, panic disorder and social phobia, chronic fatigue, gradually developing to asthma and cardiovascular problems and even self-injurious or suicidal behaviors.

Is there a possibility for a sexual abuse survivor to use this experience in a positively transformative way? Scientists today say yes. You can find an analytical explanation of this approach in the pages of this book.

Prisons are places where extremely valuable information can be collected. The largely neglected prison population is thoroughly analyzed and the information is shared with us in this book.

The traumatic experiences in childhood may be converted to organic diseases later in life and the problem is that sexual assault survivors are generally resistant to any kind of treatment because they believe that they do not deserve such care. Thus we have to find ways to approach them effectively. This book, in its second section, deals with this physiological aspect of sexual abuse.

You will find the Zambian approach in this book interesting which includes different risk factors like possible HIV infection following sexual assault. The female children that are considered to be the most vulnerable individuals for sexual assault also have a high risk of HIV infection. This brings about a serious public health problem.

We also have to have in mind that cultural differences require different strategic plans for coping with this issue. Cultural factors influence individuals' worldviews and shape the way they see the world and their place in it. It shapes the way meanings are given to experiences and they are passed between individual groups and generations. One solution may not necessarily be suitable for all cases. The attitude of different communities may lead to the cover-up of sex crimes at the expense of victims. The third section of this book includes different attitudes in coping with sexual assault based on different cultural backgrounds.

We all hope that this book will open a debate on sexual assault for future practice and policy and that it will be a step forward to 'break the silence'.

Ersi Abacı Kalfoğlu
Dean of the Faculty of Health Sciences,
Yeni Yüzyil University,
Turkey

Rehat Faikoğlu
Director of the Sexual Assault Crisis Center,
Director of the Department of Nursing,
Yeni Yüzyil University,
Turkey

Part 1

The Psychology of Sexual Victimization

1

A Review of Childhood Abuse Questionnaires and Suggested Treatment Approaches

Donald J. Levis
Binghamton University (SUNY)
USA

1. Introduction

The focus of this chapter is on providing a review of childhood sexual abuse, physical abuse and combined abuse assessment questionnaires. Prevalence rates of childhood abuse in the United States will also be provided along with symptom and diagnostic correlates found to be associated with a childhood history of abuse. The following seven abuse screens are reviewed. (1) The Rape Aftermath Symptom Test; (2) The Scarlett O'Hara v. MMPI Configuration; (3) The Child Abuse and Trauma Scale; (4) The Childhood Trauma Questionnaire; (5) The Trauma Symptom Checklist; (6) The Trauma Symptom Inventory; and (7) The Binghamton Abuse Screen. Finally, a brief discussion of two recommended adult childhood abuse survivor treatment approaches, cognitive behavior therapy and prolonged exposure techniques will be provided.

2. The prevalence of childhood abuse

Demause (1991) found following a comprehensive review of the literature that agreement exists between social scientists and historians that probation against incest within the immediate family can be found in every known culture. He concluded that it is incest and related forms of childhood abuse itself, not the absence of incest, which represents the true universal statement. Demause's review found that statistical reviews of child molestation in the United States only go back to 1929. He noted that the official incidence figures from the American Humane Association, working from reports from child protective agencies, estimated only 7,000 incidents of child abuse occurred in the United States for 1976. These estimates rose steadily to 113,000 incidents for 1985, which at that time, represented under one percent of American children. It was not until the late 1970's and early 1980's that careful studies began to emerge with samples large enough to warrant statistical analysis.

Once these studies were published, the mental health field was altered to the alarming, frequent and disturbing prevalence rates of childhood sexual abuse (CSA) and physical abuse (CPA) in our society. Estimates were made that one in five women and one in eleven men had experienced some form of childhood abuse (CA) prior to the age of eighteen (Doyle-Peters, Wyatt & Finkelhor, 1986; Wyatt & Doyle-Peters, 1986; Martin, Jesse, Romans, Mullen, & O'Shea, 1993). The magnitude of these earlier reported (CA) prevalence rates were confirmed by later research. For example, Finkelhor, Hotaling, Lewis & Smith (1990) suggested that as many as 27% of all women and 16% of men have experienced some form of childhood abuse. Additional data estimated the prevalence rate of (CSA) in outpatient populations to be 28% (Coverdale & Turboth, 2000) and 40% of in-patient populations (Jacobson 1990). More recent data from the Fourth National Incident of Child Abuse and Neglect found that 58% of the 533,300 children studied suffered from childhood physical abuse (CPA) and 24% from CSA. The projection was made that one out of 58 children in the U.S. will experience some form of maltreatment within a given year (Sedlak, Mittenberg, Basina, Petla, McPherson, Green & Li, S., 2010).

Additional reports on the prevalence of CPA suggest that 10 to 20% in non-clinical community samples experience physical abuse (Gelles & Straus, 1987), while in a clinical population, CPA prevalence has been estimated at 38% in outpatient populations and 49% in inpatient populations (Jacobson, 1989). These findings were supported by Macmillan et. al (1997) findings that 21% of women and 31.2% of men have experienced some form of CPA. Furthermore, it appears that despite changes in social policy aimed at combating incidences of CPA, the prevalence of CPA is not evidencing any significant change (Kunston & Selner, 1994).

It should be recognized that CPA and CSA often co-exist simultaneously and that there are commonalities associated with CPA and CSA (Briere & Runtz, 1990; Browne & Finklehor, 1986; Rosenberg 1987. Most types of maltreatment do occur in the presence of other types of abuse, especially among those who request services as adults (Briere, 1992b). In a study by Surrey, Swett, Michael & Levin (1990), fifty-six (74%) of the seventy-six outpatient women reported an episode of either CPA or CSA before the age of 18. Of these participants, twenty-eight (37%) reported both kinds of abuse compared to twelve (16%) women who reported CSA only and sixteen women (21%) who reported CPA only. In other studies, the occurrences of combined abuse in families in treatment for CSA, was estimated to be 19.7% (Daro, 1988). Similarly, combined abuse prevalence in female non-clinical populations has been estimated to be 17% (Wind & Silvern, 1992). It is evident from these data that it is not uncommon for the occurrence of CSA and CPA to occur in the presence of each other.

3. Symptom and diagnostic correlates with a history of childhood abuse

The association between long-term psychological problems and CSA and CPA has also been well documented. A comparison between individuals with a reported history of childhood abuse with those who reported no history of abuse, indicate that those with a history of abuse are at greater risk for developing psychological disorders (Mullen, Martin, Anderson, Romans, and Herbson, 1996; Polusny, & Follett, 1995; Malinowsky-Rummel & Hansen 1993; Wind & Silvern 1992), for developing more severe symptomatology (Surrey, Swett, Michaels, & Levin, 1990) and for receiving multiple diagnosis (Briere & Runtz, 1990).

Childhood abuse has been associated with the development and diagnosis of Post Traumatic Stress Disorder (PTSD) (Kendall-Tachett 2000); Zlotnick, Mattia, & Zimmerman 2001). In a study examining adults with CSA histories, Rodriguez, Ryan, Rowan & Foy (1996) reported that 72% of their sample met full DSM-III criteria for current PTSD, while 86% met criteria for lifetime PTSD. Rowan, Foy, Rodriguez, & Ryan (1994) found that of 47 adults who disclosed histories of CSA, 69% met full DSM-III criteria for PTSD, while another 19% met criteria for partial PTSD. Furthermore, CSA has been associated with mood disorders, anxiety disorders, conduct disorders, substance abuse disorders, suicidal behaviors (Fergusson, Horwood & Lynesky, 1996); and with borderline personality disorder

(Zlotnick, Mattia, & Zimmerman, 2001), chronic headaches (Domino & Haber, 1987), maladaptive sexual behavior (Briere & Runtz, 1990); irritable bowel syndrome (Walker, Katon, Roy-Byrne, Jemelka & Russo 1993), dissociative behaviors (Lipschitz, Kaplan, Sorkenn, Chorney, & Asnis, 1996), depression, alcoholism, panic disorder, and social phobia (Dinwiddle et al, 2000), chronic, fatigue, asthma, and cardiovascular problems (Romans, Belaise, Martin, Morris & Raffe, 2002), increased pain and more surgical procedures (Finestone, et al., 2000).

Similarly, CPA has been associated with an increase in long-term symptomatology, including self-injurious and suicidal behaviors and physiological and emotional problems such as somatization, anxiety, depression, dissociation, and psychoses (Malinoskey-Rummell & Hansen, 1993). Physical abuse has also been associated with more pain, increased incidence of non-GI-somatic symptoms, more surgeries, and poorer functional status (Lesserman et al. 1996). Additionally, it has been associated with mental retardation (Buchanan & Oliver, 1997), chronic headache (Domino & Haber, 1987), aggression toward others (Briere & Runtz, 1990), substance abuse (Westermeyer J., Wahmanholm, K., & Turas, 2001) and purging (Perkins, Luster, & Jank, 2002).

Given the above established findings, it is disconcerting that many clinicians still fail to adequately assess and consider in their development of a treatment plan that a potential link between the patient's presenting problem and a history of childhood abuse may exist (Agar, Read, & Bish, 2002; Lothian & Read, 2002). Even if an assessment of CSA or CPA is conducted in the initial intake, too often the response of "no abuse" by the patient is accepted as being accurate, despite the clinical findings from delayed memory recovery patients that evidence for an abuse history often does not emerge until extensive treatment has been conducted (Bell & Belicki, 1998).

Adding to the difficulty of obtaining an accurate initial assessment of CSA or CPA is the finding that adult survivors of childhood abuse often are reluctant to be honest due to their concern regarding the social stigma attached to their abuse or the feeling of guilt or intense fear associated with revealing the secret and not being believed (Curtis, 1976; Layman, Gidy, & Lynn 1996). Other inhibiting factors impeding abuse, the victim's memory recall is the presence of a strong cognitive defense structure of denial, including amnesia (Briere, & Contes 1991; Herman & Schatnow 1987; Williams (1994) and malingering (Briere, 1989, 1992a, 1992b).

Finally, some resistance by practitioners to deal with the content of abusive trauma may exist because of the difficulty of having to witness the patient's pain in re-experiencing their historical trauma or in their concerns that the memories uncovered are false and may subject them to legal ramifications.

Clinicians should not be overly concerned about the elicitation of false memories, (Robbin 1995) reports that 75% of the studies on false memory did not manufacture false memories in the experimental situation despite the implicit pressure to produce one. From the present authors' viewpoint, the abundance of cognitive research on the false memory topic has little bearing on the clinical field, largely because experimental studies on false memories have not been conducted with a clinical abuse population (see Levis 1999).

However, as Briere (1992a) warned, the possibility exists that abuse reports could reflect fantasies, delusions, or intentional misinterpretations for secondary gain. Nevertheless, it is this author's opinion that if abuse trauma memories are forthcoming, one should never agree they are factual. This responsibility must be left up to patients to decide what's true and what's not true. The key responsibility of the therapist is to determine whether the release and extinction of the affect associated with a reported trauma leads to therapeutic gains. It has been my extensive experience (30 years) from providing treatment for adult survivors of childhood abuse that it does, a finding I am sure can be confirmed by many other therapists who treat abused patients. Finally, Briere's (1992b) conclusion is correct that most researchers in the area of child abuse agree that only a small proportion of people who describe abuse experiences make them up.

Although the establishment of external corroboration of reported abuse memory recovery is desirable, it is difficult to achieve (Briere, 1992a), some success in achieving this objective has been reported (e.g., Herman & Schatzow 1987); Feldman-Summers & Pope 1994). For example, Herman & Schatzow (1987) had a group therapy treatment of CSA survivors and encouraged them to obtain corroborating information from internal sources (e.g., sibling, family memories, medical records, court proceedings, etc.). They found that 39 out of their 53 group participants (74%) found some external confirmatory evidence. Although such evidence is not definitive, it represents a first step in the attempt to provide some form of external corroboration.

4. Childhood abuse assessment questionnaires

To encourage the practitioners to further explore the possibility that an abuse history may exist in a given patient, a number of time efficient childhood abuse instruments have been developed to facilitate this objective. Unfortunately, the vast majority of the childhood trauma questionnaires reviewed provide either no or limited psychometric support. Of the numerous questionnaires reviewed, seven were selected for review which have been frequently adopted and have provided adequate psychometric support. They are as follows: (1) The Rape Aftermath Symptom Test; (2) The Scarlett O'Hara VMMPI Configuration; (3) The Child Abuse and Trauma Scale; (4) The Childhood Trauma Questionnaire; (5) The Trauma Symptom Checklist; (6) The Trauma Symptom Inventory; and (7) The Binghamton Childhood Abuse Screen.

The first two of the above inventories were not specifically designed to assess childhood abuse, but rather were designed to assess events frequently associated with a history of abuse (e.g., rape and parental alcoholism). The remaining five questionnaires were specifically designed to assess an abusive childhood history. In the conduction of this review, I would like to acknowledge the review contribution provided by two of my former students, Timothy Lock (1997) and Brian Castelda (2003).

The format adapted for these reviews is to first provide a basic description of the questionnaire, followed by an assessment of the inventories reliability, criterion related validity, convergent validity, discriminate validity, and criterion validity.

1. The Rape Aftermath Symptom Test (RAST)

This test constructed by Kirpatrick (1988) is a 70 item self report inventory comprising items designed to assess the presence of psychological symptoms and potentially fear producing stimuli. The RAST was developed using a limited sample size of 137 rape survivors and 139 non-abused victims. According to standards suggested by Devellis (1991), a sample size greater than 300 participants is needed. Nevertheless, the RAST has provided good test-retest reliability with non-rape victims (r = .95 at 2.5 month intervals) and good internal consistency reliability (α = .95). Criterion related validity was determined by discriminating statistically between scores of non-rape victims and rape victims at 6 to 21 days, 3 months, 6 months, and at 1, 2, and 3 years past the rape experience (Kirpatrick 1988; Resnick, Kirpatrick, & Lizovashky, 1991).

The psychometric properties of the RAST could be improved by increasing its validation size and by establishing convergent and discriminatory validity. Since the RAST, items are related to a rape experience, it directs relevance to the assessment of childhood abuse is somewhat limited.

2. The Scarlett O'Hara VMMPI Configuration

Goldwater & Duffy (1990) found that their Minnesota Multiphasic Inventory (MMPI) V configuration is suggestive of parental alcoholism which is frequently found in the history of childhood abused victims. Their "V" configuration refers to the MMPI scales 4 and 6 being elevated with T-scores of 65 or above, and scale 5 falling at least 30 T-scores below scales 4 and 6.

The test-retest reliability of the subscales used in the Scarlett O'Hara V configuration are as follows: Scale 4 r = .79, α = .60, 5 r = .73; α = .37; scale 6 r = .58, α = .34 (Hathaway McKinley, 1989). Criterion related validity was determined by the test ability to discriminate between participants with a history of abuse (or an alcoholic parent) and non-abuse. Histories of abuse or parental alcoholism were extracted from patients' hospital charts after discharge. The sample size evaluated consisted of 79 adult female inpatients. A key advantage of the Scarlett O'Hara V MMPI configuration is the ability to add additional information on personality structure and psychopathology. However, the test was developed using a small and restricted sample size. Further, the test-retest and/or internal consistency reliability for some of the scales are lower than desired. Finally, the presence of a parental history of alcoholism does not in and of itself provide any direct confirmation that the parental offspring have been subjected to an abusive childhood history. It simply represents a hypothesis in need of further confirmation.

3. The Childhood Abuse and Trauma Scale (CAT)

This questionnaire, developed by Sanders & Becker-Lausen (1995), was initially created as a research scale but later it was considered to be a useful tool in clinical assessment as an initial screening instrument. The scale consists of thirty-eight items to assess various forms of childhood physical, sexual, and maltreatment abuse. Part of the research objective of the scale was to combat respondent tendencies toward giving socially desirable responses. To achieve this objective, the scale was made up of general questions about the frequency of different childhood abuse experiences while allowing the respondent to determine his own evaluation of the severity of the stress experiences. Internal consistency of the entire CAT, as reflected in Cronbade's alpha was established to be .90. Test-retest reliability, determined over 6-8 weeks intervals, was .89. Besides measures of reliability, convergent validity of the CAT has been demonstrated in establishing correlations with dissociation (r = .29). The CAT also scored higher when a group diagnosed with Multiple Personality Disorder was compared to a normative sample (Sanders & Becker-Lausen, 1995).

The examination of the factor structure of the CAT revealed three factors; negativity of the home environment, sexual abuse; and punishment which accounted for 38% of the overall variance. Test-retest reliability of the subscales proved moderate with measures ranging from $\underline{r}$ = .71 to $\underline{r}$ = .91. However, males and females responded with significant differences on the sexual abuse subscale with females scoring twice as high which may reflect an over sensitivity to female responses. Furthermore, Kent & Waller (1998) reported that the inter-correlations between the scores on the subscales were strong with exception to the associations between abuse score and other scales. These correlations suggest that the CAT's subscales are not measuring entirely different constructs. Despite the CAT establishment of good reliability and other supporting psychometric data, to the author's knowledge, no studies have established criterion-related validity or have established its relationship to other abuse measures. Finally, the questionnaire items are relatively face-valid and susceptible to malingering.

4. The Childhood Trauma Questionnaire (CTQ)

The primary objective of the CTQ was to design an instrument which would allow for a comparison for both clinical and research purposes of a broad range of abuse and neglect experiences (Bernstein, Fink, Handelsman, Foote, Lovejoy, Wenzel, Sapareto & Ruggiero, 1994). The CTQ is a 70-item self-report questionnaire constructed from the author's extensive review of the literature which assess retrospectively childhood experience of abuse and neglect including aspects of their childhood rearing environment. Items are rated using a 5-point Likert-type scale.

The CTQ test-retest reliability was found to be .88 after an average interval of 3.6 months. A factor analysis of the CTQ yielded four factors accounting for 47.6% variance which were labeled physical and emotional abuse, emotional neglect, sexual abuse, and physical abuse. Convergent validity was assessed by correlating the CTQ with the Childhood Trauma Inventory (CTI) (Bernstein et al., 1994). After controlling for the effects of general maltreatment, the relation between the two sets of abuse rating was highly specific: CTQ sexual abuse was associated only with CTI sexual abuse and CTQ physical and emotional abuse was associated only with CTI physical abuse.

The CTQ has also shown good discriminent validity with measures of verbal intelligence and social desirability ($r < .10$ for all correlations; Bernstein et al., 1994) and convergent validity with the Traumatic Events Questionnaire - Adolescents (Weinzer & Lipshitz, 1997); the Traumatic History Screen (Allen, Huntoon & Evans, 1999); and other instruments designed to identify childhood maltreatment (Lipshitz, Bernstein, Wagner, & Southwick, 1999).

In addition, Bernstein, Ahluvalia, Pogge & Hanedelsman (1997) reported that CTQ cut-off scores have been devised for identifying cases of childhood abuse and neglect. In an adolescent psychiatric sample, a cut-off score of 9 on the Sexual Abuse factor had a sensitivity of .86 and specificity of .76 when therapists' ratings of sexual abuse were used as a criterion measure. Similarly, when using therapist's ratings of physical abuse as a criterion measure, a cut-off score of 12 on the physical abuse factor had a sensitivity of .82 and as specificity of .73.

Despite the widespread use of the CTQ and its supporting psychometric data, critics have pointed out that the original validation study examining convergence between the CTQ and CTI has shortcomings. For example, Bursten (1995) highlights the relative unimportance of the correlation between two forms of almost identical abuse measures and points out that these correlations tell us little of the questionnaire's ability to discriminate abuse victims. Bursten also criticized Bernstein et al. (1994) study for the author's use of the CIQ in their validation study because it was experimental and undergoing validation. Lastly, Bursten notes that aside from adolescent psychiatric patients, no normative data exists for the CTQ that would allow for its use in a clinical setting. Nevertheless, the CTQ shows considerable promise and would profit from further validation.

5. The Trauma Symptom Checklist TSC-40

The TSC-40 appears to be the most popular childhood abuse questionnaire available (Castelda, 2003) perhaps in part because of extensive research history and strong psychometric support. TSC-40 was developed from the Trauma symptom Checklist - TSC-33 (Briere & Runtz, 1989) which was developed to assess the impact of trauma especially the long-term effects of CSA. The emphasis was on gaining a more complete understanding of the precise patterns of symptomatology associated with a history of CSA (Gold, Milan, Mayall & Johnson, 1994). Participants respond to items by rating how often they had experienced each in the last two months (0 = never, 4 = very often. In a sample of woman at a crisis intervention clinic, TSC-33 was found to be internally consistent, alpha = .89 capable of correctly identifying 79% of self-reported CSA survivors. Twenty-three of these items discriminated between abused and non-abused participants. The TSC-33 consists of five subscales labeled Dissociation, Anxiety, Depression, Post-Sexual Abuse Trauma, Hypothesized and Sleep Disturbance. CSA has found to be associated with elevated scores on all of these subscales (Briere, Evans, Runtz & Wall, 1988). In addition, clinical samples report higher TSC scores than those based on non-clinical samples (Elliott & Briere, 1991).

Seven items were added to the TCS-33 to create the TSC-40, which lead to the development of six subscales: Dissociation, Anxiety, Depression, Sexual Abuse Trauma Index, Sexual Problems and Sleep Disturbance. The TSC-40 was administered to a national stratified sample of professional women (n = 2,833; Elliott & Briere, 1990; n = 2,963; Elliott & Briere, 1992). Analyses revealed an average subscale alpha of .69 and alpha of .90 for the total measure. Thirty-six of the items discriminated between CSA victims and non-abused subjects in their non-clinical sample (Elliott & Briere, 1990). As expected, TSC-40 total scores correlate highly with the TCS-33 scores (r = .99; Elliott & Briere, 1991) and repeatedly discriminate between CSA survivors and non-survivors as indexed by verbal self-report and by therapist reports (Whiffen, Benazon & Bradshaw, 1997); Elliott & Briere, 1990; Elliott & Briere, 1992). The Sexual Abuse Trauma Index (Elliott & Briere, 1990) and Dissociation subscales (Elliott & Briere, 1992) were found to be the most predictive of sexual abuse history and is according to Elliott & Briere (1990) essentially equivalent to total TSC scores in terms of responsiveness to a history of CSA. In clinical and non-clinical samples, some abuse characteristics correlated significantly with total and subscale scores, and with the duration and frequency with which the abuse occurred (Elliott & Briere, 1991). Convergent validity of the TSC-40 has been established in its relationship to other measure of CSA and Trauma (Brandyberry & MacNair-Semands, 1998; Gold & Cardena, 1998).

Despite its seemingly strong psychometric properties, the TSC-40 suffers some pitfalls. In one study, Whiffen, Benazon & Bradshaw (1997) found that the TSC-40 was no better at discriminating CSA than the SCL-90-R, a generic measure of symptomatology. In fact, for each measure (the SCL-90-R and TSC-40) the best predictors of CSA were the Anxiety subscale and the PSAT, respectively. They point out that the PSAT subscale, which is made of only a few generally worded items, includes items relating to nightmares and fears of men, suggesting that both subscales tap PTSD symptoms. They suggest the existing TSC-40 PSAT subscale items be put into more specific terms and that more items be added to the TSC-40 PSAT subscale to allow for a better characterization of CSA survivors (Whiffen, Benazon & Bradshaw, 1997). Other studies have shown that the TSC-40 not only discriminates between those with a history of CSA but also adult-experienced sexual abuse (Gold, Milan, Mayall & Johnson, 1994). Similar to the above findings, these results suggest that the TSC-40 is not entirely sensitive to the sequelae of CSA; rather it appears to tap into the trauma associated with sexual abuse in general.

The validity of the TSC-40 may also be improved by addressing some psychometric problems. One such issue is the inclusion of items in more than one subscale, thereby inflating intercorrelations. Whiffen, Benazon & Bradshaw (1997) suggest that by confirming the hypothesized structure through factor analysis, items could be independently assigned to appropriate subscales, and therefore purifying the subscales and improving the validity of the instrument.

Other criticisms of the TSC-40 have focused on the standardization sample which consists exclusively of professional women, limiting the generalizability of scores to men, minority women, and women with annual incomes under $30,000 (Lock, Levis & Rourke, 2003). Further deficiencies include: a lack of test-retest reliability estimates, overlapping standard deviations of abused and non-abused individuals which limits the interpretability of total scores; and a lack of external corroboration for the self-reported CSA criterion (Lock, Levis & Rourke, 2003).

6. The Trauma Symptom Inventory (TSI)

The TSI, developed by Briere (1995) is a 100-item, structure, self-report inventory designed for general clinical use in the assessment of the psychological sequelae of potentially traumatic events, including physical violence and sexual assault (Briere & Elliot, 1997). Its construction was in response to the paucity of standardized, clinically useful measures of posttraumatic symptomatology (Briere, Elliott, Harris & Cotman, 1995). Items were developed from an expansion of the TSC-40 and from clinical hypotheses. The test items are rated according to the frequency of symptoms over the prior six months on a four-point scale ranging from 0 ("never") to 3 ("often"). The TSI uses ten clinical scales and three validity scales. The clinical scales include: Anxious Arousal, Depression, Anger/Irritability, Intrusive Experiences, Defensive Avoidance, Dissociation, Sexual Concerns, Dysfunctional Sexual Behavior, Impaired Self-Reference, and Tension-Reduction Behavior. The validity scales include: Response Level, Measuring General Under-endorsement, Atypical Response, Evaluating Over-endorsement, and Inconsistent Response which measures inconsistent responses between similar TSI items-pairs (Briere, 1995).

The TSI was standardized using a random sample of 828 people representative of the United States and using 3,659 military recruits. Norms are available for four combinations of sex and age (Briere, 1995). The clinical scales of the TSI are relatively consistent (α = .84 - .87) and exhibit reasonable predictive and incremental validity (Briere, 1995). The TSI total scores also demonstrate good convergent validity with independently assessed PTSD status with a specificity of .92 and sensitivity of .91 (Astin, Lawrence & Foy, 1993). Briere (1995) found that total TSI scores have been found to be predictive of Borderline Personality Disorder as well as PTSD.

In a regression analysis it was shown that CSA was strongly associated with all ten subscales. CPA was the next best predictor of TSI scores, predicting all scales but the two involving sexual difficulties (Briere et al., 1994). Furthermore, the TSI show promise as a means for identifying persons motivated to exaggerate or fabricate symptomatology as well as malingering responses styles among those claiming psychological damage resulting from a traumatic experience (Edens, Otto, Dwyer, 1998).

7. The Binghamton Childhood Abuse Screen (BCAS)

Although the focus on symptom correlates of CSA has proven to be a valuable approach in the attempt to assess the presence of a CSA history, it does not directly address the methodical concerns raised above which inhibit the detection of a CSA history.

Over the past fifteen years, our laboratory has been devoted to the development of an alternative non-symptom childhood abuse questionnaire designed to increase the sensitivity of the measure's ability to detect a history of CSA. The goal was to develop a time efficient non-face-valid screen via the selection of questions that primarily query sequelae and correlates of CA. The items selected for testing were primarily selected from the present author's research data base of over 5000 treatment transcripts of adult delayed memory recall CA patients (Levis, 1995; Levis & Brewer, 2001). For example, true/false items such as "I have not had a happy childhood"; "at times I have had the feeling that I have fallen into a black hole or cloud"; and, "I am much lonelier than most people".

The first attempt to implement the above strategy consisted of a 103 true-false item screen, referred to as the Sexual Abuse Questionnaire (SAQ-I). To insure the functional utility of the SAQ, the initial validation was conducted with non-clinical undergraduates population who self-reported a history of CSA prior to the age of 15 on Part II of the SAQ which consisted of a number of open-ended questions designed to establish the presence of a history of CSA. Alexander (1993) provided support for the initial use of a non-clinical research population. He reported that the symptomatology of his non-clinical population of women who self-reported a history of incestuous abuse was comparable to that reported by a clinical population.

Lock, Levis, and Rourke (2005) provided the initial evaluation of the SAQ-I. Study I (N=548) established the SAQ's test-retest reliability, internal-consistency and convergent validity by comparing it to Eliot & Briere's (1992) Trauma Symptom Checklist (TSC-40) and to the MMPI subscale for post-traumatic stress (Keane, Malloy, & Fairbank, 1984). SAQ-I demonstrated good reliability (r=.84) and adequate internal consistency (KR-20=.89). Convergent validity was also established with the TSC-46 and Keane's MMPI subscale. After removing similar items, the SAQ correlated moderately with the TSC-40 (r=.63) and the Kean's PTSD subscale (r=.68). Thirty-nine percent of the SAQ-I items discriminated between abused and non-abused groups, compared to 35% of the TSC-40 items. Using a cutting score of 41 for males, the SAQ-I correctly classified 68% of the sample (63% of the abused participants and 69% of the non-abused sample. For women, a cutting score of 42 was established which correctly classified 67% of the sample (64% of the abused participants and 68% of the non-abused sample). The SAQ-I was able to discriminate between abused and non-abused females and males while the TSC-40 failed to discriminate between the reported abused and non-abused males. An exploratory factor analysis that utilized a maximum likelihood extraction and orthogonal rotation suggested a one-dimensional structure. Based on an item analysis of SAQ-I, 78 items were retained for the second version of the SAQ.

Study II (N=533), in addition to examining the psychometric properties of SAQ-II, also assessed the discriminant validity using the Beck Depressive Inventory (Beck, Steer, & Garbin, 1988) and the trait component of the State-Trait Anxiety Inventory (Spielberger, 1983). The SAQ-II correctly identified 86% of the male sample (73% of the abused participants and 86% of the non-abused participants). For women, 73% of the sample was correctly identified (64% of the abused participants and 74% of the non-abused participants). The SAQ-II was found to be a better post-dictor of abuse than the other two measures combined. The SAQ-II also yielded convergent validity with the TSC-40 (r=.67) and Keane's PTSSD subscale (r=.66). An exploratory factor analysis again suggested a one dimensional structure (see Lock, Levis, & Rourke, 2005). Item analysis of the SAQ-II resulted in the development of SAQ-III, a 45 item questionnaire. The SAQ-III was found to correctly identify a participant abuse history. Eighty-nine percent of the sample tested (83% of the male participants and 91% of the female participants were correctly identified (see Krantweiss, 2001, 2004).

Castelda (2006) provided an examination of the relationship between the SAQ-III and the complex post-traumatic disorder (Lenzenweger, Loranges, Korfine, & Neff, 1997). Results showed that those scoring high on the SAQ reported more incidence of childhood abuse, greater levels of PTSD and Axis II psychopathology, and displayed smaller heart rate changes during an auditory startle test than those scoring low on the SAQ.

Evidence has also been found which suggested the SAQ-III is also capable of identifying survivors of childhood physical abuse (see Krantweiss, 2004). Castelda (2003) confirmed Krantweiss's findings along with providing support for SAQ-III's ability to identify survivors of combined CSA and CPA histories. These findings are reconfirmed in Experiment I of Castelda, Levis, Rourke, and Coleman (2007) publication using a large sample of participant (N=3,505). Experiment II of this study evaluated the effectiveness of a newly developed 36 item abuse screen which was renamed the Binghamton Childhood Abuse Screen (BCAS). An ROC survey analysis was provided for determining the sensitivity and specificity indices for all possible BCAS cut-off scores across all abuse types, enabling examiners to choose cut-off scores that are suitable for their purposes. Additional criterion validity for the BCAS was established via the use of a modified Stroop task by Coleman, Rourke, and Levis (2008).

Finally, the issue of malingering regarding the BCAS has been evaluated and support for the BCAS claim that it represent a non-face valid screen, has been obtained (Levis, Rourke, Bovier, Coleman, Heron, Castelda, and Esch, 2011). Although the BCAS has received sufficient support for its use with an undergraduate college population, it has yet to be validated on an out-patient population. However, some support for its use with an in-patient population has been recently obtained (Rowland, Ocelnik, Berryman, and Levis, 2011). Although the BCAS shows promise, it still remains a work in progress.

The previous review of the prevalence rates of childhood abuse in our society and the existing established link between childhood abuse and clinical symptomatology clearly points to the need to assess the possibility that a history may exist when developing a treatment plan. The use of one of the reviewed abuse assessment inventories should not only facilitate this assessment goal but it also helps communicate to the patient the willingness of the therapists to deal with this topic. It is surprising to me that a large number of patients who I have seen have reported their previous therapist never raised the issue of childhood abuse. It is unfortunate that too many of our mental health workers are still in a state of denial regarding the impact an abuse history can have on the client's behavior. If no support for a history of abuse is found, this possibly should remain open given the finding of delayed memory recall.

If a history of childhood abuse is self-reported, the issue of treatment selection becomes paramount. Unfortunately, a review of all the existing treatment approaches would require another chapter. Nevertheless, I will briefly discuss two approaches that have yielded some experimental support.

5. Cognitive Behavioral Therapy (CBT)

The first technique to be discussed is the technique of Cognitive Behavior Therapy (CBT). The technique of CBT was designed to be used to treat a wide variety of clinical symptoms including cases with a history of childhood abuse. CBT has been subjected to experimental validations (see Lynch, Lowe & McKenna, 2010) for a review of supporting data.

CBT has been defined as an intervention whose core elements include the recipient establishing links between their thoughts, feelings and actions and targeting symptoms correcting misperceptions, irrational beliefs, and reasoning biases related to these target symptoms, involving monitoring of one's own thoughts, feelings and behaviors with respect to the symptom; and/or the promotion of alternative ways of coping with target symptoms (Lynch, Lowe & McKenna, 2010).

Although CBT is a commonly used approach, the variety of techniques used to create cognitive restriction varies from one study to the other, frequently lacking operational specificity. Given the number of strategies and approaches used to change cognitive behavior, it appears to me to be similar to the insight approaches adapted in the 1940's and 1950's, (Alexander, 1965). It can be argued that the key agent of change in CBT is the approach ability to elicit emotional affects which in turn undergoes an extinction process that in turn results in a cognitive restructuring. This hypothesis leads to the discussion of the second approach to be discussed.

6. The use of Prolonged CS Exposure (PE)

The technique of prolonged CS exposure was first developed by Thomas G. Stampfl in the late 1950's. Despite considerable pressure to publish, he refused to publish until two experimental outcome studies were conducted to support his clinical finding. They were provided by Hogan (1966) who used a psychiatric hospitalized population, and Levis & Carrera (1967) who used an outpatient population. He then published his first article (Stampfl & Levis, 1967). He labeled his new response prevention approach, Implosive Therapy (IT). He first used an in vivo extinction approach but changed to an imagery approach due to the ability to introduce hypothesized conditioned stimulus (CS) that do not lend themselves readily to in vivo exposure (e.g., the fear of bodily injury). Stampfl adapted a revision of Mowrer's two factor avoidance theory (see Levis, 1979). His theory (Stampfl, 1970, Levis, 1985) has received strong experimental support at the human and infrahuman level of analyses (Levis, 1979, 1985) including a resolution of Freud's neurotic paradox as to why clinical symptoms persist over time (Levis & Brewer, 2001). The technique has been successfully used in the treatment of obsessive compulsive behavior (Foa, 2000); in the treatment of panic disorders (Levis, 1987); phobic behavior (Stampfl & Levis, 1967) and depression (Boyd & Levis 1980). The IT technique is an operational design feedback technique capable of re-activating trauma memories. The frequent use of Stampfl's therapist directed imagery technique lead to the development of a free-recall technique (referred to as patient directed IT or brain release therapy). This approach appears capable of providing a complete re-activation of trauma experiences (Levis, 1988; Levis 1995; Kirsch & Levis, 2001).

Today, prolonged exposure therapy is perhaps the most frequent and empirically supported technique for use for patient diagnosed with PTSD including survivors of childhood abuse (see Morrison, 2011). Yet as Morrison regrettably notes, some therapists avoid its use. Part of the concern is related to the fear that the high levels of anxiety elicited may be harmful to the patent. This fear exists despite the strong experimental evidence that the approach is not harmful (see Boudewyns & Levis, 1975; Boudweyn & Shipley 1983). Another key factor in the avoidance of using PE relates to the emotional impact on the therapist who witnesses the patient's trauma as they re-experience their historical emotional trauma. Despite this difficulty, I have found the law of extinction will eventually work for both the patient and the therapist resulting in a strong positive reinforcement when a reduction for symptomatology occurs. It has also been my experience that trauma victims rarely terminate therapy prematurely or miss a session.

In closing, it is my hope this chapter will not only alert the reader to the frequent and devastating effects that childhood abuse has on the adult survivors of abuse but also serve as an alert to practitioners as to the importance of providing a comprehensive assessment of the potential presences of an abusive childhood history in their patients.

7. References

Agor, K., Read, J., & Bish, J. (2002). Identification of abuse histories in a community mental health center: The need for policies and training. *Journal of Mental Health (UK)*, (11), 533-543.

Alexander, F. (1965). The dynamics of psychotherapy in light of learning theory. *International Journal of Psychiatry*, I, 189-97.

Allen, J.G., Huntoon, J., & Evans, R.B. (1999). Self-report measures to screen for trauma history and its application to women in in-patient treatment for trauma related disorders. *Bulletin of the Menninger Clinic*, 63(3).

Astin, M.C., Lawrence, K.J., & Foy, D.W. (1993). Post-traumatic stress disorder among battered women: risk and resiliency factors. *Violence and Victims*, 8, 17-29.

Beck, A.T., Steer, R.A., & Garbin, M.G. (1988). Psychometric properties of the Beck Depression Inventory: Twenty-five years of evaluation. *Clinical Psychology Review*, 8, 77-100.

Bell, J., & Belichi, K. (1998). A community study of well-being in adults reporting childhood abuse. *Child Abuse and Neglect*, 22(7), 681-685.

Bernstein, D.P., Fink, L., Handelsman, L., Foote, J., Lovejoy, M., Wenzel, K., Sapareto, E., & Ruggerio, J. (1994). Initial reliability and validity of a new retrospective measure of child abuse and neglect. *American Journal of Psychiatry*, 151 (8), 1132-1335.

Bernstein, D.P., Abuvalia, T., Pozzi, D., & Handelsman, L. (1997). Validity of the Childhood Trauma Questionnaire in an adolescent psychiatric population. *Journal of the American Academy of Child in Adolescents Psychiatry*, 36 (3), 340-348.

Boudewyns, P.A., & Levis, D.J. 91975). Autonomic reactivity of high and low ego-strength subjects to repeated anxiety eliciting scenes. *Journal of Abnormal Psychology*, 84, 682-692.

Boudewyns, P.D., & Shipley, R.H. (1983). *Flooding and Implosive Therapy*. New York: Plenum Press.

Boyd, T.L., & Levis, D.J. (1980). Depression: In Dartzman, R.J. (Eds.), *Clinical Behavior Therapy and Behavior Modification*, New York: Garland STPM Press, pp. 301-349.

Brandyberry, L.J., & McNair-Semands, R.R. (1998). Examining the validity and reliability of childhood abuse scales: Putting the courage to heal to the test. *Child Abuse & Neglect*, 22 (12), 1253-1263.

Briere, J. (1989). Therapy for adults molested as children: Beyond survival. New York, New York: Springer Publishing Company.

Briere, J. (1992a). *Child Abuse Trauma*. Newbury Park: Sage Publications.

Briere, J. (1992b). Methodological issues in the study of sexual abuse effects. *Journal of Consulting and Clinical Psychology*, 60 (2), 196-203.

Briere, J. (1995). Trauma Symptom Inventory: Psychometrics and association with childhood and adult victimization in clinical samples. *Journal of Interpersonal Violence*, 10 (4), 387-401.

Briere, J., Evans, D., Runtz, M., & Wall, T. (1988). Symptomatology in men who were molested as children: A comparison study. *American Journal of Orthopsychiatry*, 58 (3), 457-461.

Briere, J., & Runtz, M. (1989). The Trauma Symptom Checklist (TSC-33). *Journal of Interpersonal Violence*, 4, 151-163.

Briere, J., & Conte, J. (1991). Self-reported amnesia for abuse in adults molested as children. *Journal of Traumatic Stress*, (6), 21-31.

Briere, J., Elliott, D.M., Harris, K., & Cotman, A. (1994). The trauma symptom inventory: Reliability and validity in a clinical sample. Unpublished manuscript, University of Southern California School of Medicine, Los Angeles, CA.

Briere, J., & Runtz, M. (1986). Suicidal thoughts and behaviours in former sexual abuse victims. *Canadian Journal of Behavioural Sciences*, 18, 413-423.

Briere, J., & Runtz, M. (1990). Differential adult symptomatology associated with three types of child abuse histories. *Child Abuse and Neglect*, 14, 357-364.

Briere, J. & Elliott, D.M. (1997). Psychological assessment of interpersonal victimization effect in adults and children. *Psychotherapy*, 34 (4) 353-364.

Brown, J. (1990). The treatment of male victims with mixed=-gender, short-term group psychotherapy. In M. Hunter (Ed.) *The Sexually Abused Male*, Vol. 2. Lexington: Lexington Books.

Browne, A., & Finkelhor, D. (1986). Impact of child sexual abuse: A review of the research. *Psychological Bulletin*, 99 (1), 66-77.

Buchanan, A., & Oliver, J.E. (1977). Abuse and neglect as a cause for retardation. *British Journal of Psychiatry*. 131, 459-467.

Bursten, B. (1995). Validity of child abuse measurements [letter to the editor]. *American Journal of Psychiatry*, 152 (10), 1533-1534.

Castelda, B.A. (2003). An examination of the Sexual Questionnaire-III in identifying self-reported childhood sexual, physical, and combined abuse, unpublished master thesis, Binghamton University, Binghamton, NY, USA.

Castelda, B.A. (2006). Construct validation of the Sexual Abuse Questionnaire (SAQ) using an acoustic startle procedure and measures of complex Post-Traumatic Stress Disorder (PTSD), unpublished doctoral dissertation, Binghamton University, Binghamton, New York, USA.

Castelda, B.A., Levis, D.J., Rourke, P.A.,. & Coleman, S.L. (2007). Extension of the Sexual Abuse Questionnaire to other abuse categories: The initial psychometric validation of the Binghamton Abuse Screen, *Journal of Child Sexual Abuse*, (16), 1, 207-325.

Coleman, S.L., Rourke, P.A., & Levis, D.J. (2008). Experimental and self-reported indices of childhood abuse using the Binghamton Childhood Abuse Screen. *Journal of Aggression, Maltreatment & Trauma*, 17 (4), 506-619.

Coverdale, J.H., & Turbott, S.H. (2000). Sexual and physical abuse of chronically ill psychiatric outpatients compared with a matched sample of medical outpatients. *Journal of Nervous and Mental Disorders*, 188 (7), 440-5.

Curtis, L.A. (1976). Present and future measures of victimization in forcible rape. In M.J. Walker & S.L. Brodsky (eds.) *Sexual Assault: The victim and the rapist*. Lexington, MA: Lexington Books.

Daro, D. (1988). Confronting child abuse: Research for effective program design. New York, New York. The Free Press.

Demause, L. (1991). The Universability of incest. *The Journal of Psychohistory*, 19 (2), 123-164.

DeVellis, R.F. (1991). *Scale Development: Theory and Application*. Newbury Park: Sage Publications.

Dinwiddie, S., Heath, A.C., Dunne, M.P., Bucholz, K.K., Madden, P.A.F., Slutski, W.S., Bierut, J.J., Statham, D.B., & Martin, N.G. (2000). Early sexual abuse and lifetime psychopathology: A co-twin-control study. *Psychological Medicine*, 30, 41-52.

Domino, J.V., & Haber, J.D. (1987). Prior physical and sexual abuse in women with chronic headache: Clinical correlates. *Headache*, 27, 130-134.

Doyle-Peters, S., Wyatt, G.E., & Finkelhor, D. (1986). Prevalence. In D. Finkelhor (ed.) *A Sourcebook on Child Sexual Abuse*. Beverly Hills, CA: Sage Publications.

Edens, J.F., Otto, R.K., & Dwyer, T.J. (1998). Susceptibility of the Traumatic Symptom Inventory to malingering. *Journal of Personality Assessment*, 71 (3), 379-392.

Elliot, D.M., & Briere, J. (1990, April). *Predicting molestation history in professional women with the Trauma Symptom Checklist-40 (TSC-40)*. Paper presented at the annual meeting of the Western Psychological Association, Low Angeles.

Elliot, D.M., & Briere, J. (1991). Studying the long-term effects of sexual abuse: The trauma symptom checklist (TSC) scales. In A.W. Burgess (ed.), *Rape & Sexual Assault III: A Research Handbook* (pp. 55-74), New York, NY: Garland.

Elliott, D.M., & Briere, J. (1992). Sexual abuse trauma among professional women: Validating the trauma symptom checklist-40 (TSC-40). *Child Abuse & Neglect*, 16 (3), 391-398.

Feldman-Summers, S., & Pope, K.S. (1994). The experience of "forgetting" childhood abuse: A national survey of psychologists. *Journal of Consulting and Clinical Psychology*, 62, 636-639.

Fergussen, D.M., Lynskey, M.T., & Harwood, L.J. (1996). Childhood sexual abuse and psychiatric disorder in young adulthood: Prevalence of sexual abuse factors associated with sexual abuse. *Journal of the American Academy of Child and Adolescent Psychiatry*, 34 (10).

Finkelhor, D., Hotaling, G., Lewis, I.A., & Smith, C. (1990). Sexual abuse in a national survey of adult men and women: Prevalence, characteristics and risk factors. *Child Abuse and Neglect*, 14, 19-28.

Finestone, H.M., Stenn, P., Davies, F., Stalker, C., Fry, R., Koumanis, J. (2000). Chronic pain and health care utilization in women with a history of childhood sexual abuse. *Child Abuse & Neglect*, 24 (5) 547-556.

Foa, E.B. (2000). Psychosocial treatment of post-traumatic stress disorder. *Journal of Clinical Psychiatry*, 61, 43-53.

Gelles, R.J., & Straus, M.A. (1987). Is violence toward children increasing? A comparison of 1975 and 1985 national survey rats. *Journal of Interpersonal Violence,* 2 (2), 212-222.

Gold, S.R., Milan, L.D., Mayall, A., & Johnson, A.E. (1994). A cross-validation study of the trauma symptom checklist: The role of mediating variables. *Journal of Interpersonal Violence, 9, 12-26.*

Gold, J.W., & Cardena, E. (1998). Convergent validity of three post-traumatic symptom inventories among adult abuse survivors. *Journal of Traumatic Stress*, 11 (1), 173-180.

Goldwater, L., & Duffy, J.F. (1990). Use of the MMPI to uncover histories of childhood abuse in adult female psychiatric patients. *Journal of Clinical Psychology*, 46, 392-398.

Hathaway, S.R., & McKinley, J.C. (1989). *The Minnesota Multiphasic Personality Inventory II*, Minneapolis, MN: University of Minnesota Press.

Herman, J.L., & Schatzow, E. (1987). Recovery and verification of memories of childhood sexual trauma. *Psychoanalytic Psychology*, 4 (1), 1-14.

Hogan, R.A. (1966). Implosive therapy in the short term treatment of psychotics. *Psychotherapy, Theory, Research & Practice*, 25-31.

Jacobson, A. (1989). Physical and sexual assault histories among psychiatric out-patients. *American Journal of Psychiatry*, 146, 755-758.

Jacobson, A. (1990). The relevance of childhood sexual abuse to adult psychiatric in-patient care. *Hospital Community Psychiatry*, 41 (7), 807.

Kean, T.M., Malloy, P.F., & Fairbank, J.A. (1984). Empirical development MMPI subscale for the assessment of combat-related post-0traumatic stress disorder. *Journal of Consulting and Clinical Psychology*, 52, 888-891.

Kendall-Tackett, K.A. (2000). Physiological correlates of childhood abuse: chronic hyperarousal in PTSD, depression and irritable bowel syndrome. *Child Abuse & Neglect*, 24 (6), 799-810.

Kent, A., & Waller, G. (1998). The impact of childhood emotional abuse: An extension of the child abuse and trauma scale. *Child Abuse and Neglect*, 22 (5), 393-399.

Kilpatrick, D.A. (1988). Rape aftermath symptom test. In M. Herson & A.S. Bellack (eds.) *Dictionary of Behavioral Assessment Techniques*, New York: Pergamon Press.

Kirsch, M.V., & Levis, D.J. (2001). An assessment of the accuracy of two clinical procedures to elicit in a non-patient population recall of a reportedly forgotten long-term memory: An exploratory study. *Journal of Mental Imagery*, 25, 63-78.

Knutson, J.F., & Selner, M. (1994). Punitive childhood experiences reported by young adults over a 10-year period. *Child Abuse & Neglect*, 18 (2), 1155-166.

Krantweiss, A. (2001). The utility of video film clips of sexual abuse in assessing SAQ-III and gender differences via a multi-modal assessment procedure. Unpublished master's thesis, Binghamton University, Binghamton, NY, USA.

Krantweiss, A. (2004). The utility of video film clips of sexual and physical abuse in assessing SAQ-IIIR and gender differences via a multi-modal assessment procedure. Unpublished doctoral dissertation, Binghamton University, Binghamton, NY, USA.

Layman, M., Gidycz, C., & Lynn, S.J. (1996). Unacknowledged versus acknowledged rape victims: Situational factors and post-traumatic stress. *Journal of Abnormal Psychology*, 105, 124-131.

Lesserman, J., Drossman, D.A., Li, Z., Toomey, T.C., Nachman, G., & Glogau, L. (1996). Sexual and physical abuse history in gastrointesterology practice: How types of abuse impacts health status. *Psychometric Medicine*, 58, 4-15.

Lenzenweger, M.F., Loranger, A.W., Korfine, L., & Neff, C. (1997). Detecting personality disorder in a non-clinical population. *Archives of General Psychiatry*, 54 (4), 345-351.

Levis, D.J. & Boyd, T.L. (1979). Symptom maintenance: An infrahuman analysis and extension of the conservation of anxiety principle. *Journal of Abnormal Psychology*, 88, 107-120.

Levis, D.J. (1985). Implosive theory: A comprehensive extension of conditioning theory of fear/anxiety to psychopathology. In S. Riess & R.R. Bootzin (eds.), *Theoretical issues in behavior therapy* pp. 49-82). New York: Academic Press.

Levis, D.J. (1987). Treating anxiety and panic attacks: The conflict model of implosive therapy. *Journal of Integrative and Eclectic Psychotherapy*, 6, 4, 450-461.

Levis, D.J. (1988). Observation and experience from clinical practice: A critical ingredient for advancing behavior theory and therapy. *Behavior therapist*, 11, 95-99.

Levis, D.J. (1995). Decoding traumatic memory: Implosive theory of psychopathology. In W. O'Donohue & L. Krasner (eds.). *Theories in behavior therapy* (pp. 173-207). Washington, D.C.: American Psychological Association.

Levis, D.J. (1999). The traumatic memory debate: A failure in scientific communication and cooperation. *Applied & Preventive Psychology*, 8, 71-76.

Levis, D.J., & Carrera, R. (1967). Effects of ten hours of implosive therapy in the treatment of out-patients: A preliminary report. *Journal of Abnormal Psychology*, 72, 504-508.

Levis, D.J., & Brewer, K.E. (2001). Two-factor fear theory to areas of psychopathology and trauma memory recovery. In R.R. Mowrer & S.B. Klein (eds.). *Handbook of Contemporary Learning Theories*. New Jersey: Erlbaum Associates, pp. 561-593.

Levis, D.J., Rourke, P.A., Wagner, K., Bovier, E., Coleman, S.L., Heron, K., Castelda, B.A., and Esch, R.D. (2011). Further evaluation of the Binghamton Abuse Screen (BCAS: An assessment of malingering and the screen's non-face valid status (unpublished manuscript).

Lipschitz, D.S., Kaplan, J.L., Sorkenn, J., Chorney, P., Asnis, G.M. (1996). Childhood abuse, adult assault, and dissociation. *Comprehensive Psychiatry*, 37 (4), 261-266.

Lipschitz, D.S., Bernstein, D.P., Winegar, R.K., & Southwick, S.M. (1999). Hospitalized adolescents' reports of sexual and physical abuse: A comparison of two self-reported measures. *Journal of Traumatic Stress*, 12 (4), 641-654.

Lock, T.G. (1997). Development of the Sexual Abuse Questionnaire: An examination of behavioral, emotional, memorial, and cognitive correlates of childhood sexual abuse in self-identified adult survivors. Unpublished master thesis, Binghamton University, Binghamton, NY.

Lock, T.G., Levis, D.J., & Rourke, P.A. (2005). The Sexual Abuse Questionnaire: A preliminary examination of a time and cost efficient method of evaluating the presence of childhood sexual abuse in adult patients. *Journal of Child Sexual Abuse*, (14), 1, 1-26.

Lothian, J., & Read, J. (2002). Asking about abuse during mental health assessments: Clients' views and experiences. *New Zealand Journal of Psychology*, 31, 98-103.

Lynch, D., Lowe, R.R., & McKenna, J. (2010). Cognitive behavioral therapy for major psychiatric disorders: Does it really work? A meta-analytical review of well controlled trials. *Psychological Medicine*, 40, 9-24.

Macmillian, M., Flemming, J., Trocme, N., Boyle, M.H., Wong, M., Racine, O.A., Beardslee, W.R., & Offord, D.R. (1997). Prevalence of child physical and sexual abuse in the community, results from the Ontario Health supplement. *Journal of the American Medical Association*, 278 (2), 131-135.

Malinosky-Rummell, R., & Hansen, D.J. (1993). Long-term con sequences of childhood physical abuse. *Psychological Bulletin*, 114 (1), 68-79.

Martin, J., Anderson, J., Romans, S., Mullen, P., & O'Shea, M. (1993). Asking about child sexual abuse: Methodological implications of a two stage survey. *Child Abuse & Neglect*, 17, 383-392.

Morrison, J.A. (2011) The Therapeutic relationship in prolong exposure therapy for post-traumatic stress disorder: The role of cross-theoretical dialogue in dissemination. *Behavior Therapist*. Vol.34, No.2.

Mullen, P,.E., Martin, J.L., Anderson, J.C., Romans, S.E., & Herbison, G.P. (1996). The long-term impact of the physical, emotional, and sexual abuse of children: A community study. *Child Abuse & Neglect*, 20 (1), 7-21.

Perkins, D.F., Luster, T., & Jank, W. (2002). Protective factors, physical abuse, and purging from community-wide surveys of female adolescents. *Journal of Adolescent Research*, 17 (4), 377-400.

Polusny, M.A., & Follette, V.M. (1995). Long-term correlates of child sexual abuse: Theory and review of the empirical literature. *Applied and Preventative Psychology*, 4, 143-166.

Resnick, H., Kilpatrick D., & Lipovsky, J. (1991). Assessment of rape-related post-traumatic stress disorder: Stressor and symptom dimension. *Psychological Assessment*, 3, 561-572.

Robbins, A.D. (1995). False memories or hidden agendas? *Journal of Psychohistory*, 27 (3), 305-311.

Rodriguez, N., Ryan, S.W., Rowan, A.B., & Foy, D.W. (1996). Post-traumatic stress disorder in a clinical sample of adult survivors of childhood sexual abuse. *Child Abuse & Neglect*, 20 (10), 943-952.

Romans, S., Belaise, C., Martin, J., Morris, E., Raffi, A. (2002). Childhood abuse and later medical disorders in women. *Psychotherapy and Psychosomatics*, 71, 141-150.

Rosenberg, M.A. (1987). New directions for research on the psychological maltreatment of children. *American Psychologist*, 42 (2), 166-171.

Rowan, A.B., Foy, D.W., Rodriguez, N., & Ryan, S. (1994). Post-traumatic stress disorder in a clinical sample of adults sexually abused as children. *Child Abuse & Neglect*, 18, 51-61.

Rowland, M., Ocelnik, E., Berryman, J.P., Levis, D.J. (2011). Psychometric validation of the Binghamton Abuse Screen among an in-patient population (unpublished manuscript).

Sanders, B., & Becker-Lausen, E. (1995). The measurement of psychological maltreatment: Early data on the child abuse and trauma scale. *Child Abuse & Neglect*, 19 (3), 315-323.

Sedlak, A.J., Mettenberg, J., Basena, M., Petta, I., McPherson, K., Green, A., & Lis (2010. *Fourth National Incidence Study of Child Abuse and Neglect (NIS-4)*. Report to Congress, executive summary, Washington, D.C.: US7 Department of Health and Human Services for Children and Families.

Spielberger, C.D. (1983). *Manual for the State-Trait Anxiety Inventory (STAI)*, Palo Alto, CA: Consulting Psychological Press.

Stampfl, T.G. (1970). Implosive therapy: An emphasis on covert stimulation. In D>J. Levis (ed.), Learning Approaches to therapeutic behavior change. Chicago: Aldine.

Stampfl, T.G., & Levis, D.J. (1967). Essentials of implosive therapy. A learning-based psychodynamic behavior therapy. *Journal of Abnormal Psychology*, 72, 496-503.

Surrey, J., Swett, C., Michaels, A., & Levin, S. (1990). Reported history of physical and sexual abuse and severity of symptomatology in women with psychiatric outpatients. *American Journal of Orthopsychiatry*, 60 (3), 412-417.

Walker, E.A., Katon, W.J., Roy-Byrne, P.P., Jemelka, R.P., & Russo, J. (1993). Histories of sexual victimization in patients with irritable bowel syndrome or inflammatory bowel disease. *American Journal of Psychiatry*, 150, 10, 1502-1506.

Westermeyer, J., Wahmanholm, K., Thuras, P. (2001). Effects of childhood physical abuse on course and severity of substance abuse. *The American Journal on Addictions*, 10, 101-110.

Whiffen, V.E., Benazon, N.R., & Bradshaw, C. (1997). Discriminate validity of the TSC-40 in an out-patient setting. *Child Abuse & Neglect*, 21 (1), 107-115.

Williams, L.M. (1994). Recall of childhood trauma: A prospective study of women's memories of child sexual abuse. *Journal of Consulting and Clinical Psychology*, 62, 1167-11786.

Wind, T.W., & Silvern, L.E. (1992). Type and extent of child abuse as predictors of adult functioning. *Journal of Family Violence*, 7 (4), 261-268.

Winegar, R.W., & Lipschitz, D.S. (1997). The reliability of adolescents' reports of maltreatment and a comparison of different inquiry formats. Paper presented at the 5th International Family Violence Research Conference, Durham, N.H.

Wyatt, G.E., & Doyle-Peters, S. (1986). Methodological considerations in research on the prevalence of child sexual abuse. *Child Abuse and Neglect*, 10, 241-251.

Zlotnick, C., Mattia, J., Zimmerman, M. (2001). Clinical features of survivors of sexual abuse with major depression. *Child Abuse & Neglect*, 25, 357-367.

2

Sexual Abuse Histories Among Incarcerated Older Adult Offenders: A Descriptive Study

Mary Beth Morrissey, Deborah Courtney and Tina Maschi
Fordham University, Graduate School of Social Service
USA

1. Introduction

In the United States today, there are over 2.2 million incarcerated adults held in custody in U.S. state or federal prisons or local jails (Glaze, 2010). Prison facilities are oftentimes filled to capacity or in some cases, so overcrowded that conditions violate the constitutional rights of adults in prison (Brown v. Plata, 2011; Sabol & West, 2009; West & Sabol, 2008). Official statistics paint a contemporary portrait of the 1.5 million adult sentenced prisoners under state or federal jurisdiction who are mostly male (93%) and from diverse racial and ethnic backgrounds including Black American (36%), Caucasian (31%), and Latino (20%)(West & Sabol, 2008). Black males continue to have the highest incarceration rates across all age categories compared to White or Latino males (Sabol & Couture, 2008). There is a growing number of older adults in both state and federal prisons, approaching nearly 5% of inmates 55 and older in custody of state prisons in 2007, and over 7% of inmates 56 and older in federal prison in 2009 (Cox & Lawrence, 2010; Sabol & Couture, 2008). This aging prisoner population, which is five times larger than in 1990, presents a significant public health challenge that the correctional system is not adequately equipped to address (Falter, 1999; Reimer, 2008). Moreover, the high prevalence of trauma among older adults in prison and psychological distress associated with trauma experiences raise serious concerns about the well-being of this population (Krause, 2004). Studies have shown that approximately 93% of juvenile and adult prisoners have had prior exposure to trauma, such as being a victim of and/or witness to sexual abuse (Harlow, 1999).

The high prevalence of trauma histories, especially earlier life sexual victimization, within the incarcerated older adult offenders is a major concern. If these traumatic histories go unidentified and untreated, it is likely that unresolved subjective distress about these past events may be heightened, resulting in persistent or resurfacing of post-traumatic stress symptoms or increased likelihood of criminal offending including the perpetration of sexual abuse (Leach, Burgess, Holmwood, 2008). Identifying the types of traumatic experiences, particularly sexual abuse histories, experienced by older adult offenders is important to developing comprehensive approaches to assessment, treatment and program planning for older adults in prison (Dawes, 2009; Rikard & Rosenberg, 2007; Shimkus, 2004). While there are various types of traumatic and stressful experiences in the lives of incarcerated older adults, sexual victimization is an area that demands individualized attention, especially given the high rates of sexual victimization histories prior to prison that occur within this population. For instance, traumatic sexual victimization experiences among offenders occur at much higher rates than in the general population (Teplin, 1990). Individuals who experienced traumatic experiences prior to prison have a greater likelihood of experiencing revictimization while in prison (Struckman-Johnson, Struckman-Johnson, Rucker, Bumby, and Donaldson, 1996). Failure to recognize and design appropriate responses and interventions to address sexual abuse and the cycle of "retraumatization" and its concomitant risks of sexual abuse perpetration, may result in ongoing uninterrupted trends of trauma experiences among older adults in prison who themselves are victims in urgent need of specialized care (Maschi, Gibson, Zgoba, & Morgen, 2011).

2. Trauma, sexual abuse, and life course consequences

Research indicates that childhood or adult trauma, such as being a victim or witness to sexual abuse, may have a persistent or intermittent mental or physical effect, such as continued revictimization, psychiatric disorders, maladaptive stress responses, physical disabilities, and even early death (Acierno, Hernandez, Amstadter, Resnick, Steve, Muzzy, & Kilpatrick, 2010; Gagnon & Hersen, 2000; Maschi, 2006). The type and timing of symptoms may vary. For example, subjective traumatic experiences that first occur in childhood may be accompanied by feelings of intense fear, helplessness, or horror (APA, 2000; Hiskey, Luckey, Davies, & Brewin, 2008). These feelings may occur immediately following the childhood traumatic event or remain dormant and then resurface in later life (Hiskey, Luckey, Davies, & Brewin, 2008). Evidence also suggests that when a traumatic experience is marked by intensity, duration, and chronicity, such as a prolonged exposure to sexual abuse, the likelihood of post-traumatic stress symptoms is prolonged, and may extend into later years in life (Neal et al., 1995). Research on the temporal effects of childhood trauma, especially on later life functioning, has been minimally explored. While the data are scant, findings indicate that childhood trauma exposure may result in minor psychological distress or lead to more severe mental health consequences, such as posttraumatic stress disorder (PTSD), depression, anxiety, and cognitive impairment (Maschi et al., 2011, Neal et al., 1995; Shmotkin & Litwin, 2009). It is important to note that age plays a significant role in this relationship, as older adults with earlier life trauma have been shown to have a higher risk of revictimization for elder abuse, especially if their social support network is limited (Acierno et al., 2007). Evidence suggests that older adults in prison are at an even increased risk of sexual victimization by other prisoners or staff (Dawes, 2009).

These types of childhood experiences have been found to have pronounced and long-lasting effects, especially among criminal justice populations (Abram et al., 2007; Ford et al., 2004; James & Glaze, 2006). Several mental health theoreticians have explanations for the impact of psychosocial stressors (such as being a victim and/or witness to violence, or losing a loved one) on mental health and aggressive and self-destructive behaviors (van der Kolk, McFarlane, & Weisaeth, 1996). Bessel van der Kolk (1987) offers a biopsychosocial explanation for the impact of psychosocial stressors on mental health. He sees mental health disorders as more complex than the diagnostic label given to the client. In other words, mental health disorders are not interpreted as solely biologically or genetically driven, but in fact are understood as multidimensional in nature and influenced by one's ability to cope with adverse life experiences. Van der Kolk (1987) asserts that when children experience trauma they can be deeply affected and develop jaded expectations about the world and the safety and security of their lives, and such experiences and responses may compromise their psychological, emotional, social and behavioral functioning (van der Kolk & Fisler, 1994). More specifically, van der Kolk et al. (1996) explained that traumatic experiences can consequently impact individuals' ability to regulate affect and control impulse, manifesting in symptoms of mental health disorders. It is imperative to consider such theoretical understandings of trauma in the discussion of incarcerated offenders as difficulty regulating affect and inability to control impulse can lead to many illegal behaviors and consequently a prison sentence.

3. Sexual abuse among older adults in prison and the community

More recent studies have begun to expose the life course experience of older adults in the criminal justice system (Maschi, Dennis, Gibson, MacMillan, Sternberg, Hom, 2011). For example, in a review of case records, Haugebrook, Zgoba, Maschi, Morgen, & Brown (2010) found upwards of 80% of older males in prison had documented histories of one or more traumatic or stressful life events that occurred during childhood and/or adulthood. About 20% had childhood sexual or physical assault histories. These traumatic experiences ranged from a single event to multiple traumatic and related stressful life events. Being a victim of childhood physical or sexual abuse is an example of a singular traumatic event of significant magnitude that has been linked to later life adverse mental and physical health among older adults (Lamet, Szuchman, Perkel, & Walsh, 2009; Shmotkin & Barilan, 2002). Other studies with incarcerated women find an even higher rate of sexual abuse histories (McDaniel-Wilson & Belknap, 2008). For example, McDaniels-Wilson and Belknap (2008) found that 70% of their sample of 391 incarcerated women had been raped at least once, while half of them endorsed a history of childhood sexual abuse. Not only do many prisoners come into the system with a history of sexual abuse, but there are also frequent reports of sexual violence occurring within the prison systems (Maschi et al., 2011).

For trauma victims in prison, the prison environment itself is an additional source of trauma and stress, especially among older offenders (Goff. Rose, Rose, & Purves, 2007; Stojkovic, 2007). Struckman-Johnson and colleagues (1996) report that in a sample of 1,800 adult offenders (in which 8% of the sample was aged 48 and older), 1 out of 5 were found to have been pressured or forced to have at least one unwanted sexual contact, including anal, vaginal, or oral intercourse, or being a victim of gang rape. The agency, Stop Prisoner Rape, also reports that there were frequent rapes and other forms of sexual abuse being perpetrated by correction officers within the prisons (Stop Prisoner Rape Report, 2003). In addition, offenders with histories of sexual abuse compounded with other traumas are more vulnerable while in prison. For example, Hochstetler, Murphy, and Simons (2004) found that prior victimization experiences predicted revictimization in prison.

It is imperative to consider the additional risk that older age places on incarcerated offenders with regard to past and present sexual victimization. For instance, incarcerated older adults are considered at the highest risk for victimization because of their decreasing ability to defend themselves against younger prisoners or staff (Dawes, 2009). Along the same lines older adults in frail health are at higher risk of all forms of elder abuse, which could include sexual assaults, in prison (Goff et al., 2007; Stojkovic, 2007). Furthermore, older adult offenders also have additional age specific stressors, such as concerns over failing health and the fear of dying in prison (Aday, 2006; Marushak, 2008), in addition to the physical vulnerabilities presented by the aging process. This cumulative effect of trauma and stress can have a significant adverse effect on their physical and mental well-being (Maschi et al., 2011).

These age related health and mental health factors are extremely important to consider for a number of reasons. First, Draper and colleagues (2008) found that older adults in the community with childhood physical and sexual abuse histories were at the highest risk of later poor physical health and mental health compared to those who did not have these experiences. Second, Yehuda and colleagues (1995) found a positive association between childhood trauma combined with current experiences of age-related stress and the severity of post-traumatic stress symptoms among older adults in the community. Third, Hiskey and colleagues (2008) report that older adults older adults in the community, who were childhood trauma survivors, experienced later life reactivation of traumatic memories, which had intense and vivid aspects with the same subjective potency as the original traumatic event. In sum, the age-related stressors that incarcerated adults are coping with while in prison, such as increased risk of sexual victimization, can likely trigger earlier traumatic memories and experiences leading to significant impairment and potential post-traumatic stress symptoms.

4. Purpose of book chapter

Research on trauma in the criminal justice population has commonly examined sexual victimization (e.g., Harlow, 1999; Maschi et al., 2011). These prior studies primarily document whether or not a sexual victimization has occurred or not. We lack information about the various types of sexual victimization (from minor to severe types), and the age or developmental period at which it occurred. There has been little exploration of older adults' life-course subjective experiences at the time of occurrence of sexual victimization and currently while living through later life in prison. There also is a dearth of knowledge on how these different types of sexual victimization are related to sexual offending among older adults in prison.

Therefore, the purpose of this descriptive study is to examine patterns of sexual abuse over the life-course, and temporal subjective experiences, both past and present, of sexual abuse among a sample of incarcerated older adults. It also provides a preliminary analysis of the data that examines the relationship between the different subtypes of trauma and sexual offendings. Research in this area can help expose the unexplored dimensions of sexual abuse in this largely neglected population. These findings have significance for improving trauma-informed responses among older adults, especially while in prison. As a result of examining this data, the need for effective trauma assessment in the correctional system, including specific sexual victimization assessment, along with efficacious trauma treatment modalities, is underscored. The urgency and magnitude of this public health problem is highlighted and the promise of treatment that can be used to interrupt the cycle of revictimization among these vulnerable older adults in prison.

5. Study methods

This cross-sectional correlational design used a stratified random sample of older (age 50 and above) offenders drawn from a state correctional department's administrative databases. There were 667 participants that completed a self report mail survey that used a modified version of the Life Stressors Checklist-Revised (LSC-R).

5.1 Research design

This study was conducted in September 2010 in 13 prison facilities across a statewide department of correction (DOC) located in the northeast United States. Of approximately 25,000 prisoners housed in this correctional system in January 2010, approximately 6% (n=1,500) were aged 50 and older. Information to create the sampling frame included the DOC administrative records data for State Bureau of Identification (SBI) number and age.

The DOC generated the sampling frame for the study with a list of names, so that invitations and anonymous surveys could be mailed to potential participants and return correspondence could be received.

The final sample size consisted of 667 English-speaking prisoners (aged 50 and older) who responded to the survey, which resulted in a response rate of 43%. This estimate falls within the higher range of expected mail response rates, which are 20-40% for prison populations (Hochstetler et al., 2004). The project was part of the Hartford Geriatric Social Work Faculty Scholars Program Award, which is funded by the Gerontological Society of America and the John A. Hartford Foundation. The study was approved by the Fordham University Institutional Review Board (IRB) and met the standards for conducting research with a special population of older prisoners and on sensitive topics.

5.2 Data collection

The Dillman et al. (2009) method for mailed surveys was used to maximize response rates. Specifically, potential participants received: (1) a letter of invitation; (2) a packet with a cover letter, consent form, survey, and a self-addressed electronically stamped envelope (SASE) seven days later; (3) two thank you cards and reminders sent seven days apart that included an enclosed self-addressed envelope to request a survey replacement.

5.3 Constructs and study measures

Sexual victimization was measured using the 5 item subscale of the 31-item Life Stressors Checklist (LSC-R) (McHugo et al., 2005). The LSC-R sexual abuse subscale estimates the frequency of lifetime sexual abuse which is consistent with DSM IV-TR Criterion A for post trauma stress symptoms (APA, 2000). The LSC-R has good psychometric properties, including for use with diverse age groups and criminal justice populations. Researchers have reported that the LSC-R has demonstrated good criterion-related validity for detecting traumatic events, such as sexual abuse, among prisoners (McHugo et al., 2005). For example, McHugo et a1. (2005) collected data on 2,729 women in which a test-retest sample was completed on a subset of 186 women who completed the measure on average 7 days later. Kappa's range averaged .70 for different items.

5.3.1 Objective occurrences of sexual victimization

The LSC-R enables the measurement of 'objective' sexual abuse, which is defined in this study as whether or not one or more types of sexual abuse have occurred. Sexual abuse experiences are defined as those objective events that are consistent with DSM IV-TR Criterion A for PTSD (APA, 2000). Participants endorsed across 5 items as to whether or not each of these events occurred (0 = no; 1 = yes). These items included sexual touch before and after the age of 16, sexual harassment, and sexual assault before and after the age of 16 and were operationalized as follows.

1. Sexual touch before the age of 16 - "Before age 16, were you ever touched or made to touch someone else in a sexual way because he/she forced you in some way or threatened to harm you if you didn't?"
2. Sexual assault before the age of 16 – "Before age 16, did you ever have sex (oral, anal, genital) when you didn't want to because someone forced you in some way or threatened to hurt you if you didn't?"

3. Sexual harassment – "Have your ever been bothered or harassed by sexual remarks, jokes, or demands for sexual favors by someone at work or school (for example, a coworker, a boss, a customer, another student, a teacher)?"
4. Sexual touch after the age of 16 – "After age 16, were you ever touched or made to touch someone else in a sexual way because he/she forced you in some way or threatened to harm you if you didn't?"
5. Sexual assault after the age of 16 – "After age 16, did you ever have sex (oral, anal, genital) when you didn't want to because someone forced you in some way or threatened to harm you if you didn't?"

5.3.2 Age of occurrence and subjective experiences of sexual victimization

If participants endorsed 'yes' to an objective occurrence of traumatic or stressful life experiences, three follow-up items asked participants about their age and related post traumatic stress symptoms. As for age, it was measured as a continuous variable and participants were asked, "How old were you when this happened?" As for post traumatic stress symptoms, participants were asked: (1) "at the time of the event did you believe that you or someone else could be killed or seriously harmed?" (2) At the time of the event did you experience feelings of intense helplessness, fear, or horror?" Participants could respond yes or no to these two questions and they were measured as dichotomous/nominal level variables.

The LSC-R also includes a subscale for participants' 'subjective' impressions of sexual abuse victimization. For each of the types of sexual victimization experienced, participants were asked their current subjective impression of these events by asking them to rate each type of traumatic and stressful life event on the degree to which it was bothersome within this past year. Each item was measured using a five point Likert scale from 1 = not at all to 5 = extremely.

5.3.3 Sexual offense history

Sexual offense history was measured using the following self-report survey item: "Have you ever been charged with a sexual offense?" Participants could respond 'yes' or 'no'.

5.4 Data analysis

Descriptive statistics were used to examine the sociodemographic characteristics of sexual assault. A series of chi square analyses also were conducted to explore whether earlier life sexual abuse victimization (e.g., sexual touch before age 16, sexual assault before age 16, sexual touch after age 16, sexual assault after age 16, and sexual harassment) was related to the older adults' self-report sexual offense histories. All variables were dichotomous consisting of yes or no response categories.

6. Major findings

6.1 Sample description

The sample consisted of 667 adults (607 males and 24 females) serving prison sentences in a state correctional system in the north east United States in September 2010. The mean age of participants was 56.47 (sd = 6.31). The participants' racial ethnic backgrounds consisted of African-American (45%), White (36%), Hispanic/Latino (10%), and Other (9%). Only 10%

reported having no high school diploma and 30% reported serving in the military. As for family, about 24% of participants reported currently being married or partnered. Furthermore, most participants reported having children (80%), and over half reported having grandchildren (62%).

About one third of participants reported having a mental health diagnosis (36%) or a drug or alcohol problem (36%). The majority had serious offenses, including sex offenses (26%) and violent offenses (64%). On average participants served 132 months (or 11 years). Over half of the participants were expected to be released from prison within one year (37%) or 2 to 5 years (26%); while approximately 10% were expected to be released within 6 to 10 years and 17% after eleven or more years.

6.2 Sexual victimization: Objective and subjective experiences

Table 1 presents the findings on the sexual victimization experience of the study sample. Both inappropriate sexual touch and assault were found to be twice as common before the age of 16 compared to after the age of 16. More specifically, descriptive analyses revealed that 21.9% of the participants reported being a victim of inappropriate sexual touch before the age of 16 compared to 9.4% of the participants reported experiencing inappropriate sexual touch after the age of 16. Similarly, 18.5% reported forced sexual assault before the age of 16, while 9.1% reported sexual assault after the age of 16. The lifetime occurrence of sexual harassment was reported by approximately 1 out of 10 participants. That is, 12.9% of participants endorsed having experienced sexual harassment in their lifetime.

As for age of sexual victimization, the data revealed that childhood sexual abuse began at an average age of 10 with a standard deviation of 4.4 for sexual touch and 3.6 for sexual assault. The average age reported for sexual harassment was 18.6 (sd = 12.4). With regard to the subjective experiences of sexual touch or assault before or after age 16, most participants reported experiencing 'horror felt at the time' (ranging from 79.2%-89.1%). Furthermore, prior sexual touch and sexual assault appeared to have a lingering psychological effect. Many participants also reported that in the past year they felt 'moderately to extremely bothered by the incident in the past year' (ranging from 61.8% - 75.4%). In comparison to sexual touch and victimization, slightly less participants who experienced sexual harassment reported that they perceived that someone could have gotten hurt at the time (36.5%), felt horror at the time (62.7%), and were moderately to extremely bothered by it in the past year (55.1%).

	Objective Occurrences		Average Age First Occurred		Believe Someone Could Get Hurt		Horror Felt at Time		Moderately to Extremely Bothered in Past Year	
Traumatic Events	%	N	M	SD	%	N	%	N	%	N
1. Sexual Touch < age 16	21.9	132	10.1	4.4	56.9	74	85.5	106	65.2	86
2. Sexual Assault < age 16	18.5	117	9.9	3.6	62.1	72	86.7	98	69.0	80
3. Sexual Harassment	12.9	78	18.6	12.4	36.5	27	62.7	47	55.1	43
4. Sexual Touch > age 16	9.4	57	16.6	9.5	64.9	37	89.1	49	75.4	43
5. Sexual Assault > age 16	9.1	55	19.6	11.1	62.7	32	79.2	42	61.8	34

Table 1. Descriptive statistics for the Occurrence of Trauma and Mean Scores for Age First Occurred, Believe Someone would get hurt, Felt Horror at the Time, Moderately to Extremely Bothered by it Past Year

6.3 Chi square results

The results from the series of chi square tests that were run indicate that there is a significant relationship between having a sexual offense history and each of the sexual victimization variables (sexual touch before age 16 ($X^2 = 26.32$, $df = 1$, $p = .001$), sexual assault before age 16 ($X^2 = 8.16$, $df = 1$, $p = .001$), sexual touch after age 16 ($X^2 = 6.0$, $df = 1$, $p = .02$), sexual assault after age 16 ($X^2 = 7.9$, $df = 1$, $p = .01$), and sexual harassment ($X^2 = 10.5$, $df = 1$, $p = .001$). These findings suggest that there is a relationship between prior sexual victimization and sexual offending.

7. Conclusion

7.1 Overview of purpose and major findings

The purpose of this chapter was to explore patterns of sexual abuse over the life-course among incarcerated older adult offenders and the relationship to sexual offense histories, and their temporal subjective experiences of trauma. This study corroborates prior results that find high prevalence rates of trauma among juvenile and adult prisoners (Abram et al., 2007). However, this study makes a number of significant contributions to the field. Firstly, it focuses in on traumatic experiences specific to sexual victimization. Secondly, it not only examines the objective occurrence of such experiences, but also examines incarcerated older adults' past year subjective impressions of these events, indicating significant present distress from past sexual abuse experiences. Thirdly, it examined and found support for a positive and significant relationship between having committed a sexual offense and experiences of sexual victimization.

7.2 Implications

Currently, the sexual abuse victimization experiences of older adults who also are incarcerated offenders have been largely ignored. This is a serious oversight since prison systems are known for being highly stressful environments in which older adults are at greater risk for the onset or resurfacing of post traumatic stress symptoms (Maschi, Gibson, Zgoba, & Morgen, 2011). In court or prison intake assessment and pre-parole evaluations, subjective experiences, especially psychological distress related to past events, and sexual victimization, are not assessed. Without proper assessment, can older adults in prison access the types of services to help process unresolved sexual abuse experiences and take responsibility for their offenses?

In addition to adjustment to prison, about half of the incarcerated older adults are expected to be released to the community. There is potential for new federal proposals to aid in improving both advancing the discourse about these issues and improving practices for older adults in prison facilities. For example, in America, the Substance Abuse and Mental Health Services Administration (SAMHSA, 2011) recently created eight new initiatives (2011-2014), including trauma and justice. Programs that provide sexual abuse and sex offender specific treatment are warranted. Treatment options should be available from the point of entry into the correctional system, in preparation for re-entry into the community, and care after release.

As the findings suggest, significant differences were found between objective and subjective experiences of sexual abuse in this population. Understanding these differences and the more significant role that subjective experience plays for these participants, are essential in understanding, developing, and refining, effective screening instruments and implementing appropriate, trauma-informed interventions. This study supports the notion that assessing for objective and subjective distress related to these events also may be essential.

Along the same lines, evidence-based assessment and interventions must be in line with the finding of how significant the subjective impressions of sexual assault are for incarcerated older adults in treatment. A promising intervention that is being piloted in the criminal justice system with younger age groups is Eye Movement Desensitization and Reprocessing (EMDR). EMDR specifically targets change in subjective units of distress among trauma survivors, particularly sexual abuse survivors, which in turn reduces post traumatic stress symptoms (Kitchiner, 2000). Moreover, previous research with incarcerated juvenile offenders shows that EMDR can work in reducing post traumatic stress reactivity resulting in less violent behavior and conduct problems among samples. Its utility for older adults, especially those with histories of sexual assault victimization and perpetration is perhaps a promising intervention. The use of evidence-based practices suggests that untreated trauma and grief are related to increased adult recidivism rates (Leach et al., 2008). Therefore, treating psychological distress and untreated symptoms effectively, which involves both screening and treatment that captures subjective experiences, may help to break the cycle of recidivism and in some case sexual offending.

7.3 Limitations and future research directions

This study has notable limitations. First, the study used a cross-sectional design thus precluding causal inferences about the relationship between sexual victimization and sexual offending. The study sample from a northeast state prison system may not be representative of and generalizable to prisoners in other geographic locations and non-English speaking participants. Using a mailed self-administered survey may be another limitation because of possible low response rates and possible limited literacy levels.

Perhaps most importantly, while the data found in this study related to sexual abuse are slightly higher than in the general public, it is imperative to consider that these numbers are still not representative of the actual rates of sexual victimization in older prisoners. Offenders often do not endorse a history of sexual abuse even if it is present. For instance, research shows that 40% of randomly selected male inmates met the criteria for being a victim of sexual abuse. However, 41% of those people did not consider themselves to have been sexually abused (Fondacaro, Holt & Powell, 1999). Similarly, results from a large study by the Alaska Department of Corrections (1998) of prisoners in Alaska reveal that while 70% of respondents endorsed a history of sexual acts prior to the age of 12, all of which would indicate sexual abuse, only 12% of them considered the experiences to be sexual abuse (Langworthy, Barnes, & Curtis, 1998). As a result, it must be considered a possibility that these numbers are lower than actuality.

The findings of this study support the need for future research to examine the relationship between sexual offending and sexual victimization among incarcerated older offenders. This includes studies that examine a broad range of sexual victimization and how these experiences influence subjective physical and mental well-being and criminal offending, including sexual offending. A longitudinal study examining reactivity among ex-offenders after reentry would greatly benefit the field and provide evidence for policy makers to implement such trauma-informed treatments within the prison system and community correctional programs.

7.4 Conclusion

In conclusion, this study attempted to fill a gap in the literature about earlier sexual abuse victimization experiences among incarcerated older adults and the relationship to sexual offending histories. Overall, the plight of older adults in the criminal justice system has largely been ignored. Continuing to neglect the later life aftermath of earlier life sexual abuse experiences may have detrimental effects on the individual experiencing them then and now.

8. Acknowledgment

The project was part of the Hartford Geriatric Social Work Faculty Scholars Program Award, which is funded by the Gerontological Society of America and the John A. Hartford Foundation.

9. References

Abram, K. M., Washburn, J. J., Teplin, L. A., Emanuel, K. M., Romero, E. G., & McClelland, G. M. (2007). Posttraumatic stress disorder and psychiatric comorbidity among detained youths. *Psychiatric Services, 58(10)*, 1311–1316.

Acierno, R, Hernandez, M.A., Amstadter, A.B., Resnick, H.S, Steve, K; Muzzy, W; & Kilpatrick, D. (2010). Financial abuse and potential neglect in the united states: The national elder mistreatment study. *American Journal of Public Health, 100*(2),292-297.

Acierno, R, Lawyer, S.R, Rheingold, A, Kilpatrick, D.G, Resnick, H.S; & Saunders, B.E. (2007). Current psychopathology in previously assaulted older adults. *Journal of Interpersonal Violence, 22*(2), 250-258.

Aday, R. H. (2003). *Aging prisoners: Crisis in American corrections.* Westport, CT: Praeger.

Aday, R. H. (2006). Aging offenders' concerns toward dying in prison. *OMEGA: Journal of Death and Dying, 52(3)*, 199–216.

American Psychiatric Association. (2000). Diagnostic and statistical manual of mental disorders (TR). Washington, DC: Author.

Brown, *Governor of California, et al. v. Plata et al.*, 2011.

Cauffman, E., Feldman, S., Waterman, J & Stiener, H. (1998). Posttraumatic stress disorder among female juvenile offenders. *Journal of the American Academy of Child and Adolescent Psychiatry 37*: 1209-216.

Cox, J. F. & Lawrence, J.E. (August 2010). *Planning services for elderly inmates with mental illness.* (Library ID. 024489.) National Institute of Corrections.

Dawes, J. (2009). Ageing Prisoners: Issues for social work. *Australian Social Work, 62*(2), 258-271.

Draper, B., Pfaff, J., Pirkis, J., Snowdon, J., Lautenschlager, N., Wilson, I., et al. (2008). Long-term effects of childhood abuse on the quality of life and health of older people: Results from the depression and early prevention of suicide in general practice project. *Journal of the American Geriatrics Society, 56*(2), 262-271.

Falter, R.G. (2006). Elderly inmates: An emerging correctional population. *Correctional Health Journal, 1*, 52-69.

Fondacaro, K., Holt, J. & Powell, T. (1999). Psychological impact of childhood sexual abuse on male inmates: The importance of perception. *Child Abuse and Neglect, 23*, 361 – 369.

Ford, J. D., Hartman, K., Hawke, J., & Chapman, J. F. (2008). Traumatic victimization, posttraumatic stress disorder, suicidal ideation, and substance abuse risk among juvenile justice-involved youth. *Journal of Child and Adolescent Trauma, 1*, 75-92.

Gagnon, M., & Hersen, M. (2000). Unresolved childhood sexual abuse and older adults: Late-life vulnerabilities. *Journal of Clinical Geropsychology, 6*(3), 187-198.

Glaze, L.E. (2009). Correctional population in the US, 2009. (NCJ Publication No. 231681). Washington, DC: US Department of Justice.

Goff, A., Rose, E., Rose, S., & Purves, D. (2007). Does PTSD occur in sentenced prison populations? A systematic literature review. *Criminal Behavior & Mental Health, 17(3)*, 152–162.

Harlow, C. W. (1999). Prior abuse reported by inmates and probationers. (NCJ Publication No. 172879). Rockville, MD: U.S. Department of Justice.

Haugebrook, S., Zgoba, K., Maschi, T., Morgen, K., & Brown, D. (2010). Trauma, stress, health, and mental health issues among ethnically diverse older adult prisoners. *Journal of Correctional Health Care, 16*(3), 220-229.

Hiskey, S., Luckie, M., Davies, S., & Brewin, C. (2008). The phenomenology of reactivated trauma memories in older adults: A preliminary study. *Aging & Mental Health, 12*(4), 494-498.

Hochstetler, A., Murphy, D. S., & Simons, R. L. (2004). Damaged goods: Exploring predictors of distress in prison inmates. *Crime & Delinquency, 50(3)*, 436–457.

James, D. J., & Glaze, L. E. (2006). Mental health problems of prison and jail inmates. (NCJ Publication No. 213600). Rockville, MD: U.S. Department of Justice.

Kitchiner, N. J. (2000, February). Using EMDR to treat post-traumatic stress disorder in a prison setting. *British Journal of Community Nursing, 5*(1), 26-31.

Krause, N. (2004). Lifetime trauma, emotional support, and life satisfaction among older adults. *The Gerontologist, 44*(5), 615-623.

Lamet, A., Szuchman, L., Perkel, L., & Walsh, S. (2009). Risk factors, resilience, and psychological distress among holocaust and nonholocaust surviviors in the post-9/11 environment. *Educational Gerontology, 35*(1), 32-46.

Langworthy, H., Barnes, R, & Curtis, R. (1998). Results From the Long-Term Inmate Survey: Focus on Child Abuse Histories. Report prepared for the Alaska Department of Corrections. Anchorage, AK: Justice Center, University of Alaska Anchorage.

Leach, R.M., Burgess, T., & Holmwood, C. (2008) Could recidivism in prisoners be linked to traumatic grief? A review of the evidence. *International Journal of Prisoner Health, 4*(2), 104-119.

Maruschak, L. M. (2008). Medical problems of offenders. (NCJ Publication No. 221740). Rockville, MD: U.S. Department of Justice.

Maschi, T. (2006). Exploring the link between trauma and delinquency: The cumulative versus differential risks. *Social Work, 1,* 59–75.

Maschi, T., Dennis, K., Gibson, S., MacMillan, T., Sternberg, S., & Hom, M. (2011). Trauma and stress among older adults in the criminal justice system: A review of the literature with implications for social work. *Journal of Gerontological Social Work, 54,* 347-360.

Maschi, T., Gibson, S., Zgoba, K.M., & Morgen, K. (2011). Trauma and life event stressors among young and older offenders, *Journal of Correctional Healthcare, 17*(2), 160-172.

Maschi, T., Morgen, K., Zgoba, K., Courtney, D., & Ristow, J. (2011). Trauma, stressful life events, and post traumatic stress symptoms: Do subjective experiences matter? *The Gerontologist.* doi:10.1093/geront/gnr074

McDaniels Wilson, C. & Belknap, J. (2008). The extensive sexual violation and sexual abuse histories of incarcerated women. *Violence Against Women, 14,* 1090-1127.

Neal, L., Hill, N., Hughes, J., Middleton, A., & Busuttil, W. (1995). Convergent validity of measures of PTSD in an elderly population of former prisoners of war. *International Journal of Geriatric Psychiatry, 10*(7), 617-622.

Reimer, G. (2008). The graying of the U.S. offender population. *Journal of Correctional Health Care, 14*, 202-208.

Sabol, W.J. & West, H.C. (2009). *Prisoners in 2008*. (NCJ Publication No. 228417). Washington, DC: U.S. Department of Justice.

Sabol, W. J., & Couture, H. (2008). Prison inmates at midyear 2007. (NCJ Publication No. 221944). Rockville, MD: U.S. Department of Justice.

Shmotkin, D., & Barilan, Y. (2002). Expressions of Holocaust experience and their relationship to mental symptoms and physical morbidity among holocaust survivor patients. *Journal of Behavioral Medicine, 25*(2), 115-134.

Shmotkin, D., & Litwin, H. (2009). Cumulative adversity and depressive symptoms among older adults in Israel: the differential roles of self-oriented versus other-oriented events of potential trauma. *Social Psychiatry & Psychiatric Epidemiology, 44*, 989–997. doi:10.1007/s00127-009-0020-x

Shimkus, J. (2004). The graying of America's prisons: Corrections copes with care for the aged. Retrieved July 2007 from http://www.ncchc.org/pubs/CC/aging_inmates.html

Stesssman, J., Cohen, A., Hammerman-Rozenberg, R., Bursztyn, M., Azoulay, D., Maaravi, Y., et al. (2008). Holocaust survivors in old age: The Jerusalem Longitudinal Study. *Journal of the American Geriatrics Society, 56*(3), 470-477.

Stojkovic, S. (2007). Elderly offenders: A growing and forgotten group within correctional systems vulnerable to elder abuse. *Journal of Elder Abuse & Neglect, 19(3/4)*, 97–117.

Stop Prisoner Rape. (2003). The sexual abuse of female inmates in Ohio. Retrieved from http://www.justdetention.org/pdf/sexabuseohio.pdf

Struckman-Johnson, C., Struckman-Johnson, D., Rucker, L., Bumby, K., & Donaldson, S. (1996). Sexual coercion reported by men and women in prison. *Journal of Sex Research, 33(1)*, 67–76.

Substance Abuse and Mental Health Services Administration [SAMHSA] (2011). *Leading change: A plan for SAMHSA's roles and actions.* Retrieved May 7, 2011 from http://store.samhsa.gov/shin/content//SMA11-4629/04-TraumaAndJustice.pdf

Teplin, L.A. (1990). "The prevalence of severe mental disorder among male urban jail detainees: Comparison with the epidemiologic catchment area program." *American Journal of Public Health, 80*, 663-669.

van der Kolk, B. A., & Fisler, R.E. (1994). Child abuse and neglect and loss of self-regulation. *Bulletin of the Menninger Clinic, 58*, 10-23.

van der Kolk, B.A. (Ed.). (1987). *Psychological trauma*. Washington, DC: American Psychiatric Association.

van der Kolk, B.A., McFarlane, A.C., & Weisaeth, L. (Eds.). (1996). *Traumatic stress: The effects of overwhelming experience on mind, body, and society*. New York: Guildford Press.

West, H. C., & Sabol, W. J. (2008). Prisoners in 2007. (NCJ 224280). Rockville, MD: U.S. Department of Justice.

Widom, C. (1989). Does violence beget violence? A critical examination of the literature. *Psychological Bulletin, 106*, 3–28

Yehuda, R., Kahana, B., Schmeidler, J., Southwick, S., Wilson, S., & Giller, E. (1995). Impact of cumulative lifetime trauma and recent stress on current postraumatic stress disorder symptoms in Holocaust survivors. *American Journal of Psychiatry, 152*(12), 1815-1818.

3

A Salutogenic Approach to Healing Following Child Sexual Assault

Sheryle Vilenica and Jane Shakespeare-Finch
School of Psychology and Counselling, Institute of Health and Biomedical Innovation, Queensland University of Technology, Brisbane, Australia

1. Introduction

Decades of research has now produced a rich description of the destruction child sexual assault (CSA) can cause in an individual's life. Post-Traumatic Stress Disorder (PTSD), Dissociative Identity Disorder, Borderline Personality Disorder, depression, anxiety, Panic Disorder, intimacy issues, substance abuse, self-harm, and suicidal ideation and attempts, are some of the negative outcomes that have been attributed to this type of traumatic experience. Psychology's tendency to dwell within a pathological paradigm, along with popular media who espouse a similar rhetoric, would lead to the belief that once exposed to CSA, an individual is forever at the mercy of dealing with a massive array of accompanying negative effects. While the possibility of these outcomes in those who have experienced CSA is not at all denied, it is also timely to consider an alternative paradigm that up until now has received a paucity of attention in the sexual assault literature. That is to say, not only do people have the ability to work through the painful and personal impacts of CSA, but for some people the process of recovery may provide a catalyst for positive life changes that have been termed post-traumatic growth (Tedeschi & Calhoun, 1995).

To begin with in this chapter, the negative sequale' of childhood sexual assault it discussed. Inherent to this discussion are questions of measurement and definitions of sexual assault. The chapter highlights ways in which the term CSA has been defined and hence operationalised in research, and the myriad problems, confusions, and inconclusive findings that have plagued the sexual assault literature. Following this is a review of the sparse literature that has conceptualised CSA from a more salutogenic (Antonovsky, 1979) theoretical orientation. It is argued that a salutogenic approach to intervention and to research in this area, provides a more useful way of promoting healing and the gaining of wisdom, but importantly does not negate the very real distress that may accompany growth. This chapter will then present a case study to elucidate the theoretical and empirical literature discussed using the words of a survivor. Finally, the chapter concludes with implications for therapeutic practice, which includes some practical ways in which to promote adaptation to life within the context of having survived this insidious crime.

1.1 The impact of child sexual abuse: An overview of the pathological paradigm

For those who work therapeutically with individuals who have a history of child sexual abuse (CSA) there is no difficulty in understanding just how impactful this particular type of trauma can be on a person. The elements that CSA consist of in the context of traumatic events are remarkably unique. With few exceptions, such as war, persecution, and slavery, most traumatic events are just that, single episode events that occur unexpectedly and are unpredictable. With CSA however, the 'event' is something that often, though not always, occurs over and over again, with a certain amount of predictability. Furthermore, the person responsible for committing CSA acts is resoundingly more often someone the child knows, loves, and often depends on for survival (Fanslow et al., 2007; Kouyoumdjian et al., 2009). That is to say, more frequently than not, offenders are either related to the child directly or are closely involved with the child's family; trusted, influential, and deeply imbedded within the child's support network. The betrayal of trust, abuse of the child's love for, and devotion to, the offender, and confusion caused by being both hurt and loved by a trusted adult is in and of itself damaging to the child's emerging sense of self and their intrinsic worth. This in turn greatly influences the child's working models of relationships and their place within these relationships. A further unique aspect of CSA is the secrecy that surrounds this issue. With other traumatic events often the event is well known to others, and support is available to the aggrieved party. However, when a child is sexually assaulted, more often than not the child suffers in silence, feeling alone and isolated (Isely et al., 2008). In addition to the emotional isolation is fact that CSA is an offence that happens *within* the child's body. Even acts of physical violence occur *to* an individual; with CSA the violation physically crosses the line from outside to within, and there is nowhere to escape. All this can happen at a time when the child has limited resources, or recourses, open to them, due to developmental stages associated with childhood (e.g., cognitive development, dependence). It is little wonder that so many individuals who have experienced this particular interpersonal trauma are often left with deep psychological scars that resound through so many domains within their lives (Nelson et al., 2002).

The field of psychological enquiry has long been aware of the devastating effects CSA leaves in its wake. In the three decades since CSA was first brought openly into the light of scientific investigation much has been learned not only in relation to the myriad negative impacts that follow CSA, but also regarding the array of mediating and moderating factors found to contribute to the increase or decrease of the subjective impact felt. Overwhelmingly, the focus of psychological investigation has been through the lens of a pathological paradigm. The focus of the pathological paradigm is on the origins of ill-health in the form of diagnosable psychological disorders, in the process of seeking to understand what contributes to worse outcomes so that one can identify and alleviate distressing symptoms. The overarching intention is to identify ways to alleviate suffering. With this framework of investigation, the field of psychological research has provided a rich description of the pathology that often occurs as a result of a child being sexually assaulted.

Of all areas studied pertaining to CSA, the area given most attention has been that of the negative outcomes experienced by victims of this crime. Consistently, research has continued to show the direct link between CSA exposure and negative outcomes (e.g. Molnar et al., 2001; Nelson et al., 2002; O'Leary et al., 2010). Of the diagnosable disorders, major depressive disorder (Nelson et al., 2002), anxiety disorders (Calam et al., 1998), suicide attempts (Belik et al., 2009), sexual dysfunction (Gold et al., 1999), post-traumatic stress disorder (PTSD) (Shakespeare-Finch & De Dassel, 2009), and other psychopathology (Molnar et al., 2001) are commonly studied, demonstrating that those who have experienced CSA are at a significantly greater risk of developing these impairments. Even amongst sufferers of other tragedies and traumas, those who have experienced CSA show higher levels of impairment (Shakespeare-Finch & Armstrong, 2010), a testament to the highly invasive, personal, and damaging nature of the experience of sexual abuse in childhood.

The intrapersonal impact of CSA is perhaps the most pronounced and enduring of all the potential outcomes that can stem from a history of sexual abuse. Pervasive feelings of shame, guilt, and responsibility plague many of those who have endured this experience (Coffey et al., 1996). These particular effects show enduring consistency in those who have experienced repeated abuse over many years, through to those who have experienced one intrusive contact abuse act (Isley et al., 2008; Molner et al., 2002). Feelings of shame and responsibility permeate to the core of how an individual feels about themselves, not only as a person, but as a person within the abuse dyad. For a great many abuse survivors, a feeling of complicity exists, particularly if the offender is older, stronger, and in a position of authority over the child, and the abuse was not overtly challenged by the child. Survivors then take on the responsibility of the abuse, either in part or in full, believing had they said something, done something different, or been in some way different, this would not have happened to them. Through this process, core beliefs are formed about the self that often reflect worthlessness, hopelessness, or inherent 'badness'. Unfortunately, even therapeutic intervention has done little to create a shift in the global, negative way that individuals *feel* about who they are, as well as what they are worth as a person (Lev-Wiesel, 2000). From the vantage point of holding such a negative self-image, it is not difficult to understand how the interpersonal and social difficulties that can stem from CSA are encountered.

In the search for understanding the sources of difficulty and distress in survivors of CSA, the pathological paradigm has provided a rich description of the vast spectrum of potential negative outcomes that often follow sexual abuse. Adding to the understanding of pathology are an array of established mediating and moderating variables known to increase the risk of harm and suffering after experiencing CSA. Abuse-specific variables of a longer duration (Reyes, 2008), a familial offender (Zinzow et al., 2010), more intrusive abuse (Nelson et al., 2002), and subjective distress at time of abuse (Briere & Elliott, 2003) have all been shown to cause more distress and impairment. When an individual discloses their abuse, as well as how it is responded to, makes a difference to psychological outcomes. Often it is found that children who's abuse is disclosed or discovered in childhood fare much worse than those who choose to wait until adulthood (O'Leary et al., 2010), although the reverse has also been found (Ullman, 2007). If disclosure is met with silence, or worse, with condemnation of the victim, poorer outcomes are likely to follow (Del Castillo & O'Dougherty, 2009). Attachment has been shown to be an important variable in outcomes, as children who report having one non-offending parent who provides them with belief and support fare better than those who do not report such a relationship (Bolen & Lamb, 2007). In adulthood, support appears to be just as important; women with CSA histories have reported the often transformative act of being believed and accepted by another through the process of disclosure, if the disclosure is met with acceptance and validation (Del Castillo & O'Dougherty, 2009), while the damaging effects of stigma and judgement after disclosure has been reported as an area of further distress and isolation (Jonzon & Lindblad, 2004).

With what is already known through exploration using the pathological paradigm it can be said definitively and conclusively that CSA causes harm, and that a direct link exists between CSA and risk for adverse outcomes (Molar et al., 2001; Nelson et al., 2002; Wiffen & MacIntosh, 2005). With this being said, due to the heterogeneity of CSA experiences, individual differences in coping strategies during and after abuse, the interplay of the various mediating and moderating variables, as well as a host of other factors, a simple cause and effect model cannot be created to account for the myriad adverse outcomes that co-occur with the often traumatic experience of CSA (Putnam, 2003). This disparity not only exists among the types of experiences or environmental conditions that make up the population of those exposed to CSA; discrepancy and contradictions exist within the CSA literature itself.

2. CSA research and the plague of null findings

Despite robust and consistent findings throughout the CSA literature, research has also been plagued with null findings. It seems for any measured variable found to show an association with negative outcomes, another study will show the opposite. Age at the beginning of abuse, a closely related offender, longer duration of abuse, the use of force to elicit abuse acts, and a lack of support following disclosure, have all been shown to be related to greater levels of symptomology at time of measurement (O'Leary et al., 2010; Reyes, 2008; Zinzow et al., 2010). However, studies can also be found that show no such associations (see Paolucci et al., 2001). The one finding that maintains consistency however is that of intrusion: more intrusive, invasive, penetrative abuse acts have repeatedly been associated with worse outcomes for individuals (Nelson et al., 2002; Ullman, 2007).

Although consistency in research findings far outweighs the discrepancies, the fact that null findings continue to arise has led some to believe CSA is not as harmful as first thought (Rind et al., 1998). It can be argued, however, that the reason so many inconsistencies are found within the research base is not due to the possibility that CSA is not severe or damaging, but instead the ways in which research into this area is conducted is in and of itself problematic. For example, the choices of populations to study, a lack of standardisation in the definition of CSA, and the vast catch-all approach to including any form of sexual exposure of an individual during childhood in research samples, are all areas that contribute to the inconsistencies identified in the literature.

2.1 Populations

Population estimates of the prevalence of CSA among the general community in Western societies indicate an estimated 9% - 35% of women and 4% - 19% of men have experienced some form of sexual abuse in childhood (Pereda et al., 2009; Putnam, 2003). These figures themselves, though alarmingly high, are cautioned to be conservative estimates due to a combination of the sensitive and personal nature of CSA, the relatively high rates of non-disclosure (McGregor et al., 2010), and the likelihood that the data contains a healthy percentage of false-negatives (Nelson et al., 2002). These estimates are testament to the fact that a substantial percentage of functioning, non-clinical men and women in the general community have been affected by CSA. However, beginning research into CSA was often conducted on clinical female populations, with many participants being in-patients within psychiatric facilities (Gold et al., 1999). In general psychological clinical samples the rate of CSA is remarkably high and the type of abuse reported is often intrusive, enduring, and severe (Calam et al., 1998; Gold et al., 1999). The outcome of these investigations clearly showed the severe and lasting effects of the impact of CSA, with high impairments found across a number of domains within these women. However, clinical populations do not provide a representative picture of the majority of those who have experienced CSA, as evidenced by the large number of people within the general community who report experiencing abuse.

The rise of university student samples has been a popular choice for researchers for some time now (see Finkelhor & Browne, 1986). The benefit of using university students as research populations is that it provides researchers with access to large numbers of easily accessible participants. Although ease of gathering information with the use of this population is enticing, there are also inherent problems with the use of university student samples. First, within university samples, CSA prevalence rates have been shown to be lower than what is found within the general community, and the types of offences reported show a disproportionately higher percentage of non-contact abuse (exposure, pornography), and single-episode, non-penetrative abuse (Ullman, 2007; Zinzow et al., 2010) than those found within the general public (McGregor et al., 2010). A further limitation in utilising university students is that they often consist of relatively young people, the majority of whom are in their late teens to early thirties, who most often are not married and have no children (Harding et al., 2010; Zinzow et al., 2010). What this means in practice is that the sample consists largely of individuals who would be considered high-functioning, as evidenced by the fact they have met requirements to enter tertiary education, and who are also yet to go through significant life stages of partnering, marriage, and child rearing; stages that often cause one to think about the impacts of their own childhood on the way in which one conducts themselves as a spouse, mother or father (O'Dougherty et al., 2007). Not surprisingly then, university populations have been found to show less impairment than that found when studying individuals within the general population (Molner et al., 2001; Rojas & Kinder, 2009).

In reality, neither of these sample bases can be considered truly representative to the scope of individuals affected by CSA. With estimates of one in four women and one in seven men experiencing some form of CSA in childhood (Finkelhor, 1994) we only need to look at our workplaces, the local community, and indeed our own families, to see that if we have a mother, sister, aunty, and grandmother, the likelihood exists that one of these women have been affected (not withstanding familial correlates of CSA incidents). Similarly, a company board meeting consisting of 25 men could mean three or more of these men have also experienced CSA. What this means for research is that in order for our results to be truly meaningful, and to encapsulate the spectrum of individuals affected by this experience, broadening the use of general population samples would provide a more representative view of CSA and arguably, a reduction of null findings would also follow.

2.2 Definitions and measurement

Other problematic issues within research lays both within the way CSA is defined and measured. As it stands, no universal definition exists as to what actually constitutes CSA. This alone is contentious, as an obvious question is then of how is it possible for contradictory findings *not* to emerge if there is yet to be an agreement on what CSA actually is. Definition and measurement discrepancies lay within the types of experiences classified as abuse, the age of the victim at time of the assault, and a lack of enquiry into the subjective distress of the individual at the time of the experience. These factors are expanded on in the following sections.

Definitions of what constitutes CSA vary widely between studies. Some studies use questionaries from previous research (Rojas & Kinder, 2009; Ullman, 2007), others choose to use a more legal definition (see Paolucci et al., 2001) and some researchers use no definition at all, choosing to simply ask if participants had experienced sexual abuse in childhood (O'Leary et al., 2010; Phanichrat & Townshend, 2010). The latter approach in directly asking participants if they have experienced sexual abuse in childhood appears to be in the minority, with researchers often framing questions to read more on the lines of enquiry into sexual experiences (Ullman, 2007), sexual contact (Harding et al., 2010), or sexual activities (Zinzow et al., 2010) in childhood. The problem with such varied definitions of what constitutes CSA, is the likelihood of samples being inflated with the inclusion of false-positives, because not all experiences classified as CSA by the researcher may be equally classified as abuse by the participant. This point becomes pertinent when looking at responses from men who have been designated into a 'sexually abused' group on the definition of 'sexual experiences in childhood'. By this definition, a surprising majority of these men state their experience as being 'positive' (Schultz & Jones, 1983). In their qualitative study on men who had endured sexual abuse as boys by members of the clergy, Isley et al., (2008) did not find one man who rated their experience as being 'positive'. However they did report that all the men themselves spoke of experiencing pervasive feelings of inadequacy, shame, isolation, and a belief they were 'damaged' by the abuse. In contrast, for a man who, at 15 had a sexual encounter with a woman in her 20's, the likelihood of that man rating his experience as 'positive' is substantially greater. However, all too often both of these men would likely be grouped together as being 'abused'. When the operational definitions of abuse vary so greatly, it is hardly surprising that such discrepancies exist within research findings.

Age of the victim at time of abuse is another area that varies widely between studies, and has the potential to contribute to inconsistent findings. Common cut-off ranges for age at beginning of abuse or abusive episodes are 14 years (Ullman, 2007; Ullman et al., 2009), 16 years (Rojas & Kinder, 2009) and 18 years of age (Harding et al., 2010; Zinzow et al., 2010). Some studies chose to include both an upper and lower age range (Palesh et al., 2007), while others provide no age descriptors at all (Del Castillo & Dougherty, 2009; McGregor et al., 2010; O'Leary et al., 2010). The age of an individual is a potentially important factor due to the relevance of emerging sexuality and sexual experimentation that is integral to the adolescent life stage. A five-year age gap between a 16 and 21 year old is not unusual for a consenting relationship; a sexual relationship between a 17 and 22 year old is also not uncommon (Darroch et al., 1999). And within these relationships, or within other contexts that adolescents find themselves in, intrusive and unwanted sexual experiences do most certainly occur. However, these types of unwanted sexual experiences are not representative of the dynamics of what CSA is known for. The sexual abuse of a child is just that, it is an *abuse* of power, an *abuse* of trust, and an *abuse* of authority over a minor, through the *abnormal use* of a child for an adult's, or significantly older teenager's, own sexual gratification. The inclusion of age ranges that extend to 18 years of age, well above the legal age of consent of 16 years of age in many places, creates the potential for individuals being included in the cohort of those experiencing CSA, when in fact this may not be the case. Therefore, the compounding effects of the lack of an agreed-upon definition of CSA, coupled with the inclusion of unwanted sexual experiences of teenagers well into their sexual experimentation years, has the potential to confound results with the inclusion of acts that are not what would be considered to be within the realm of sexual abuse of a child, nor incorporates the relevant factors of grooming, complicity, shame, power-over, and secrecy that are important factors in the initiation and continuation of CSA.

Gaining an accurate account of subjective distress, rather than assuming inferred harm, is perhaps one avenue that could contribute to reducing null findings and inconsistencies within the literature. All too often, the phenomenological experience of the individual is overlooked within research of any description. Without an understanding of the subjective distress at the time of the abuse, there is a higher likelihood that researchers are comparing "apples with oranges". A point has been made that just because an act is considered morally wrong, that in and of itself is not enough to assume that harm has been done (Rind et al., 1998). Obviously, individual differences in coping abilities and factors associated with notions of dispositional resilience play their part, for it is not possible to know all the underlying factors that cause someone to be more or less resilient than someone else who has experienced the same type of encounter. Nor is it possible to measure in detail how any particular risk or resilience factor, let alone all of the ones currently known, may contribute to a person's perception and subsequent reaction to sexual abuse. However, it must be considered that not all incidents are experienced or interpreted equally. For instance, in relation to non-contact abuse, a pre-teen girl who was 'flashed' by a stranger in a park may show no long-term ill-effects, while a similar-aged girl who's older brother intentionally invades her privacy by leering at her whilst showering, may show more distress. Similarly, in relation to contact abuse, someone who experienced being touched on their breast over the top of their clothes by the brother of an older playmate may be less affected than someone who experienced being fondled on their genitals underneath their clothes by their uncle.

Given the above examples of areas of potential confounds within CSA research, it could be argued that research into CSA would do well to increase its rigour around these particular areas. The use of community samples as the choice of populations to study would provide a more useful participant base from which to extrapolate findings that hold more meaning across the scope of individuals who have experienced CSA. Finding an agreed-upon operational definition of what constitutes CSA, one that includes pertinent aspects of CSA such as grooming and the use of trust and/or power to gain compliance and secrecy, as well as one that is more descriptive of CSA rather than simply sexual experiences, could assist in decreasing discrepancies, by reducing confounds of false-positives through methodological wording. Finally, gaining an accurate understanding of the subjective impact CSA has had on an individual can be an avenue that reduces assumptions in research, and allows for a more authentic view of the real impact of different degrees of CSA exposure.

Yet, even with the potential areas for problems, research has provided us with a wealth of information into the serious, damaging, and pervasive negative effects that a history of sexual abuse in childhood can have on an individual. This information arms researchers and clinicians alike with a valuable knowledge base into not only the workings of CSA, but also the likely effects that may follow, and in light of this, efforts can be made to alleviate distress within individuals who have suffered this experience. However, the pathological paradigm has its limitations, and perhaps as an antidote to this, a relatively new wave of research is beginning to emerge; one that seeks to add a new body of information on CSA; a complimentary, innovative way in which we both understand and work with survivors of this particular trauma.

3. The salutogenic paradigm: Growth from the ashes

"The world breaks everyone, and afterward some are strong at the broken places" Hemmingway

In a move from the more traditional focus on pathological outcomes of trauma, and the understanding of what makes a difference in terms of reducing severity and duration of negative outcomes, research is now opening up to the broader scope of human experience and has begun to investigate factors related to more positive outcomes after trauma or severe stress. Concepts such as hardiness (Kobasa, 1979) and resilience (e.g., Bonanno, 2004; Rutter, 1987) have arisen as important determinants implicated in maintaining a person's base-line well-being in the face of traumatic or aversive life events. What these investigations have shown is that despite enduring personal traumas, some people, due to things such as favourable environmental conditions (e.g., support) and personality elements, are able to continue to function well, or are able to 'bounce back', with more ease and speed from these stressors than others. Walsh (2002) conceptualises resilience as "bouncing forward", suggesting that trauma changes a person's life and therefore "back" is not possible, and may not be desirable. Resilience and hardiness however, do not encapsulate the wide variety of ways of coping after stressors and traumas, and to this end, other investigations into how people cope with adversity and suffering have emerged in the literature.

The Salutogenic paradigm (Antonovsky, 1979) is one such reference theory that is interested in exploring the question of "What is it that keeps people well?", not only enduring personal traumas, but also within the bounds of more ordinary experiences of life stress, personal hardships, and setbacks. It was through his work with menopausal women, a sub-group of who had survived the holocaust, that medical sociologist Aaron Antonovsky began to wonder this very question. Studying these women who had endured unimaginable horrors, he discovered, to his surprise, that within the sub-group of menopausal holocaust survivors, nearly one third of the women were not only maintaining a good level of health, but were also managing to lead a fulfilling life, despite the trauma of their experiences. It was this discovery that led Antonovsky to depart from the more traditional, reductionist focus of pathology into a new paradigm of human capacity for health and wellness. Antonovsky's focus shifted to an attention on how people use their resources to remain well, even in the wake of very difficult circumstances. What he found was that the people who were able to remain relatively healthy after adversity had a certain way of looking at the world and their life, and he also noted differences in the way they coped with their life stressors. He suggested such people had a "sense of coherence".

Antonovsky's (1979) salutogenic theoretical approach views well-being as a multidimensional continuum, with health/ease on one end of the continuum, and dis-ease at the other, with fluid movement between the ends of these two poles being the normative experience. This way of thinking takes into account the very real fact that life is in and of itself inherently stressful, and that heterostasis, illness, and senescence are part of the human condition. This is a sentiment echoed by an ancient philosopher over 2 ½ thousand years ago, in the words of Buddha, *"Life is suffering"*. From this perspective, the focus is on coping resources that contribute to movement towards the healthy end of the wellbeing continuum, or at the very least, which assists in the maintenance of one's position. In this way, salutogenesis is an investigation of the total story of a person, discovering how one successfully resolves tension in their lives and maintains or enhances their position on the well-being continuum despite, or perhaps because of, their difficulties.

At the core of the salutogenic paradigm is the theory behind the perceptual differences Antonovsky discovered in individuals who were able to maintain wellness despite their previous or current circumstances, what Antonovsky coined the sense of coherence (SOC). The SOC comprises three main components across cognitive, behavioural, and emotional domains, being comprehensibility, manageability, and meaningfulness. Comprehensibility is the extent to which an individual views stressors as understandable, clear and ordered. Manageability is the extent that resources are perceived to be available to the individual, and that these resources are adequate to meet the challenges a person might face. Meaningfulness is the extent to which an individual believes their emotional life makes sense, and the emotional demands they face are worth investing energy into. Therefore, healthy coping, according to Antonovsky, is when one is able to make sense of their situation, believe they have the abilities to cope with what is in front of them, and believe that the emotional struggle to deal with their difficulties is of importance and worthy of investment (Antonovsky, 1987).

3.1 Post-traumatic growth

The overall outlook of the salutogenic orientation is to offer a theoretical perspective of successful coping. Inherent in this theory is the notion that human wellness is more than an absence of pathology, and takes into consideration the human ability to flourish and experience positive change after the experience of a major disruption or trauma. Positive changes that arise from the struggle to cope with a traumatic event have been termed *posttraumatic growth* (PTG) (Calhoun & Tedeschi, 2006; Tedeschi & Calhoun, 1996). The notion of PTG is a burgeoning field of research that takes the notion of resilience and resistance to stress to a new level. Consequently, the past 15 years of inquiry has provided research demonstrating positive post-trauma changes in individuals who have struggled with many types of trauma (Janoff-Bulman, 2006; Tedeschi & Calhoun, 1995).

One theoretical process model of the pathways to PTG asserts that the experience of trauma is so powerful that it shakes the very foundations on which we view ourselves, our world, and our place in it (Janoff-Bulman, 2006). Fundamental cognitive assumptions held about the self and one's environments, assumptions that serve to make life predictable, logical, and intelligible, and which are based on concepts such as safety, benevolence, and good things happening to good people, and bad things happening to someone else, are believed to be in dissonance with reality after a perceived traumatic event, due to the profound loss of safety, protection and certainty the experience of trauma often brings (Janoff-Bulman, 2006; Calhoun & Tedeschi, 2006). The internal disruption of one's inner world through the experience of loss of safety and security is believed to overwhelm ordinary defences, leaving one with a sense of threat, helplessness, and vulnerability. Coping, then, becomes a process of reworking internal fundamental assumptions, moving from overgeneralisation of danger and helplessness, to a place that incorporates both the new reality of the uncertainty of the world and one's own vulnerability. In other words, there needs to be a cognitive shift from being a 'victim' to being a 'survivor', while also allowing for a more positive sense of self and the world to emerge; one that is aware of, but is not defined by, vulnerability. Janoff-Bulman (2004, 2006) postulates that the path to successful coping is achieved through three psychological process; strength through suffering, psychological preparedness, and existential re-evaluation. Strength through suffering allows for knowledge gained through the struggle of coping to open an individual to a deeper understanding of themselves. Psychological preparedness is the process of the strengthening of inner resources through coping, which also makes future traumas more easily dealt with, as with experience one is more prepared for future challenges. While existential re-evaluation is the process of more fully connecting to one's life, such as developing a new-found appreciation of one's existence in the world, or developing a greater appreciation of one's life, as well as encompassing changes to one's philosophy of life and how they engage with themselves, others, and their environment on a day-to-day basis.

Theoretically however, the notion of trauma shaking the foundations of one's assumptive worlds does not entirely fit for those who experience trauma as children. Childhood and adolescence is seen as a time when one is *building* assumptive worlds about the self, others, and the world (Erikson, 1980). Therefore, it can be postulated that instead of *shaking* one's internal assumptions, childhood traumas like CSA could be seen to actually *create* assumptions about the self, as the trauma is co-occurring at a time when these attributions are being formulated. This can be seen in research findings where individuals who were abused at a later age of onset, or experienced abuse that continued into their adolescence, are found to attribute the blame for the abuse on themselves (Zinzow et al., 2010). Frequently, research and clinical practice reveals that individuals who experience CSA hold inherent perceptions of themselves based on concepts of wrongness, damagedness, and separateness (Isely et al., 2008; Zinzow et al., 2010). Perhaps growth then, for those who experience traumas at a time when they are constructing their internal assumptions, could be more of a process of uncovering the false perceptions of the self and connecting to their true nature, or the truth about who they really are. An example of this can be seen in Phanichrat and Townshend's (2010) study of men and women who regard themselves a healed from CSA. Sentiments echoed from these individuals show that the process of letting go of shame and truly accepting themselves, and shifting the way they viewed themselves in relation to the abuse, were fundamental avenues that lead to their healing. Other research has revealed that gaining an understanding of power differentials, hierarchical relationships, and personal boundaries helped women to shift their perspective of self-blame to a more realistic and healthy view that the offender was responsible for the abuse, and not them (Flynn, 2008). By these reports, shifts in self-perception are seen as important aspects that allow for an experience of inner transformation and contribute significantly to healing from CSA.

A further theoretical postulation of PTG comes from Tedeschi and Calhoun (2004) who have found that through the process of actively dealing with the experience of trauma, people often report growth and change in three major domains; in ones' sense of self, their relationships with others, and in their philosophy in life. People report feeling a greater sense of personal strength, self-reliance and competence through successfully negotiating the struggle to cope with their traumatic experience, a strengthening in their relationships with others and greater freedom of self-disclosure within personal relationships, a shift in their philosophy of life, such as greater appreciation of the 'little things', changed priorities, or changes in religious or existential beliefs (Calhoun & Tedeschi, 2006; Tedeschi & Calhoun, 1999). Calhoun and Tedeschi (2006) propose growth is both a process and an outcome, in that processes such as volition rumination, self-disclosure, and managing distress, lead to the three broad outcome domains. This is a sentiment echoed in existing theories of coping that assert the struggle to process negative events, through mechanisms such as meaning making, leads to growth outcomes of cognitive reappraisals of fundamental assumptions (Park & Folkman, 1997; Park, 2009). An example of this can be seen in Flynn's (2008) investigation of women sexually abused by members of their church clergy. Although PTG was not examined in this study, the qualitative reports reveal that the process of being believed and supported was influential in these women being able to shift their negative view of themselves to a more realistic and positive view. Further, the women in this study also reported that shifting their focus of spirituality from a hierarchical, patriarchal church structure to a more relational, spiritual connection, allowed for a deeper connection to self and inner transformation. Although the question of whether PTG is a process or an outcome is left to be answered, from a philosophical perspective, an outcome depends on only where you stand in time. There are others however, who suggest that the pathways *to* growth are not necessarily the same as the outcomes *of* growth, and that research would do well to explore further the pathways taken that result in positive post-trauma change (Janoff-Bulman, 2004; Woodward & Joseph, 2003).

Within these above-mentioned complimentary perspectives of human wellness and growth, the recurrent themes of three major processes are apparent. Antonovsky's SOC concept of manageability is echoed in Janoff-Bulman psychological preparedness and Tedeschi and Calhoun's strengthening of relationships with others, as each of these have components of being able to utilise resources, both intrapersonally and interpersonally, as that which assist in the facilitation of adaptive coping. Similarly, comprehensibility, strength through suffering, and changes in the way one views themselves all resonate with the notion that an increased knowledge and understanding of the self is important for positive change and growth. Finally, meaningfulness, existential re-evaluation, and changes in one's philosophy of life have at their core the assumption that changes in one's connection and commitment to one's life is an important determinant of growth, healing, and wellness after adversity. Reflected in these perspectives are themes such as connection, deepening of relationships, the use of knowledge as power, gratitude, and appreciation. By opening up to the whole story of the person, rather than merely focussing on negative outcomes from trauma and distress, a fuller picture of the human capacity to cope, survive, and thrive after adversity emerges.

The phenomenon of PTG has now been shown to occur after an array of traumatic events, from bereavement (Cadell, 2003) and motor vehicle accidents (Shakespeare-Finch & Armstrong, 2010), to acts of terrorism (Take et al., 2008). However, the external event in and of itself is not what 'creates' the conditions for PTG to occur, but instead, it is more the internal disruption the experience creates, the subjective experience of it, and, most importantly, the struggle engaged in to incorporate the event into life. This is demonstrated by the fact that not all witnesses or survivors of a potentially traumatic experience suffer long-term negative effects from their exposure. Indeed some people may perceive an experience to be traumatic whereas the same experience may not be perceived as traumatic by another. The majority of people exposed to any of the myriad of sudden, unexpected, negative events that could be construed as a traumatic experience tend to show initial, short-lived posttraumatic symptoms (a normal response to such an experience) however, most people will not develop PTSD (Bonanno, 2004). Although this holds for the broader scope of traumatic events, sexual trauma is significantly different. Not only are those who experience CSA at a significantly high risk of developing PTSD at some stage than survivors of other sorts of trauma, they are also more likely to endure lifetime PTSD symptoms (Rodridues et al., 1998). Another difference found when contrasting CSA survivors with other trauma populations is the trend for them to show less growth as a group compared to those who have survived serious motor vehicle accidents or sudden bereavement (Shakespeare-Finch & Armstrong, 2010). These differences could be due to the fact that CSA is often a prolonged, intentional trauma, most commonly perpetrated by a loved and trusted abuser, rather than single incident trauma, such as a car accident. Recently it has been suggested that the domains of PTG may have different values to different trauma populations, and to this end it would be wise to explore different types of trauma separately (Shakespeare-Finch & de Dassel, 2009), or with very large and tightly defined groups permitting in-depth analysis of the dimensions of growth in relation to other variables, including depression, anxiety, and PTSD.

3.2 Growth, healing, and wellness after CSA

Currently the research exploring wellness and PTG processes and outcomes on the single population of adult survivors of CSA is still emerging and is relatively scarce (Lev-Wiesel et al., 2004; Shakespeare-Finch & de Dassel, 2009; Woodward & Joseph, 2003). What research has uncovered at this point in time however, is that growth and healing after sexual abuse in childhood is possible, that the relationship between growth and distress is currently unclear, and that the traditional ways of working therapeutically with CSA survivors may not be as facilitative of growth and change as other modalities.

Contrary to historical views of outcomes of CSA, research has shown that positive change and growth can and does occur in many individuals. O'Dougherty and colleagues (2007) explored the ways in which 60 women with children found ways of positively resolving their CSA histories. In this sample almost half of the women conveyed that they perceived they had gained great benefit as a result of working through their trauma, whereas only 7% felt nothing positive had come from their experience of CSA. Resonating with PTG theory, the women who felt they had gained something reported positive changes in areas of personal strength and knowledge, changes in their relations with others, including a positive influence in the way they parented their children, and changes in their spiritual or religious domains. Where women situated themselves on their healing journey was important in relation to the amount of growth felt, as those who reported greater meaning as a result of their struggle were also more likely to report their abuse as mostly resolved. Similarly, in a study investigating turning points in men and women's lives who had experienced CSA, Woodward and Joseph (2003) also found people reported positive changes in the way they saw themselves, in their relationships with others, and in their philosophy of life. Further, their findings revealed that it was more the process of gaining a sense of mastery and control over one's life, be that by taking the offender to court, developing a kinder intrapersonal connection, or investing in nurturing relationship with others, that was seen as an important factor for health and recovery in these individuals.

Another finding from PTG research is that is that growth as a result of dealing with CSA and distress from CSA appear to be independent of each other. Lev-Wiesel and colleagues (2004) explored both PTSD and PTG in women who were abused by either a family member or a stranger. Their findings revealed a high positive relationship between PTG and PTSD. Further, those who experienced abuse at the hand of a relative were both more likely to have high levels of PTSD and were also more likely to report positive change and growth. A similar relationship between distress and growth can also be seen in the sample of women studied by O'Dougherty and colleagues (2007), although benefits reported from the struggle to cope with abuse resonated across intrapersonal, relational, and existential domains, these perceived benefits were not associated with lower depressive symptoms. What these findings suggest is that the relationship between growth and distress is not yet clear. As has been previously stated, the likelihood of growth occurring out of a traumatic experience is dependent upon both the trauma being severe enough to cause disruption to one's internal world, as well as one's active engagement in rebuilding one's self after such an experience. The process of actually facing the impact CSA has had one one's life and actively engaging in healing from this experience is in itself a process of turning *towards* the pain and working through it. With that in mind, it does make intuitive sense that growth and distress would occur at the same time.

An interesting finding from research into positive change and growth after CSA is the role of coping in healing. Qualitative research into processes that lead to positive change and growth reveal the adaptive nature of avoidant coping and how individuals often choose avoidant strategies as a way of managing overwhelming distress until the time comes when they have adequate resources to actively deal with their trauma (Phanichrat & Townshend, 2010). Expressions of avoidant coping strategies being 'best-friends' or 'life-savers' show that these ways of coping, for a time, can be highly adaptive and can allow one to function in their lives until such time that they are able to move from avoidance to active engagement (Phanichrat & Townshend, 2010). Although avoidant coping has been reported as being adaptive during a point in time in ones healing journey, staying with this way of coping is not facilitative of growth, and in fact has been shown to negatively correlate with growth (Shakespeare-Finch & De Dassel, 2009). What has been shown is that the absence of avoidant coping, and thereby implied the presence of acceptance of what has actually occurred, or successful coping, assists in the positive resolution of CSA (O'Dougherty et al., 2007). But there is perhaps an optimum time for this transition from avoidant coping to happen, which is likely to be highly individualised.

Beyond coping, Bogar and Hulse-Killacky (2006) found some similar processes of resilient women who had experienced CSA and who were actively engaged in their lives, and who rated their lives as meaningful. What these women revealed is that the processes of moving on from their old self-constructs, active participation in their healing, and achieving a sense of closure to their CSA experiences, is what made the difference to their healing. Traditionally, treatments for CSA have focussed on reducing post-traumatic symptoms in order to facilitate change and psychological improvement (Chambless & Hollan, 1998; Foa et al., 1999). As the majority of adult CSA survivors who seek therapy have experienced PTSD at some point in their lives (Rodridues et al., 1998), the most advocated approach to the treatment of PTSD in sexual trauma survivors has been through the use of cognitive-behavioural therapy (CBT), with particular emphasis on exposure and desensitisation (Foa et al., 1999). Clinical practice however, often reveals that it is precisely this focus on the constant revisiting of the trauma that causes people to terminate CBT interventions early, often with reports that range from dissatisfaction in the therapeutic process by not exploring the core issues relating to their inner experience, through to feeling more traumatised than before therapy due to the constant revisiting of the abusive acts via the process of desensitisation. Far from needing to talk about the specifics of their abuse and to de-sensitise to their traumatic memories, the well-functioning women in Bogar and Hulse-Killacky's (2006) study reveal that actively connecting to the impact the experience of CSA had on their lives and on their sense of self, and changing the way in which they viewed themselves, was the most important determinant of wellness and being able to move on.

4. A case study in growth and healing from CSA

The following story outlines some of the major themes explored in this paper, and is taken from a women in her 40's who has participated in the authors' research project looking at pathways to health and healing after CSA. Kate (not her real name) experienced on-going, intrusive, contact sexual abuse by her older brother from the age of 8 till 14. She did not disclose her abuse in childhood, and when her abuse was made known to her family as an adult, she was not believed or supported by them. The story is punctuated with reference to the themes covered in this chapter to connect the theory and research discussed to the story of one woman's journey to healing.

Secrecy and shame

The reaction to being asked by someone to come out about the abuse is often too confronting. Kate had a typical reaction to the suggestion: "NO! Imagine what that would do to the family!"

Subjective distress at the time of abuse

Kate was asked to use a five-point scale (1 = a little upsetting - 5 = extremely distressing) to describe her levels of distress at the time of the abuse. She said: "(when it was happening) I don't think I knew enough, but maybe 2 ½ - 3. Looking back now I would say a 4. I feel as a child, with more time and knowledge, and because it had carryon effects and the effects were more after then during. So then I would say 4 ½, give it a 5!!! It is interesting how it changed!"

Negative effects of the abuse

"Depression, suicidal ideation, being scared of everything in the world, headaches, low self-esteem, poor body image, fear, guilt, shame, perfectionism. It made me feel worthless, not loveable. I thought the world was scary. I had a sense that there was something wrong with me and that I was all alone. Lack of trust, I couldn't trust myself. Really, really poor self-esteem. Always wondering what people were thinking of me and did people see through me? There was just this fear that I could not cope, lack of trust in myself. Poor relationship with my mother".

On how the attachment relationship was more impactful than the abuse

"I remember before I was eight, I thought I had the best mother in the world, and there was a time when I was eight or nine when it all changed. I feel strongly that the poor relationship with my mother has had more detriment than the actual abuse, and the way she reacted to it (the abuse) too, it has a bearing on that. The first reaction (from my mother) was "No, it didn't happen", and she has said "well this is just the things that kids do". And whether it is just in my mind thinking that "your mum doesn't love you", I have learnt that this has a BIG impact; it has had one on me".

Acknowledgement of abuse started the healing process

"The first time in my adult life that I ever had talked face to face with (the offender) he said, "It was nothing", and I said "It's not like nothing happened". That was the first time that I had acknowledged it in his company. And then, because I was having flashbacks and not sleeping after that phone call, I then rang the SA (sexual assault) unit and started the first real counselling that I had". Prior to this phone call, Kate had brief discussions with her husband about her abuse, but would minimise the impact it had on her, saying: "It wasn't much; I was one of the lucky ones. I think I allayed his (her husband) anxieties by saying I was one of the lucky ones, I am fine". After verbally acknowledging the abuse to her offender, this brought to the surface all the latent emotions that were still within her and started Kate on her path to healing.

After a process of active engagement in her healing, these are some of the pathways Kate identified in her eventual resolution of the past and her new appreciation of herself and her life.

Growth as a process

"There were times (after the disclosure) when I was feeling very vulnerable with two young children and all this going on and lots to carry once it had blown up, and I stood on my own. And it was all good, for me to prove that once I am in the firing line I was able to trust my own judgement, and that helped me get through too. Circumstances transpired that put me in situations to enable me to have a chance to prove to myself that I can cope". This quote indicates the perception of manageability and also of psychological preparedness for future life experiences that may threaten her sense of self, and being able to trust that she could cope.

When describing the turning points for her that were gained through a therapeutic process, Kate said: "Something in counselling that has really helped is that I am only responsible for myself, but I AM responsible for my stuff. That was very powerful, and it helped me release old feelings of responsibility for others and for the abuse. Overcoming the mind talk, that has been a wonderful gift. Just being able to know that I am not my mind, I am not my collection of thoughts, I am so much more. I have come a long way; I was so in my head and could not get out – knowing now that I am not my collection of thoughts. I read a lot about CSA and perpetrators and got all this knowledge. I think the knowledge helped too, once I saw that it wasn't just me and I read it is NEVER YOUR FAULT - that was a turning point, once I stopped blaming myself it was a real unblocking. Also, moving from the 'victim mode' (was important). I think the victim phase served me, it helped, because if I never felt like that I would not have been able to release all the stagnant energy and toxicity in me. I had to feel it to heal it, but I didn't know that yet. And victim is not a good place to be so I wasn't going to stay there". In this quote, Kate reveals her new-found capacity for comprehensibility of her experiences. She also demonstrates that she has found a new sense of personal strength through her suffering. This quote also highlights the importance of connecting to the pain of being a victim, and how it is described as a necessary place to be, for a time. It also shows the transformative power of moving on from only seeing one's self as a victim to feeling more in control.

A very important component in growth from trauma is the notion of acceptance (e.g., Shakespeare-Finch & Copping, 2006). Acceptance does not mean that you are accepting of the abuse but rather, that it occurred: "I let myself FEEL. And there was SO MUCH STUFF IN THERE!! I felt it pushed down to my toes, burying, bottled, and pressure. And whenever I cried, it would just let it. At first I would stop it because it hurt, but I learnt very quickly that the more I let out I felt lighter and better. And rather than trying to stop it I just let more come up and I got very good at it, and it would come up and up and up, and in the end I just loved it because when I went through those periods I saw past it as another big step forward. So cry, cry, cry! It's all good" In the latter part of this quote, Kate is describing a sense of meaning that she attached to this process, and how the process of accepting the reality of the pain of her felt experience of her emotions allowed her to gain a sense of mastery.

Growth as an outcome

The following quote demonstrates a belief that Kate has; that she has changed fundamentally: "In terms of the old self-beliefs, they are non-existent now. I know they are non-truth. Now I think of myself as pure, intact, not damaged, very loving, I don't need to judge myself. The shame has gone, and the guilt. Knowing that the way I do it is right – because that is something that I grappled with from a self-esteem point of view, feeling damaged – (I felt that) everyone knew how to do it (life) right but I didn't. And I didn't trust my own intuition. But the way I do it is the way that is right". Her change in her view of herself was described as "That was amazing". Kate also expressed that she had experienced changes in relationships with others through the conscious struggle she engaged in to come to terms with her abuse: "I think my growth has affected my parenting in that my children, they have to KNOW that I love them. I also have a paradigm that I live with now, that everything is part of a perfect plan. And I have an appreciation of nature! Through healing, growth, and looking within, by connecting to self I realised I am connected to nature" This comment describes a fundamental shift in philosophy of life.

On-going healing

As we have said throughout this chapter, healing and growth do not discount elements of ongoing distress such as intrusive thoughts. However, Kate said: "Things still come in to my mind but I recognise them straight away, I am not scared of my thoughts anymore, I see the thoughts for what they are". Below is a summary of some of the pivotal points along her journey that Kate states as being the most fundamental in her healing.

"I had a Lomi Lomi massage and I think that was a big, big, big turning point, and I haven't stopped growing. I just totally opened to receiving healing **(active engagement in healing)**. I first thought 'Oh wow, spirituality', but I was ready for it. She (the Lomi Lomi therapist) also sat and talked to me first, and it was who she was, and it was just an open, non-judging relationship "**(acceptance)**.

"My husband being a supportive partner has been very significant in my healing. I really respect him and he respects me. He saw through the manifestations (negative effects of the abuse) and saw the real me. And I have had snippets of the real me throughout this time, but generally it was with people in my life that I felt real love. I felt my husband loved me for who I was underneath and it just helped me get rid of the shame, the guilt. It was acceptance" This is obviously another example of the power of acceptance, and also of validation and connection; being able to connect with the truth of herself as being worthy of love and respect.

There were also significant others who assisted Kate on her healing journey. The following quote explains the importance of emotional and instrumental support in promoting well-being: "And something significant in my healing, I had an uncle and as a young child I idolised him. I thought he was kind and gentle and handsome, strong and a man of his word, held his own. He met a partner and she and I connected, she was the most beautiful woman in the world, to me she was an angel on this earth, and I think (the relationship) had an impact on the rest of my life. It was a really significant relationship connection. I saw the love between the two of them, so I saw what was possible. That good, healthy modelling and I think it opened my eyes up and started to connect to the real me, and I resonated with that. And I would hang out every evening for hugs, because I would get a hug every evening before bed, I wished it would never stop that hug, particularly from her, but my uncle as well. I could trust, there was no mistrust there, but I did not disclose to them".

Kate continued to discuss how her uncle's partner was a pivotal person in her life. She said: "She taught me that the most simple things in life are to be celebrated. Every meal she would set the table beautifully, clean sheets on the bed, daily a fresh towel, and if it was raining she would cherish the rain. And that is with me now to this day and that has just grown bigger and bigger. Love of nature and that hope that you could have a marriage that was beautiful, happy, loving. So to me that put a standard in my head that that is what I wanted. So that was a really significant thing in my healing, she was an angel on earth and I have no doubts about that, so that bought the real me out that I knew was there. It seemed pure, clean, loving. Pure love without all the games. Trust." It was through this relationship that Kate connected with a feeling of self-love. Kate describes this particular relationship in her life as reminding her of: "A faint memory of love for myself" that she drew upon as a source of strength whilst working through her healing.

Describing processes that lead to healing, Kate said of herself: "She [the Lomi Lomi therapist] told me to do a burning ceremony and that really helped, the visualisation. She came up with good things to read. I read so much"!! Kate also engaged in journaling. "Gratitude journaling, I would highly recommend it to anybody. That got me in touch with who I am and what resonated with me. That is self-love, because it made me stop and actually think 'what do I like'? And one thing led to another and then I could see, even just sensing, what kind of things I was writing down - beauty. It showed me what was important in my life; relationships, nature. Yeah, so gratitude journal is right up there for power for me". In this quote, Kate is describing how the process of learning to connect with herself, and what is important to her, allowed for a deepening relationship to her inner life, and connected her to the truth of who she really is.

Kate was also asked to reflect upon any benefits she felt had come out of her healing journey; elements of her life that perhaps may not be there, had she not engaged in healing from her experiences of CSA. To this Kate stated: "A deep desire to be happy and content. Spiritual awareness. Spiritual development. Peace. Self-love. Living in my heart more, trusting intuition. Art, painting, that has been wonderful. I was always good at art and somewhere along the line as a child I got the message that was a waste of time, but reconnecting to that has been a big part of my healing. Improved relationships. Improved parenting. Flowing with things that are happening without reacting". In this quote, Kate clearly expresses how the struggle to heal from CSA has not only provided her with a deep and fulfilling life, but that she also feels her life has been more enriched and meaningful for the painful experiences she has actively engaged in overcoming.

5. Implications for therapeutic practice

There are many implications for main-stream therapeutic practice that can be taken from this case study. First, it is important to acknowledge that "mainstream practice" indicates the Western tendency in psychiatric and psychological literature to favour CBT as a therapeutic intervention of choice following any kind of trauma (e.g., Forbes et al., 2007). Although CBT clearly has its strengths, the processes outlined in this case study highlight aspects that speak to deep processes, such as the importance of healthy and authentic responsibility-taking, connection to inner experience, including the energy of emotions within the body, as well as the relationship one has with ones-self, including beliefs about the self and learning to trust, both in one's self, and also in others.

Feelings of responsibility and guilt for the abusive experiences, either in part or in full, are commonly experienced by those with a CSA history. In addition, there is also the assumed responsibility that survivors place on themselves in relation to the ramifications of disclosure of the abuse, which often impacts on relationships within their family of origin, particularly if the offender is intra-familial. This was highlighted in Kate's statement regarding her thoughts on disclosure "Imagine what that would do to the family". In the therapy room, assisting those who have experienced CSA to clearly understand the dynamics of abuse, including unequal power dynamics, grooming behaviours, and learned helplessness, is a most helpful way of assisting clients to begin transforming the way they see themselves within the abusive relationship. Searching for specific, concrete examples within the client's narrative that provide ways of showing how the offender is solely responsible for the abuse, and providing many opportunities to uncover the unique effects their experience has had on the way they come to terms with the issue of 'responsibility' in their day-to-day lives, can help to facilitate this change. Further to this is the importance of learning to accept a genuine and authentic measure of responsibility in order to gain control and mastery over one's life, thus facilitating the move from feeling like a victim, to knowing they can cope with what is in front of them.

Acceptance of the emotional impact of CSA, such as connecting to the often painful, physical experience of *feeling* emotions within the body and acknowledging their existence, was an important turning point for Kate. Physical detachment, or dissociation, from emotions is a common coping mechanism in those who have experienced CSA, and occurs in varying degrees of detachment. However, a common occurrence is that, with the protracted use of dissociation from inner experience as a means of coping, comes a sense of not *knowing* one's self. Further, being detached from physical experience can impair one's ability to identify emotions within the body, and as such, people often report having a sense of existing 'outside' of their bodies. This again reaffirms the important distinction of this particular trauma happening *within the body;* shutting off one's connection to felt sensations is an understandable way to deal with such an intrusive, physical experience. Within therapy, teaching modalities that assist in the development of acceptance of experience, such as breathing techniques, meditation, and tactile exercises such as body work, can all be used as ways of assisting clients to become more aware of, and comfortable with, their inner experience. Learning to reconnect with one's body through acknowledgment and acceptance of emotions is another avenue that provides opportunities to experience a sense of mastery and control. It is also of great benefit to clients if therapists have a personal and working knowledge of how the processes of meditation and breath work are both utilised and cultivated, and to this end it is suggested that therapists choosing to use such activities with clients are themselves practitioners of these things.

Learning to see the truth of who one is, distinctly from the 'un-truth' of long-held intrapersonal misconceptions, such as the negative core beliefs often held by those who have experienced CSA, is another point demonstrated in the case study as being important in healing from CSA. Core beliefs based on feelings of inherent badness, wrongness, or deficiency are commonly expressed in the therapy room by survivors of CSA, and also by Kate. As Kate expressed, "Once I stopped blaming myself; that was a real unblocking". This point speaks to the importance of assisting clients in their development of a caring, unconditional acceptance of who they are. This process allows clients to move from a place of shame and guilt to a more honest view of seeing themselves as whole and possessing self-worth.

Another aspect noted in the case study is the importance of a sense of mastery, self-efficacy, or a trust in one's own abilities; in being able to trust in one's own judgment and prove that one can cope. Being able to shed the identity of 'victim' requires a movement from helplessness into a position of knowing one can help one's self. Learning to trust one's own judgment is an essential foundation on which to begin to build, or re-build, trust in others; an issue that often is a point of difficulty for survivors of CSA, in light of the *abuse* of trust CSA often entails. Inherent within discussions of strength, mastery, and most importantly the judgment of self that occurs with such experiences, healing, as it were, is best discussed with clients as something that should be viewed as a dynamic and on-going process.

6. Summary

Research regarding the experience of negotiating childhood sexual assault has postulated numerous variables that apparently inform *outcomes*. The outcomes that research and literature have predominantly focussed on are largely deprivational, which is understandable, and arguably morally just, but are also largely void of hope, growth, or transformation. Trauma is labelled as such because it is an experience, or perhaps multiple experiences, of having one's inner core fundamentally shifted by something so profound, so threatening, and helplessness rending, that it affords significant life change. Literature has focused on the insidious impacts, overtly displayed or covertly expressed, and a number of potentially diagnosable pathological impacts of such life experiences. What is evident is that many more people than not are living *normal* lives as survivors of CSA, and other traumas, and most importantly, that one outcome measure denoting difficulty in adjustment does not negate the presence of other markers of positive development.

It is important in the pursuit of promoting mental health, to also acknowledge the many ways in which a CSA survivor may heal, learn, and/or use the experience of their lives in a positively transformative way. It is the very nature of CSA being insidious, invasive, pervasive, shameful, anxiety-provoking, soaked in self-doubt, and brimming in hypocrisy and betrayal that makes it the single (or enduring) trauma type that is constantly shown to be predictive of a higher prevalence of negative impacts than other traumatic experiences. However, there is a more holistic picture that needs to be kept in mind. Beyond the often-reported negative impacts, there are also many survivors who find a path to healing from these deleterious effects, or at the very least, find ways that allow them to be able to maintain a level of well-being and functionality that leads to productive and engaged lives. Exploring with greater scope the pathways and determinants that contribute to health, well-being, healing, and growth in individuals who have experienced CSA, could assist greatly in broadening the way therapeutic intervention is looked at and undertaken with individuals who have experienced this particular trauma.

7. References

Antonovsky, A. (1979). Health, Stress and Coping. San Francisco: Jossey:Bass

Antonovsky, A. (1987). Unraveling the Mystery of Health. San Francisco: Jossey-Bass

Beitchman, J. H., Zucker, K. J., Hood, J. E., daCosta, G. A., Akman, D., & Cassaiva, E. (1992). A review of the long- term effects of child sexual abuse. *Child Abuse & Neglect*, 16, 101–118

Belik. S.L., Stein, M. B., Asmundson, G. J. G., & Sareen, J. (2009). Relation between traumatic events and suicide attempts in Canadian military personelle. *Canadian Journal of Psychiatry (54)* 2, 93

Bogar, C. B., &Hulse-Killacky, D. (2006). Resiliency determinants and resiliency processes among female adult survivors of childhood sexual abuse. *Journal of Counselling and Development, 84,* 318 - 327

Bolen, R. M., & Lamb, J. L. (2007). Parental support and outcome in sexually abused children. *Journal of Child Sexual Abuse, 16* (2), 33 - 54

Bonanno, G. A. (2004). Loss, trauma, and human resilience. Have we lost the human capacity to thrive after extremely aversive events? *American Psychologist, 59,* (1) 20-28

Briere, J., & Elliott, D. M. (2003). Prevalence and psychological sequelae of self-reported childhood physical and sexual abuse in a general population sample of men and women. *Child Abuse & Neglect*, 27, 1205–1222

Cadell, S. (2003). Trauma and growth in Canadian carers. *AIDS Care*(0954-0121), *15*, 639.

Calam, R., Horne, L., Glasgow, D., & Cox, A. (1998). Psychological disturbance and child sexual abuse: A follow- up study. *Child Abuse & Neglect*, *22*, 901–913

Calhoun, L. G., & Tedeschi, R. G. (2006). The foundations of posttraumatic growth: An expanded framework, pp 3 - 23. In L.G. Calhoun & R.G. Tedaschi, *Handbook of Posttraumatic Growth.* Lawrence Erlbaum Associates, Inc

Chambless, D. L., & Hollan, S. D. (1998). Defining empirically supported therapies. *Journal of Consulting and Clinical Psychology, 66,* 7-18

Coffey, P., Leitenberg, H., Henning, K., Turner, T., & Bennett, R. T. (1996). Mediators of the long-term impact of child sexual abuse: Perceived stigma, betrayal, powerlessness, and self-blame. *Child Abuse & Neglect*, 20(5), 447–455

Darroch, J. E., Landry, D. J., & Oslak, S. (1999). Age differences between sexual partners in the United States. *Family Planning Perspectives, 31* (4) 160 - 167

Del Castillo, D., & O'Dougherty, W. M. (2009).The perils and possibilities in disclosing childhood sexual abuse to a romantic partner. *Journal of Child Sexual Abuse, 18* (4), 386 - 404

Erikson, E. (1980). Identity and the Life Cycle. New York: Norton & Company, Inc

Fanslow, J. L., Robinson, E. M., Crengle, S., & Perese, L. (2007). Prevalence of child sexual abuse reported by a cross-sectional sample of New Zealand women. *Child Abuse & Neglect 31,* 935 – 945

Finkelhor, D. (1994). The international epidemiology of child sexual abuse. *Child Abuse and Neglect, 18*: 409-417.

Finkelhor, D., & Browne, A. (1986). Impact of child sexual abuse: A review of the research. *Psychological Bulletin, 99,* 66-77

Flynn, K. A. (2008). In their own voices: Women who were sexually abused by members of the clergy. *Journal of Child Sexual Abuse, 17* (3), 216 – 237

Foa, E.B., Dancu, C.V., Hembree, E., Jaycox, L.H., Meadows, E.A., & Street, G.P. (1999). The efficacy of exposure therapy, stress inoculation training and their combination in ameliorating PTSD for female victims of assault. *Journal of Consulting and Clinical Psychology, 67,* 194-200

Forbes, D., Creamer, M., Phlelps, A., Bryant, R., McFarlane, A., Devilly, G., Matthews, L., Raphael, B., Doran, C., Merlin, T., & Newton, S. (2007). Australian guidelines for the treatment of adults with acute stress disorder and posttraumatic stress disorder. *Australian and New Zealand Journal of Psychiatry, 41,* 637-648

Gold, S. N., Lucenko, B. A., Elhai, J. D., Swingle, J. M., & Sellers, A. H. (1999). A comparison of psychological/psychiatric symptomology of women and men sexually abused as children. *Child Abuse & Neglect, 23,* 683–692

Harding, H, G., Zinzow, H, M., Burns, E,E., & Jackson, J.L (2010). Attributions of responsibility in a child sexual abuse (CSA) vignette among respondents with CSA histories: The role of abuse similarity to a hypothetical victim. *Journal of Child Sexual Abuse, 19* (2), 171- 189

Isely, P. J., Isely, P., Freiburger, J., &McMackin, R. (2008). In their own voices: A qualitative study of men abused as children by catholic clergy. *Journal of Child Sexual Abuse, 17* (3), 201 – 215

Janoff-Bulman, R. (2004). Posttraumatic growth: Three explanatory models. *Psychological Inquiry, 15* (1), 30-34.

Janoff-Bulman, R. (2006). Schema change perspectives on posttraumatic growth. Pp 81-99 In L.G. Calhoun & R. G. Tedaschi, *Handbook of Posttraumatic Growth.* Lawrence Erlbaum Associates, Inc

Jonzon, E., &Lindblad, F. (2004). Disclosure, reactions, and social support: findings from a sample of adult victims of child sexual abuse. *Child Maltreatment, 9* (2), 190-200

Kobasa, S. C. (1979). Stressful life events, personality and health. *Journal of Personality and Social Psychology, 37,* 1 - 11

Kouyoumdjian, H,. Perry, A.R,. & Hansen, D, J (2009). Non-offending parent expectations of sexually abused children: Predictive factors and influence on children's recovery. *Journal of Child Sexual Abuse, 18* (1), 40- 60

Lev-Wiesel, R. (2000). Quality of life in adult survivors of childhood sexual abuse who have undergone therapy. *Journal of Child Sexual Abuse*, 9, 1–13

Lev-Wiesel, R., Amir, M., & Besser, A. (2004).Posttraumatic growth among female survivors of childhood sexual abuse in relation to the perpetrator identity. *Journal of Loss and Trauma, 10* (1), 7 – 17

McGregor, K., Jülich, S., Glover, M., & Gautam, J. (2010). Health professionals' responses to disclosure of child sexual abuse history: Female child sexual abuse survivors' experiences. *Journal of Child Sexual Abuse, 19* (3), 239 – 254

Molnar, B E., Buka,S. L., & Kessler, R. C.(2001). Child sexual abuse and subsequent psychopathology: Results from the national comorbidity survey. *American Journal of Public Health*, 91, 753–760

Najman, J. M., Nguyen, M. L. T., & Boyle, F. M. (2007). Sexual abuse in childhood and physical and mental health on adulthood: An Australian population study. *Archives of Sexual Behaviour, 36,* 666 - 675

Nelson, E. C., Heath, A. C., Madden, P. A. F., Cooper, L., Dinwiddie, S. H., Bucholz, K. K., Glowinski, A., McLaughlin, T., Dunne, M. P., Statham, D. J., & Matrin, N. G. (2002). Association between self-reported childhood sexual abuse and adverse psychosocial outcomes. *Archieves of General Psychiatry, 59,* 139 – 146

O'Dougherty., Wright, M., Crawford, E., & Sebastian, K. (2007). Positive resolution of childhood sexual abuse experience: The role of coping, benefit-finding and meaning-making. *Journal of Family Violence, 22,* 597 – 608.

O'Leary, P., Coohey, C., & Easton, S. D.(2010). The effect of severe child sexual abuse and disclosure on mental health during adulthood. *Journal of Child Sexual Abuse, 19* (3), 275 – 289

Palesh, O. G., Classen, C.C., Field, N., Kraemer, H.C., & Spiegel, D. (2007).'The relationship of child maltreatment and self-capacities with distress when telling one's story of childhood sexual abuse. *Journal of Child Sexual Abuse, 16* (4), 63 – 80

Paolucci, E. O., Genuis, M. L., &Violato, C. (2001). A meta-analysis of the published research on the effects of child sexual abuse. *The Journal of Psychology, 135* (1), 17 – 36

Park, C. L. (2009). Overview of theoretical perspectives. In *Medical Illness and Positive Life Change: Can Crisis Lead to Personal Transformation?* (p. 11). Washington: American Psychological Association

Park, C., & Folkman, S. (1997). Meaning in the context of stress and coping. *Review of General Psychology, 1,* 115-144

Pereda, N., Guilera, G., Forns, M., & Gomez-Benito. (2009). The prevalence of child sexual abuse in community and student samples: A meta-analysis. *Clinical Psychology Review,29, 328- 338*

Phanichrat, T., & Townshend, J. M. (2010). Coping strategies used by survivors of childhood sexual abuse on the journey to recovery. *Journal of Child Sexual Abuse, 19,* 62 - 78

Putnam, F. W. (2003). Ten-year research update review: Child sexual abuse. *Journal of American Academy of Child and Adolescent Psychiatry, 42* (3), 269 – 278

Reyes, C. J. (2008). Exploring the relations among the nature of the abuse, perceived parental support, and child's self-concept and trauma symptoms among sexually abused children. *Journal of Child Sexual Abuse, 17* (1), 51 - 70

Rind, B., Tromovitch, P., & Bauserman, R. (1998). A meta-analytic examination of assumed properties of child sexual abuse using college samples. *Psychological Bulletin, 124,* 22-53

Rodrigues, N., Vande Kemp, H., & Foy, D. W. (1998). Posttraumatic stress disorder in survivors of childhood sexual and physical abuse: A critical review of the empirical research. *Journal of Child Sexual Abuse, 7,* (2) 17 - 45

Rojas, A., & Kinder, B. N. (2009). Are males and females sexually abused as children socially anxious adults? *Journal of Child Sexual Abuse, 18* (4), 355 - 366

Rutter, M. (1987). Psychosocial resilience and protective mechanisms. *American Journal of Orthopsychiatry, 57,* 316–331

Shakespeare-Finch J., & Armstrong, D. (2010). Trauma type and post-trauma outcomes: Differences between survivors of motor vehicle accidents, sexual assault and bereavement. *Journal of Loss and Trauma, 15,* 59 - 82

Shakespeare-Finch, J., & Copping, A. (2006). A grounded theory approach to understanding cultural differences in posttraumatic growth. *Journal of Loss and Trauma, 11,* 355-371

Shakespeare-Finch, J., & de Dassel, T. (2009). Exploring posttraumatic outcomes as a function of childhood sexual abuse. *Journal of Child Sexual Abuse, 18* (6), 623-640

Schultz, L., & Jones, P. (1983). Sexual abuse of children: Issues for social service and health professionals. *Child Welfare, 62,* 99-108

Take, K., Cann, A., Calhoun, L. G., & Tedeschi, R. G. (2008). The factor structure of the posttraumatic growth inventory: A comparison of five models using confirmatory factor analysis. *Journal of Traumatic Stress, 21,* (2) 158-164

Tedeschi, R. G., & Calhoun, L. G. (1995). *Trauma and transformation: Growing in the aftermath of suffering*. Thousand Oaks, California: Sage Publications Ltd

Tedeschi, R. G., & Calhoun, L. G. (1996). The Posttraumatic Growth Inventory: Measuring the positive legacy of trauma. *Journal of Traumatic Stress, 9*(3), 455-471

Tedeschi, R. G., & Calhoun, L. G. (2004). Posttraumatic growth: Conceptual foundations and empirical evidence. *Psychological Inquiry, 15,* 1-18

Ullman, S.E., Najdowski, C.J., & Filipas, H. H. (2009). Child sexual abuse, post-traumatic stress disorder, and substance use: Predictors of revictimization in adult sexual assault survivors. *Journal of Sexual Abuse, 18,* 367-385

Ullman, S. E. (2007). Relationships to perpetrator, disclosure, social reactions, and PTSD symptoms in child sexual abuse survivors. *Journal of Child Sexual Abuse, 16* (1), 19 - 36

Whiffen, V.,E & MacIntosh, H. B. (2005). Mediators of the link between childhood sexual abuse and emotional distress : A critical review. *Trauma, Violence, and Abuse,* 6 (1), 24 - 39

Woodward, C., & Joseph, S. (2003). Positive change processes and post-traumatic growth in people who have experienced childhood abuse: Understanding vehicles of change. *Psychology and Psychotherapy: Theory, Research, and Practice, 76,* 267 - 283

Zinzow, H., Seth, P., Jackson, J., Niehaus, A., & Fitzgerald, M. (2010). Abuse and parental characteristics, attributions of blame, and psychological adjustment in adult survivors of child sexual abuse. *Journal of Child Sexual Abuse, 19* (1), 79 - 98

4

Do Alexithymia, Dissociation, and CSA Explain the Controversial Topic of Memory Recovery?

Peter Paul Moormann[1], Francine Albach[3] and Bob Bermond[2]
[1]*Leiden University,*
[2]*University of Amsterdam,*
[3]*Private Psychotherapeutic Center in Amsterdam,*
The Netherlands

1. Introduction

In the foregoing chapter gender differences in symptomatology among victims of CSA were investigated. As alexithymia and dissociation are considered to be different manifestations of the same psychological state aiming at emotional disengagement from serious trauma first the affinity between alexithymia and dissociation will be investigated and then it will be explored whether specific abuse characteristics are related to alexithymia and dissociation. Because nowadays in the DSM the Janetian construct of dissociative amnesia instead of the Freudian construct of repression is seen as the mechanism behind recovered memories it will be tested whether dissociative amnesia is indeed related to having experienced episodes of inability to recall the traumatic event and its duration. In concreto the following research questions were posed:

- How are alexithymia and dissociation related to each other?
- Are alexithymia and dissociation affected by abuse characteristics?
- More in particular: Is the severity of abuse characteristics with or without real body contact of crucial importance for developing abuse related symptomatology?
- Is Memory Recovery associated with Dissociative Amnesia?

1.1 Dissociation and its affinity with alexithymia

Following Freud and Breuer (1893/1924) and Janet (1911), intense anxiety, one of the most painful emotions in human existence, is regarded as the impulse leading to the disruption of the normal controlling functions of consciousness. As early as 1911, Janet gave a detailed description of this disruptive power of intense emotions (p. 532):

"With respect to this subject I have demonstrated the dissolving power of emotions on voluntary decisions, feeling states, and conscious sensations, and I consider the dissociation of memories to be part of the larger group where dissociation of coherent structures is induced by emotions" (translation from French).

However although Janet considered high emotionality to be the trigger for dissociation, traumatized people are usually characterized by flatness of affect instead of high emotionality. How then can the paradox between on the one hand intense affect and on the other hand affective blocking be explained? Krystal (1988) gives the following answer (p. 151):

"The paradox in the traumatic state is that the numbing and closing off are experienced as relief from previously painful affects such as anxiety".

The affective tension is so strong that it takes the form of a blow down turned inwards, resulting in the non-feeling state that is expressed through the splitting of consciousness (dissociation), switching off feeling any emotions (alexithymia), and anaesthesia expressed through the lack of feeling any actual physical pain (Moormann et al., 2004). Such affective disruptions are very often manifested in individuals suffering from PTSD, where alexithymia and dissociation contribute to the enhancement of emotional disengagement from the traumatic event (Krystal et al., 1986; Chu & Dill, 1990; Hyer et al., 1990; Thomas et al., 1992; Zlotnick et al., 1996; Frewen et al., 2008).

Although several studies (Cloitre et al., 1997; Berenbaum, 1996; Sher & Twaite, 1999; Bermond et al., 2008) do support Krystal's (1988) view that CSA may cause alexithymia later in life, other investigations failed to come forward with empirical evidence for this notion (Paivio & McCulloch, 2004; Kooiman et al., 2004; Modestine et al., 2005). Many explanations are given for inconsistent findings (see Taylor & Bagby, 2004), such as the age of the children at the time of the abuse, the duration of the abuse, and whether or not the children developed PTSD. Frequency of the episodes seems to contribute to the form of expression of alexithymic features as well. Those victims of rape that underwent more than one episode of abuse manifested a greater degree of alexithymia compared to those that were abused only once (Zeitlin et al., 1993). Kooiman et al. (2004) suggested that less serious forms of CSA might be responsible for the lack of association between CSA and alexithymia. This idea seems to be justified by a recent study (Bermond et al., 2008) using the Bermond Vorst Alexithymia Questionnaire (BVAQ) instead of the Toronto Alexithymia Scale (TAS-20). Respondents with severe CSA did score significantly higher than matched controls on the sum-total of the BVAQ, in particular on the cognitive dimension (more precisely on the subscales reduced verbalizing and identifying). However, no significant difference was found on the affective dimension (measuring reduced fantasizing and emotionalizing).

Regarding dissociation abuse characteristics seem to play a role as well. Kisiel and Lyons, (2001) for instance revealed higher scores of dissociation for CSA children when compared to physically abused children. This seems to indicate that sexual abuse triggers dissociative tendencies stronger than physical abuse. Nevertheless, in cases where sexual abuse was combined with physical abuse the dissociative symptoms seem to be even more severe (Chu & Dill, 1990; Gold et al., 1999). Furthermore, the number of different sexual perpetrators has been positively correlated with greater scores on dissociation as well (Eliot & Briere, 1992; Zlotnick et al., 1996). In general, the prevalence of severe forms of CSA, rather than mild forms of abuse, contributes to the development and expression of consequently greater dissociation scores (Kirby et al., 1993).

Considering the findings that CSA may induce both alexithymia and dissociation and the notion that both constructs can be considered as manifestations of emotional disengagement, the strong association between alexithymia and dissociation (Berenbaum & James 1994; Zlotnick et al., 1996; Irwin & Melbin-Helberg, 1997) is from a theoretical point of view far from astonishing and has been reported within posttraumatic experiences (Frewen et al., 2008). Other commonly documented disturbances, also related to CSA, are depression, anxiety, eating disorders and self-mutilation (Parker, Bagby & Taylor, 1991; Zlotnick et al., 1996; Lipsanen et al., 2004). One common ground between the two phenomena is a displayed inability of the patients to consciously integrate segments of neuropsychological functions such as memories and feelings (Grabe et al., 2000). Elzinga et al. (2002) reported that dissociative tendencies where related to a general 'difficulty in identifying one's own feelings' as part of a response to periods of stress. Furthermore, they suggested that already existing characteristics of alexithymia might promote pathological dissociative reactions by enhancing a dysfunctional response to stress and trauma. There seems to be a displayed dissociation between the verbal processing system and the affective processes, indicating an inability to verbalize one's own affective states, not due to an actual absence of an affective vocabulary, but rather due to a general inability to access and utilize such vocabulary in order to outline emotional states (Irwin & Melbin-Helberg, 1997). Following the same line of research Mason et al. (2005) came up with a relationship between 'difficulty identifying feelings' and two subscales of dissociation on the DES, namely 'Depersonalization' and 'Absorption'. Another study comparing clinical and non-clinical subjects also came up with a strong positive correlation between alexithymia and dissociative symptomatology (Grabe et al, 2000). However, even though alexithymia and dissociation share features (for instance in the domain of fantasy) convincing evidence has been brought forward for two distinct constructs (Lipsanen et al., 2004).

1.2 Abuse characteristics and symptom reporting

The relation between abuse characteristics and psychopathology is lacking clear-cut results. In a Meta-Analytic study by Rind et al. (1998) for instance it was examined how aspects of the CSA experience moderated self-reported reactions and effects, as well as symptoms. Although these results should be viewed cautiously, because they were for a large part based on a small number of samples, it was found that only force (coercion) and incest moderated outcomes. The largest relation occurred between force and self-reported reactions or effects, but force was unrelated to symptoms. Incest moderated both symptoms and self-reported reactions and effects. Penetration, duration, and frequency did not moderate outcomes. The near-zero correlation between penetration and outcome was consistent with the multiple regression analysis finding of the same study that contact sex did not moderate adjustment. This result provided empirical support for Finkelhor's (1979) observation that our society's view of intercourse as the most damaging form of CSA is "a well-ingrained prejudice" unsupported by research. Composite measures consisting of various combinations of moderators (e.g., incest, force, penetration) showed no association with symptoms in four of five studies that constructed such measures. According to Rind et al. (1998) this finding is in agreement with the Laumann et al. 1994 study concerning a U.S. national sample, where a failure to find an association between a composite variable (consisting of penetration, number of older partners-abusers, relatedness of partner-abuser, frequency of contacts, age when having contacts, duration of contacts) and adjustment for sexually abused respondents was reported as well.

Hence, although the literature indicates that CSA is associated with alexithymia, and dissociation later in life, the impact of abuse characteristics related to single or composite variables on symptom reporting is either absent, weak or inconclusive. The data even suggest that the severity of abuse characteristics with or without real body contact is not of crucial importance for developing abuse related symptomatology.

1.3 Memory recovery and dissociative amnesia

Originally, the psychodynamic construct of repression was seen as the mechanism behind (psychogenic) amnesia for highly threatening aspects of traumatic material and its spontaneous recovery. However the impact of Janetian thinking (1889, 1911, 1928) had become so great over the last decades of the 20ieth century that the term psychogenic amnesia (based on the Freudian construct of repression) from the DSM-III-R (American Psychological Association, 1987) was replaced by the term dissociative amnesia (based on the Janetian construct of dissociation) in the DSM-IV (American Psychological Association, 1994). The logic behind this change of constructs was that Janet adepts argued that dissociated memories were related to actual traumatic events while repressed memories were related to inner conflicts resulting from unacceptable impulses and wishes, as conceptualized in psychoanalytic theory (Van der Kolk, 1987; Boon & Draijer, 1993). The introduction of a Janetian construct within a psychodynamic frame of PTSD (based on Freud (1939) and Horowitz (1976)) is not only highly confusing, but it implied that from then on dissociation became the explanatory mechanism behind forgetting painful traumatic material and its subsequent recall (dissociated memories). In the updated, newest DSM V proposal, available through the internet (February-8-2011) Dissociative Amnesia is defined as the inability to recall important personal information, usually of a traumatic or stressful nature, that is inconsistent with ordinary forgetting. Two primary forms of Dissociative Amnesia are distinguished: (1) Localized amnesia for a specific event or events, and (2) Dissociative Fugue: generalized amnesia for identity and life history. Fugue may be accompanied by either purposeful travel or bewildered wandering. Even though Dissociative Amnesia and Psychogenic amnesia both deal with memory deficits it should be noted that Dissociative Amnesia primarily deals with Identity Disorders, e.g. with disorders such as Dissociative Fugue, while localized amnesia in fact is what was formerly called psychogenic amnesia.

1.4 Hypotheses

Research by Vorst and Bermond (2001) on the validity and reliability of the BVAQ demonstrated that the Principal Component Analysis of subscale interrelations yields a clear-cut two-factor structure. One comprises an affective component (reduced Emotionalizing and Fantasizing) and the other a cognitive component (reduced Identifying, Verbalizing, and Analyzing emotions). By combining extreme scores on the two alexithymia components four alexithymia types can be distinguished: (1) *Type I alexithymia,* characterized by low emotionality and a poor fantasy life in combination with poorly developed cognitions accompanying the emotions; (2) *Lexithymia,* characterized by both high emotionality and an enriched fantasy-life in combination with very well-developed cognitions accompanying the emotions; (3) *Type II alexithymia,* characterized by high emotionality and a rich fantasy-life in combination with poorly developed cognitions accompanying the emotions; and (4) *Type III alexithymia*, characterized by a low emotionality and a poor fantasy-life, but with very well-developed cognitions accompanying the emotions. Based on confirmatory validity principles only subjects with an impaired cognitive component (e.g. Type I and Type II alexithymia) are considered to be alexithymic, while subjects with an unimpaired cognitive component (Lexithymics and Type III alexithymia) are seen as non-alexithymic, even though Type III alexithymics have an impaired affective component (the lack of emotionality and fantasy makes them stress resistant - see Moormann & Pijpers, 2004). Another argument for considering an impaired cognitive alexithymia component as indicative for the label 'alexithymic' is that Vorst and Bermond (2001) reported that the sum total of the TAS-20 was comparable with the cognitive component of the BVAQ, as both alexithymia measures were found to be highly interrelated (r = .80). Furthermore recent research on alexithymia types (Moormann et al., 2008) indicated that persons experiencing problems with the cognitive component of alexithymia (Type I and Type II) displayed a wide array of psychological problems, whereas more healthy personality profiles can be seen in persons where the cognitions accompanying the emotions were highly articulated (Lexithymia and Type III). Considering the above it is **hypothesized** that:

1. CSA subjects with an impaired cognitive alexithymia component (Type I and Type II) will have significantly higher dissociation scores than subjects with a very well developed cognitive alexithymia component (Lexithymia and Type III). The association between the impaired cognitive alexithymia component and dissociation would also find its expression in positive correlations.
2. Furthermore within the group with an impaired cognitive component it is hypothesized that Type II alexithymia (unimpaired affective component) will have significantly higher dissociation scores than Type I alexithymia (impaired affective component), based on Janet's assertion (1911) that highly painful, intense emotions (Type II) will lead to a splitting of consciousness. The association between the unimpaired affective alexithymia component and dissociation would then find its expression in negative correlations, in particular with the subscale Emotionalizing.

The alternative hypothesis, based on Krystal's Paradox of the traumatic state (1988) implies affect intolerance or psychic numbing (Type I), as a protection device against re-experiencing the traumatic events. Then, from Krystal's emotional disengagement point of view Type I alexithymics would have significantly higher dissociation scores than Type II alexithymics. The association between the impaired affective alexithymia component and dissociation would then find its expression in positive correlations, in particular with the subscale Emotionalizing.

However if both Type I and Type II alexithymia would display high dissociation scores, and if no significant differences between the two types can be demonstrated, then both affect intolerance and affective flooding are involved in dissociation. This line of reasoning is in agreement with the perspective of PTSD where the avoidance component is represented by affect intolerance while the re-experiencing component is represented by affective flooding (startle responses). From the point of view of individual differences in personality, where coping with stressful events has become a personality trait, victims of CSA may have either affect intolerance or affective flooding as their predominant personality trait. Hence, with the introduction of alexithymia types individual differences in emotional reactivity are assumed.

In the **explorative part** it will be investigated whether:

a. Alexithymia types differ on abuse characteristics.
b. Abuse characteristics are related to alexithymia and dissociation.
c. The impact of the abuse is greater (regarding alexithymia, dissociation, and memory recovery) when it happened before ten years of age.
d. Dissociative Amnesia is related to memory recovery and its duration.

2. Method

For this section we refer to the foregoing chapter, because, the subjects, procedure, and instruments are identical.

2.1 Statistical analyses

Conducting *One-Way Anovas with planned comparisons,* where alexithymia types act as the independent variable and dissociation as dependent variable is used for testing **Hypothesis 1 and 2**.

For the association between alexithymia and dissociation *Pearson Product-Moment Correlation Coefficients* will be applied. The same procedure will be done in the **explorative part** when the association between abuse features, alexithymia, and dissociation is investigated. Running Independent-Samples t Tests will be used to identify whether the impact of the abuse is greater (alexithymia, dissociation, and memory recovery act as dependent variables) when it happened before the age of ten (independent variable). Conducting *One-Way Anovas with post hoc comparisons,* where alexithymia types act as the independent variable and abuse characteristics as dependent variables, is used for exploring whether alexithymia types differ on abuse characteristics.

3. Results

3.1 Hypotheses

In **Hypothesis 1** it is stated that CSA subjects with an impaired cognitive alexithymia component (Type I and Type II) have significantly higher dissociation scores than subjects with a highly articulated cognitive alexithymia component (Lexithymia and Type III).

The results of the *One-way ANOVAS* with the dissociation variables as dependent variables and alexithymia types as independent variable (see Table 1) were significant (2-tailed) for 'Absorption and Imaginative Involvement' $(F(2,32) = 3.67^{*})$, for 'Depersonalization and Derealization' $(F(2,32)=7.75^{**})$, and for 'DES/28' $(F(2,32)= 4.62^{*})$. However not significant for 'Activities of Dissociated States' or 'Dissociative amnesia' $(F(2,32) = 1.34, p = .28)$. *Levene's Tests* were not significant and consequently equal variances were assumed. The effect size or strength of the relationship between alexithymia types and dissociation variables, as assessed by *Partial Eta Squared* $(P\eta^2)$, was very large for 'Absorption and Imaginative

Involvement' *(0.17)*, 'Depersonalization & Derealization' *(0.33)*, and DES/28 *(0.22)*, and medium for 'Activities of Dissociative States' *(0.08)*.

The *contrast coefficients* for Hypothesis **1** were *1, 1, and -2* for Type I, Type II, and the combined group of Type III & Lexithymia respectively. Except for 'Activities of Dissociated States' or amnesia *(t(32) = 1.49; p = .07 (1-tailed))*, indicating a trend (but it should be noted that the main Anova already was not significant), all remaining results of the contrast tests clearly confirmed hypothesis 1: (*t(32) = 2.17, p = .02 (1-tailed))* for 'Absorption & Imaginative Involvement'), *(t(32) = 3.80, p = .001 (1-tailed))* for 'Depersonalization & Derealization', and finally *(t(32) = 2.75, p = .003 (1-tailed))* for the 'DES/28'.

The outcomes above come forward with *substantial support for Hypothesis 1.*

The *contrast coefficients* for **Hypothesis 2**, stating that Type II alexithymia (unimpaired affective component) has significantly higher dissociation scores than Type I alexithymia (impaired affective component), were *-1, 1, and 0* for Type I, Type II and the combined group of Type III & Lexithymia respectively. Even though all mean scores of the DES were higher for Type II than Type I alexithymia, the differences were too small to reach significance: a) *(t(32) = 1.33, p= .10 (1-tailed))* for 'Absorption and Imaginative Involvement', b) *(t(32) = 0.47, p = .37 (1-tailed)* for 'Activities of Dissociative States' or dissociative amnesia, c) *(t(32) = 0.51, p = .31 (1-tailed))* for 'Depersonalization & Derealization', and finally *(t(32) = 0.93, p = .18 (1-tailed))* for the DES/28. Therefore *Hypothesis 2 was rejected.*

	Type I alexithymia (14%)			Type II alexithymia (26%)			Type III & Lexithymia (10%)		
	M	SD	N	M	SD	N	M	SD	N
Absorption	487.10	214.77	10	595.60	203.88	18	350.04	205.38	7
Amnesia	160.50	143.58	10	184.71	120.49	18	90.29	132.74	7
Dep & Der	332.30	176.87	10	363.03	158.52	18	98.71	87.24	7
DES/28	35.00	17.02	10	40.83	15.66	18	19.25	15.00	7

Table 1. Differences between the alexithymia types on mean, standard deviation, and number of subjects for each dissociation variable (DES).

The distribution of gender over the types was as follows: 4 males and 6 females in Type I, 4 males and 14 females in Type II, and 6 males and only 1 female in the combined group of Type III and Lexithymia. Because of the small number of males or females within some cells no gender x type Anovas could be performed. In total 40% of the 70 respondents who completed the BVAQ fell in the alexithymia range (14% Type I and 26% Type II). From the remaining 60% of non-alexithymics only 10% possessed a highly articulated cognitive component. This outcome further supports the notion on the devastating effect of CSA on psychological health. However it should be noted that alexithymia was defined as having an impaired cognitive dimension, implying that respondents with an impaired cognitive & an average affective component (not involved in the Anovas) should be added to the number of Type I and II alexithymics from Table 1 as well, when defining the incidence of alexithymia. A closer inspection of the data-file didn't reveal such subjects.

Considerable support was demonstrated for the intricate relation between alexithymia and dissociation (see Table 2).

	DES /28	a. Absorption	b. Amnesia	c. Dep & Der
ALEX Total N=69	0.43**	0.34**	0.36**	0.49**
a. Verbalizing N=70	0.46**	0.41**	0.33**	0.52**
b. Identifying N=70	0.59**	0.51**	0.50**	0.61**
c. Analyzing N=69	0.16	0.12	0.15	0.19
d. Fantasizing N=70	- 0.32*	- 0.32**	- 0.27*	- 0.24*
e.Emotionalizing N=70	0.30*	0.25*	0.32*	0.29*

Table 2. Pearson correlation coefficients between alexithymia and dissociation (*: p< 0.05 (2-tailed); **: p< 0.01 (2- tailed)). Positive correlations with alexithymia mean a reduced while negative correlations mean an augmented ability to …

Nearly all alexithymia subscales (except Analyzing) did show robust significant correlations with the DES/28 and its three subscales. Alexithymia total and the cognitive component are, as expected, positively correlated with dissociation. The negative correlation between Fantasizing and dissociation (Absorption & Imaginative involvement) supports the notion about dissociation and fantasy-proneness. The positive correlation between Emotionalizing and dissociation favours the emotional disengagement hypothesis.

3.2 Explorative part

3.2.1 Alexithymia types and abuse characteristics

Moreover it was explored whether the characteristics of CSA would be associated with particular alexithymia types. Because the literature on the impact of specific abuse features on the development of alexithymia is equivocal, *one-way Anovas* with *post hoc* instead of planned comparisons were performed. Significant differences between the alexithymia types were only found for Duration *($F(2, 29) = 4.15$, $p = .03$; 2-tailed)*. The Mean duration for Type I, Type II and Type III & Lexithymics were 4.56, 4.25, and 2.57 years respectively. The effect size (*Partial* $\eta^2 = .22$) was large. The *Bonferroni Test*, assuming equal variances, revealed a significant difference between Type I and Type III & Lexithymia *(p = .04; 2-tailed)* and between Type II and Type III & Lexithymia *(p = .05; 2-tailed).*

3.2.2 Onset before the age of 10 and abuse characteristics, alexithymia, and dissociation

None of the *t-tests* did reach significance on dissociation as dependent variable. However respondents abused before the age of 10 displayed significantly more *($t(64) = -2.27$, $p = .03$; 2-tailed)* Fantasizing (M = 24.00; SD = 7.24) than respondents abused after the age of 10 (M = 28.75; SD = 7.51). Furthermore respondents abused before the age of 10 reported significantly more *($t(64) = 2.59$; $p = .01$; 2-tailed)* problems with Verbalizing emotions (M = 29.72; SD = 7.26) than respondents abused after the age of 10 (M = 24.19; SD = 7.96). Finally respondents abused before the age of 10 not only reported significantly more *($t(29,06) = 2.61$, $p = .02$; 2-tailed)* Memory Recovery (M = 0.60; SD = 0.50)) than respondents abused after the age of 10 (M = 0.25; SD = 0.45), but they also reported significantly longer *($t(30,38) = 2.25$, $p = .03$; 2-tailed)* episodes of inability to recall the traumatic event (M = 12.47 years; SD = 13.54) than respondents abused after the age of 10 (M = 4.80 years; SD = 10.64).

Assuming that retrieval of abuse in adults is dependent upon the ability to verbalize emotions would imply a relation between problems with verbalizing emotions and memory recovery, but this hypothesis was rejected because of the low non-significant correlation between verbalizing emotions and memory recovery *($r = -0.07$, $N = 62$)*. An alternative hypothesis dealing with false memories, stating that memory recovery is due to fantasy proneness had to be rejected as well, because the correlation between fantasy and memory recovery was low and non-significant *($r = -0.18$, $N = 62$)*. In fact memory recovery correlated significantly neither with alexithymia, nor with dissociation, but both having experienced episodes of inability to recall the traumatic event *($r = 0.26^*$, $N = 61$)* and the duration of those episodes *($r = 0.33^*$, $N = 60$)* did correlate significantly with the father being the perpetrator.

3.2.3 Correlations between abuse characteristics and alexithymia total, and dissociation

However Alexithymia Total turned out to be significantly correlated with a few abuse characteristics: with Frequency *($r = 0.31^*$, $N = 56$)*, Position of Power *($r = 0.33^{**}$, $N = 64$)*, and Emotional Pressure *($r = 0.28^*$, $N = 62$)*.

The DES/28 score also correlated with some abuse characteristics: with Duration *($r = 0.30^*$, $N = 62$)*, Frequency *($r = 0.37^{**}$, $N = 57$)*, Attempted Coitus *($r = 0.28^*$, $N = 61$)*, Threatening *($r = 0.47^{**}$, $N = 66$)*, and Physical Violence *($r = 0.33^{**}$, $N = 65$)*.

3.2.4 Correlations between Activities of Dissociated States (Dissociative Amnesia) and Memory Recovery

Neither Dissociative Amnesia and Memory Recovery (r = -0.12, N = 63), nor Dissociative Amnesia and the duration of Memory Recovery (r = -0.07, N = 62) did correlate significantly. These results suggest that Dissociative Amnesia and Memory Recovery are separate entities, where Dissociative amnesia is related to alexithymia (see Table 2), duration (*r = 0.31*, N = 62*), frequency (*r = 0.28*, N = 57*), attempted coitus (*r = 0.26*, N = 61*), threatening (*r = 0.39**, N = 66*) and physical violence (*r = 0.30*, N = 65*), while memory recovery is only associated with the father being the perpetrator and an onset < 10 years (for correlations see above).

4. Discussion

4.1 Primary and secondary alexithymia

Although it can be argued that suffering from alexithymia is a trait, primarily based on inherent malfunctions of the brain or neurobiological deficits (called primary alexithymia by Sifneos, 1988), others have reported (Berenbaum, 1996; Cloitre et al., 1997; Sher & Twaite, 1999; Bermond et al., 2008) that alexithymia can also be induced by situational factors such as massive psychological trauma in childhood or later in life (called secondary alexithymia, for descriptions see Taylor et al., 1997; and Krystal, 1988). When looking at the present alexithymia and dissociation scores it could be argued that the interaction between trait and situation components in combination with plasticity and critical periods in brain maturation has led to what has been measured with the self-report questionnaires administered in our research. Therefore in adulthood it remains difficult to disentangle neurobiological deficits from deficits due to adverse situational forces in childhood. However, if situational factors were really crucial then an extensive pattern of substantial correlations between abuse characteristics and alexithymia ought to be found. These were not found, as alexithymia turned out to be significantly correlated with only a few abuse characteristics: with frequency, position of power, and emotional pressure. These outcomes make sense for the aetiology of alexithymia where situational forces are involved, because CSA is surrounded by secrecy, and therefore victims are withheld from both expressing their negative emotions (Miller, 1981) and learning to attach a verbal label to the emotional experience. Being abused at a young age is another important situational factor. Subjects abused before the age of 10 were more fantasy prone and displayed significantly more problems with verbalizing emotions. This result is in agreement with more recent neurobiological investigations suggesting that paediatric post traumatic stress disorder is associated with adverse brain behaviour (De Bellis & Keshavan, 2003), including those areas related to emotional behaviour (see also Bermond et al., 2006). Moreover CSA victims with an impaired (Type I and Type II) cognitive alexithymia component reported significantly longer abuse durations than CSA victims with a well-developed (Type III and Lexithymia) cognitive alexithymia component. From the above it is concluded that some situational factors indeed seem to enhance the development of alexithymia. However, it is striking that despite these harmful situational factors still 10% of the CSA victims did not display any signs of alexithymia (6 males and only 1 female). Our results on alexithymia types suggest that the abuse duration seems to be a crucial factor in the development of alexithymia types, as the average abuse duration of non-alexithymics lasted 'only' 2.57 years as opposed to 4.56 years for Type I and 4.25 for Type II alexithymics. The adverse effects of the duration of CSA on affect regulation may be due to retarded brain maturation as research on brain structures of PTSD subjects demonstrates that intracranial and cerebral volumes each correlated negatively with the duration of the maltreatment experience in years (De Bellis & Keshavan, 2003). Supporting parental styles such as unconditional positive regard (Rogers, 1951) and healthy personality traits such as emotional stability (lack of neuroticism) are likely to act as a buffer against the adverse effects of CSA.

4.2 Dissociation, alexithymia and sexual assaults

Dissociation correlated with some abuse characteristics as well: with duration, frequency, attempted coitus, threatening, and physical violence. It is striking that only one assault (e.g. attempted coitus) turned out to be correlated with dissociation. None was related to alexithymia. Therefore our results support Finkelhor's (1979) observation that our society's view of intercourse as the most damaging form of CSA is "a well-ingrained prejudice" unsupported by research.

4.3 Dissociation can be related to both a numbing (emotional disengagement) and a startle response (dissolving power of emotions)

Another interesting general finding concerns the association between alexithymia and dissociation. Substantial support was found for the hypothesis stating that alexithymics (subjects with an impaired cognitive alexithymia component, e.g. Type I and Type II) have significantly higher dissociation scores than non-alexithymics (subjects with a highly articulated cognitive alexithymia component, e.g. Lexithymia and Type III). Furthermore the cognitive alexithymia component and as a consequence nearly all its subscales (except Analyzing) did show robust significant correlations with the average DES and its three sub-scales. In non-clinical samples alexithymia is characterized by paucity of fantasies. Here we find fantasy-proneness, which is in accordance with the notion that dissociative subjects score high on 'Absorption & Imaginative involvement', another fantasy measure. Moreover the valence of the correlation between Emotionalizing and dissociation was positive, indicating that dissociation is related to reduced emotionality or flatness of affect and supports the point of view that both alexithymia and dissociation contribute to the enhancement of emotional disengagement.

At first sight the last outcome is puzzling, as it does not correspond to the view Janet (1911) originally had on the dissociative impulse. Janet (1911) emphasized the dissolving power of emotions on voluntary decisions, feeling states, and conscious sensations, e.g. intense anxiety, one of the most painful emotions in human existence was regarded as the impulse leading to the disruption of the normal controlling functions of consciousness. In the literature on dissociation this inconsistency with Janet's theory is captured by making a distinction between the acute dissociative response (peritraumatic dissociation) and the persistent dissociation which presence is more likely to be linked to pertinent psychopathological characteristics, among others affect intolerance (Foa & Hearst-Ikeda, 1996; Gershuny et al., 2003; Panasetis & Bryant, 2003). However none of these studies tried to solve this problem by looking at individual differences in emotional reactivity associated with contrasting dissociative states (based on animal studies), such as for instance Kretschmer (1961) did when explaining war neuroses. On the one hand animals are found to show a 'death feint' (Totstellreflex), also called an immobilization reflex or freezing response, and on the other hand an 'instinctive flurry' (Bewegungssturm) or startle response when exposed to an intensely stressful event. In competitive sports such different dissociative responses have been described when explaining performance deterioration in serious competition (Moormann, 1994), and empirical evidence for such dissociations have been brought forward in figure skating, swimming and cycling (Moormann & Pijpers, 2004). The distinction between alexithymia types, e.g. when comparing Type I with Type II alexithymia allows for the investigation of differences between alexithymics with a numbing response (Type I - emotional flatness) versus alexithymics with a startle response (Type II – emotional flooding). A recent study on psycho-physiological correlates of the alexithymia components of the BVAQ (Bermond et al., 2010) demonstrates that, when comparing GSR responses in neutral versus fear inducing conditions, Type I alexithymics hardly respond to fear stimuli, while Type II alexithymics display longer lasting and strong responses. Both reactions can be found in traumatized people and are part of the alternating system within PTSD (Horowitz, 1976), consisting of avoidance (numbness) and re-experiencing components in combination with hyper-arousal (startle responses). As research on alexithymia types indicates that Type II alexithymics (impaired cognitive & unimpaired affective component) suffer from the greatest array of psychological problems (Moormann & Pijpers, 2004; Moormann et al. 2008) it was also tested whether Type II had significantly higher dissociation scores than Type I. Even though all mean scores of the DES were higher for Type II (Average DES = 40.84) than Type I (Average DES = 35.00), the differences were not large enough to reach statistical significance (it should be noted that both dissociation scores were very high and fell in the DID range). This result implies that in 26% of all CSA cases dissociation was associated with high emotionality (instinctive flurry - support for Janet's original view where intense emotions act as the dissociative impulse), while in 14% of all CSA cases dissociation was associated with low emotionality (freezing - support for the emotional disengagement hypothesis or persistent dissociation). This new approach in the study of alexithymia and dissociation not only allows for a more refined differential diagnosis, but has therapeutic implications as well, because it seems likely that Type I will benefit most from interventions used in the autistic spectrum (full blown alexithymia - Schizoid features), whereas therapeutic approaches used in Borderline PD will be more suited for the treatment of Type II (emotional roller coaster, see Moormann et al., 2008). The results can be criticized on the small number of subjects in the non-alexithymic cell, but it should be noted that the effect size was very large (*Partial* $\eta^2 = .22$).

Future research with alexithymia types within CSA should be directed at larger cell numbers.

4.4 No empirical support for the notion of dissociative amnesia as the explanatory mechanism behind memory recovery

In the explorative part analyses on the onset of the abuse before the age of ten revealed some interesting outcomes. Respondents abused before the age of ten reported both significantly more memory recovery and significantly longer episodes of inability to recall the traumatic event than respondents abused after the age of ten. Furthermore they reported significantly more problems with verbalizing emotions and significantly more fantasy-proneness. Therefore it is tempting to argue that memory recovery is associated with not being able to verbalize emotions or making up the abuse and eventually believing that it really happened (e.g. implanted memories). However no support was found for the hypothesis that retrieval of abuse in adults is hampered by problems with verbalizing emotions. The alternative hypothesis dealing with false memories (Loftus, 1997), stating that memory recovery is due to fantasy proneness, had to be rejected as well. What then is crucial in memory recovery? According to the current DSM dissociative amnesia is held responsible for having experienced episodes of inability to recall the traumatic event. However, despite the very high average DES scores in our present research, indicating DID, the DES subscale 'Activities of dissociated states' (e.g. Dissociative Amnesia) did not correlate significantly with a) having experienced episodes of inability to recall the traumatic event and b) its duration. Apparently more mechanisms than dissociation alone can be held responsible for memory recovery. In an earlier study on memory recovery, based on in-depth interviews (Albach et al., 1996), initially the role of peridissociation was investigated as well. In the first draft a table was included where CSA women who dissociated at the time of the traumatic event (37% reported peridissociation) were compared with CSA women who did not dissociate at the time of the event (27%) on having experienced an episode of inability to recall the event as dependent variable. The result from the Chi-square test was not significant ((1, N = 74) = 0.32). Although this table has not been published in the final version the results indicate clear-cut that other mechanisms than dissociation alone must be involved in memory recovery. If dissociation is not the crucial mechanism behind memory recovery what then is important? In the current study it turned out that memory recovery was only associated with the abuse onset before the age of ten and with the father being the perpetrator. If the father has been the perpetrator the child becomes confused. Fathers love you, show attention, affection and tenderness, but don't hurt, manipulate or threaten you. In psychodynamic thinking this ambivalence towards the father causes an inner conflict in the child and repression is seen as seen as one of the many active defences against this inner conflict. The abuse is banned out of consciousness. That an inner conflict may hamper recall is in line with the findings of Browne and Finkelhor (1986) who indicated that abuse by fathers or stepfathers has a more negative impact than abuse by other perpetrators. It is also in line with the results of Williams' prospective study (1994), noting that sexual abuse by a perpetrator with a close relationship to the child is likely to combine elements of betrayal, fear, and conflict, which may cause the victim to be confused about the nature of the abuse and to experience problems with the memory of it. From a neurobiological point of view it can be argued that, when the brain matures, material stored in memory needs constant re-elaboration (new updates) to remain accessible for retrieval. Memory material not subjected to regular updates, especially when it has been banned out into the periphery of attention and consciousness, becomes extremely difficult to retrieve. The avoidance component in PTSD ensures that the traumatic events are kept out of the focus of attention. The avoidance component collapses (decompensation) as soon as unforeseen stimuli appear that act as abuse-related triggers leading to a complete re-experiencing of the traumatic event, a so-called amnestic turning point (see Albach, 1993; Albach et al., 1996).

5. Conclusions

1. New insights were obtained by introducing the distinction between alexithymia types in the complicated relation between alexithymia and dissociation, as both a high affective alexithymia component (Janet's original view of intense emotion as the dissociative impulse) and a low affective alexithymia component (the emotional disengagement hypothesis) turned out to be related to very high average DES scores (>

25), indicating DID. In 26% of all CSA cases dissociation was associated with Type II alexithymia (implying startle responses - support for Janet's original view), while in 14% of all CSA cases dissociation was associated with Type I alexithymia (implying psychic numbing - support for the emotional disengagement hypothesis or persistent dissociation).

2. Our results support Finkelhor's (1979) observation that our society's view of intercourse as the most damaging form of CSA is "a well-ingrained prejudice" unsupported by research. The severity of sexual assaults with or without real body contact was not of crucial importance for developing alexithymia and dissociation in adulthood.
3. No empirical evidence could be brought forward for the DSM notion that dissociative amnesia (Activities of dissociative states) is the mechanism behind memory recovery. Instead our results favour the Freudian construct of repression in combination with an early onset (support for Freud's Seduction theory, which he later abandoned in favour of Psychoanalysis; see Albach, 1993) as memory recovery was only related to the father being the perpetrator (implying an inner conflict) and an abuse onset < 10 years of age.

6. References

Albach, F. (1993). *Freud's Verleidingstheorie: Incest, trauma en hysterie* [Freud's seduction theory: Incest, trauma and hysteria]. PhD thesis, University of Amsterdam, Stichting Petra, ISBN 90-74214-04-5, Middelburg, The Netherlands

Albach, F.; Moormann, P.P., & Bermond, B. (1996). Memory recovery of childhood sexual abuse. *Dissociation*, Vol.9, pp. 258-269

American Psychiatric Association (1987). *Diagnostic and statistical manual of mental disorders, DSM-III*, The American Psychiatric Association, Washington

American Psychiatric Association (1994). *Diagnostic and statistical manual of mental disorders, fourth edition, DSM-IV*, The American Psychiatric Association, Washington

American Psychiatric Association (2011). *DSM-5 Development.* Available from: http://www.dsm5.org/Pages/Registration.aspx

Berenbaum, H. (1996). Childhood abuse, alexithymia and personality disorder. *Journal of Psychosomatic Research*, Vol.41, pp. 585-595

Berenbaum, H. & James, T. (1994). Correlates and retrospectively reported antecedents of alexithymia. *Psychosomatic Medicine*, Vol.56, pp. 353-359

Bermond, B.; Vorst, H.C.M. & Moormann, P.P. (2006). Cognitive neuropsychology of alexithymia: Implications for personality typology. *Cognitive Neuropsychiatry, Vol.11*, No.*3*, pp. 332 – 360

Bermond, B.; Moormann, P.P.; Albach, F. & Dijke, A. van (2008). Impact of severe childhood sexual abuse on the development of alexithymia in adulthood. *Psychotherapy and Psychosomatics*, Vol.77, pp. 260-261

Bermond, B.; Bierman, D.J.; Cladder, M.A.; Moormann, P.P. & Vorst, H.C.M. (2010). The cognitive and affective alexithymia dimensions in the regulation of sympathetic responses. *International Journal of Psychophysiology*, Vol.75, pp. 227-233

Boon, S. & Draijer, N. (1993). *Multiple personality disorder in the Netherlands: A study on reliability and validity of the diagnosis*, Zwets & Zeitlinger, Lisse

Browne, A. & Finkelhor, D. (1986). Impact of child sexual abuse: A review of the research. *Psychological Bulletin*, Vol.99, No.1, pp. 66-77

Chu, J.A. & Dill, L.D. (1990). Dissociative symptoms in relation to childhood physical and sexual abuse. *American Journal of Psychiatry, Vol.147*, pp. 887-892

Cloitre, M.; Scarvalone, P. & Difede, J. (1997). Posttraumatic stress disorder, self- and interpersonal dysfunction among sexually retraumatized women. *Journal of Traumatic Stress*, Vol.10, pp. 437-442

De Bellis M.D. & Keshavan, M.S. (2003). Sex differences in brain maturation in maltreatment-related pediatric posttraumatic stress disorder. *Neuroscience and Biobehavioral Reviews*, Vol.27, pp. 103-117

Eliot, D.M. & Briere, J. (1992). Sexual abuse trauma among professional women: Validating the Symptom Trauma Checklist-40 (TSC 40). *Child abuse and Neglect*, Vol.16, pp. 391-398

Elzinga, B.; Bermond, B. & Van Dyck, R. (2002). The relationship between dissociative proneness and alexithymia. *Psychotherapy and Psychosomatics*, Vol.71, pp. 104-111

Finkelhor, D. (1979). *Sexually victimized children*, The Free Press, New York

Foa, E.B. & Hearst-Ikeda, D. (1996). Emotional dissociation in response to trauma: An information processing approach. *Handbook of dissociation: Theoretical and clinical perspectives*, In: L.K. Michelson & W. J. Ray (Eds.), pp. 207-222, Plenum, New York

Freud, S., & Breuer, J. (1893). On the physical mechanism of hysterical phenomena. *Collected papers, Vol. 1*, In: Freud, S., International Psychoanalytic Press (1924), London

Freud, S. (1939). Moses and monotheism. *The standard edition of the complete psychological works of Sigmund Freud*, In: J. Strachey (Ed. and Trans.), Vol.23, pp. 3-137, Norton, New York

Frewen, P.A.; Dozois, D.J.A.; Neufeld, R.W. & Lanius., R.A. (2008). Meta-analysis of alexithymia in Post Traumatic Stress Disorder. *Journal of Traumatic Stress*, Vol.21, pp. 243-246

Gershuny, B.S.; Cloitre, M. & Otto, M. (2003). Peritraumatic dissociation and PTSD severity: Do event related fears about death and control mediate their relation? *Behaviour Research and Therapy*, Vol.41, pp. 157-166

Grabe, H.J.; Rainermann, S.; Spitzer, C.; Gansicke, M. & Freyberger, H.J. (2000). The relationship between dimensions of alexithymia and dissociation. *Psychotherapy and Psychosomatics*, Vol.69, pp. 128-131

Gold, S.N.; Hill, E.L.; Swingle, J.,M. & Elfant, S.A. (1999). Relationship between childhood abuse characteristics and dissociation among women in therapy. *Journal of Family Violence*, Vol.14, pp. 157-17

Horowitz, M.J. (1976). *Stress response syndromes* (2nd. Ed.), Jason Aronson, Northvale, NJ

Hyer, L.; Woods, G.; Summers, M.N.; Boudewyns, P. & Harrison, W.R. (1990). Alexithymia among Vietnam veterans with Post Traumatic Stress Disorder. *Journal of Clinical Psychiatry*, Vol.51, pp. 243-246

Irwin, H.J. & Melbin-Helberg, E.B. (1997). Alexithymia and dissociative tendencies. *Journal of Clinical Psychology*, Vol.53, pp. 159-166

Janet, P. (1889). *L'automatisme psychologique* [The psychological automatism], Félix Alcan, Paris

Janet, P. (1911). *L'état mental des hystériques. [The mental state of hysterics, 2nd. Ed.]*, Félix Alcan, Paris

Janet, P. (1928). *De l'angoisse à l'extase, études sur les croyances et les sentiments. [From fear to ecstacy, studies on credibility and feeling]*, Félix Alcan, Paris

Kirby, J.S.; Chu, J.A. & Dill, D.L. (1993). Correlates of dissociative symptomatology in patients with physical and sexual abuse histories. *Comprehensive Psychiatry*, Vol.34, pp. 258-263

Kisiel, C.L.L. & Lyons, S.J. (2001). Dissociation as a mediator of psychopathology among sexually abused children and adolescents. *American Journal of Psychiatry*, Vol.158, pp. 1034-1039

Kolk, B.A. van der (1987). *Psychological trauma*, American Psychiatric Press, Inc., Washington DC

Kooiman, C.G.; Rees Vellinga, S van; Spinhoven, P., Draijer, N.; Trijsburg, R.W & Rooijmans, H.G.M. (2004). Childhood adversities as risk factors for alexithymia and other aspects of affect dysregulation in adulthood. *Psychotherapy & Psychosomatics*, Vol.73, pp. 107-116

Kretschmer, E. (1961). *Hysteria, reflex, and instinct*, Peter Owen, London

Krystal, J. H.; Giller, E. L. & Cichetti, D. V. (1986). Assessment of alexithymia in post traumatic stress disorder and somatic illness: Introduction of a reliable measure. *Psychosomatic Medicine*, Vol.48, pp. 84-94

Krystal, H. (1988). *Integration and self-healing: Affect, trauma and alexithymia*, Analytic Press, Hillsdale, NY

Larsen, J.K.; Brand, N.; Bermond, B. & Hijman, R. (2003). Cognitive and emotional characteristics of alexithymia: A review of neurobiological studies. *Journal of Psychosomatic Research*, Vol.54, pp. 533-541

Laumann, E.O.; Gagnon, J.H.; Michael, R.T. & Michaels, S. (1994). *The social organization of sexuality: Sexual practices in the United States*, University of Chicago, Chicago

Lipsanen, T.; Saarijärvi, S. & Lauerma, H. (2004). Exploring the relations between depression, somatization, dissociation and alexithymia – Overlapping or independent constructs? *Psychopathology, Vol.37*, pp. 200–206

Loftus, E.F. (1997). Creating false memories: Researchers are showing how suggestion and imagination can create "memories" of events that did not actually occur. *Scientific American*, September, pp. 50-55

Mason, O.; Tyson, M.; Jones, C. & Potts, S., (2005). Alexithymia, its prevalence and correlates in a British undergraduate sample. *Psychology and Psychotherapy: Theory, Research and Practice, Vol.78*, pp. 113-125

Miller, A. (1981). *In den beginne was er opvoeding* [First there was education], Wereldvenster, Bussum

Modestine, J. ; Furrer, R. & Malti, T. (2005). Different traumatic experiences are associated with different pathologies. *Psychiatry Quaterly*, Vol.76, pp. 19-32

Moormann, P.P. (1994). *Figure skating performance: A psychological study*. Dissertation, Leiden University, ISBN 90-9006862-7, The Netherlands

Moormann, P.P. & Pijpers, J.R. (2004). *Scoren tussen de oren: De theorie en praktijk van individuele mentale* training [Achieving is believing: Theory and practice of individual mental training], Harcourt, ISBN 90 265 1735 1 NR 770 , Lisse

Moormann, P.P.; Bermond, B. & Albach (2004). The Reality Escape Model: The intricate relation between alexithymia, dissociation, and anesthesia in victims of child sexual abuse, In: *Emotional Expression and Health,* Ivan Nyklicek, Ad Vingerhoets, & Lydia Temoshok (Eds), 82-98, Brunner Routledge, Hove

Moormann, P.P.; Bermond, B.; Vorst, H.C.M.; Bloemendaal, A.; Teijn, S. & Rood, L. (2008). New avenues in alexithymia research: The creation of alexithymia types. In: *Emotion Regulation: Conceptual and Clinical Issues,* Johan Denollet, Ivan Nyklicek, & Adrianus Vingerhoets (Eds.), 27-42, Springer, New York

Paivio, S.C. & McCulloch, C.R. (2004). Alexithymia as a mediator between childhood trauma and self-injurious behaviors. *Child Abuse and Neglect,* Vol.28, pp. 339-354

Panasetis, P., & Bryant, R.A. (2003). Peritraumatic versus persistent dissociation in acute stress disorder. *Journal of Traumatic Stress,* Vol.16, Nr.6, pp. 543-566

Parker J.,D.A; Bagby R.M, & Taylor G.J. (1991). Alexithymia and depression: Distinct or overlapping constructs? *Comprehensive Psychiatry,* Vol. *32,* pp. 387–394

Rind, B.; Tromovitch, P. & Bauserman, R (1998). A meta-analytic examination of assumed properties of child sexual abuse using college samples. *Psychological Bulletin,* Vol.124, Nr.1, pp. 22-53

Rogers, C. (1951). *Client Centered Therapy,* Houghton Mifflin, Boston

Sher, D. & Twaite, J.A. (1999). The relationship between child sexual abuse and alexithymic symptoms in a population of recovering adult substance abusers. *Journal of Child Sexual Abuse,* Vol.8, pp. 25-40

Sifneos, P.E. (1988). Alexithymia and its relationship to hemispheric specialization, affect, and creativity. *Psychiatric Clinics of North America,* Vol.11, Nr.3, pp. 287-292

Taylor, G.J.; Bagby, R.M. & Parker, D.A. (1997). *Disorders of affect regulation: Alexithymia in medical and psychiatric illness,* Cambridge University Press, Cambridge

Taylor, G.J. & Bagby, R.M. (2004). New trends in alexithymia research. *Psychotherapy and Psychosomatics,* Vol.73, pp. 68-77.

Thomas, R.K.; Krystal, J.H.; Giller, E.L.; Frank, J. & Dan., E. (1992). Alexithymia as a predictor response in post traumatic stress disorder. *Journal of traumatic stress,* Vol.5, pp. 563- 573

Vorst, H.C.M. & Bermond, B. (2001). Validity and reliability of the Bermond-Vorst Alexithymia Questionnaire. *Personality and Individual Differences,* Vol.30, pp. 413-434

Williams, L. Meyer (1994). Recall of childhood trauma: A prospective study of women's memories of child sexual abuse. *Journal of Consulting and Clinical Psychology,* Vol.62, pp. 1167-1176

Zeitlin, S.B.; McNally, R.J. & Cassiday, K.L. (1993). Alexithymia in victims of sexual assault: An effect of repeated traumatization? *American Journal of Psychiatry,* Vol.150, pp. 661-663

Zlotnick, C.; Shea, M.T.; Pearlstein, T.; Simpson, E.; Costello, E. & Begin, A. (1996). The relationship between dissociative symptoms, alexithymia, impulsivity, sexual abuse, and self-mutulation. *Comprehensive Psychiatry*, Vol.37, pp. 12-16

5

Gender Differences in the Impact of Child Sexual Abuse on Alexithymia, Dissociation and Self

Peter Paul Moormann[1], Francine Albach[3], Bob Bermond[2], Annemieke van Dijke[4], Jakob de Jong[1], Jaco Wineke[1], Kalliopi Metta[1] and Argyro Karanafti[1]

[1]*Leiden University,*
[2]*University of Amsterdam,*
[3]*Private Psychotherapeutic Center in Amsterdam*
[4]*Delta Psychiatric Center,*
The Netherlands

1. Introduction

Childhood Sexual Abuse (CSA) is a topic with a long history in both psychiatry and psychology. In fact grand old theories such as Freud's Psychodynamic Theory, its predecessor the Seduction Theory, and Janet's Dissociation Theory were based on the investigation of hysteria in cases of sexual abuse. In those days sexual abuse primarily concerned women. The recent attention in the media for male victims of sexual abuse, particularly young boys having been molested by Catholic priests and very young children having been abused in crèches and being exposed on the secret internet websites of paedophile networks, has led after the second feministic wave to a renewed interest in CSA and its adverse effects. Therefore in the forthcoming research the following questions will be raised:

What is the impact of severe CSA on alexithymia, dissociation and self?
Do female subjects differ from male subjects on the impact of CSA?

In the theoretical part first the issue of credibility in relation to gender will be briefly discussed in a historical perspective. Sexual abuse is a criminal act and the credibility of a victim who accuses a perpetrator of sexual abuse has always been, and still is, a delicate subject in court. After having dealt with the literature on the impact of CSA upon alexithymia, dissociation and self the theoretical part will be concluded with some general findings on how the sexes cope with CSA, as no systematic studies have been conducted yet on gender differences in alexithymia, dissociation and self in CSA.

2. Gender and the issue of credibility

In contrast with female victims of sexual abuse from the 19th century on up to the recent case of DSK (Dominique Strauss-Kahn) the credibility of war victims in the 1st World War was not an issue of importance. There were no doubts on what had happened to them, because quite often there was a whole regiment of witnesses. However doubts existed on whether soldiers were really ill as they displayed a wide array of behavior that nowadays would be classified as conversion hysteria. Since Horowitz's (1976) introduction of the Theory of Stress Response Syndromes there has been a growing interest in the effects of exposure to traumatic events, and the systematic investigation of complaints reported by male survivors of war resulted in the description of Post Traumatic Stress Disorder (PTSD). However it took much longer before reports of CSA in women were taken seriously. Already from the end of the 19th century reports on female sexual abuse were considered to be false sexual allegations ('sexuelle Falschanschuldigungen' in German, see Birnbaum, 1915) and in France it was called the phenomenon of the 'accusatrices hystériques' (see Garnier, 1903). This tradition was kept alive when Psychoanalysis dominated the academic scene, as accounts of sexual abuse were simply treated as 'Oedipal Fantasies'. Hence, the term 'pseudologia phantastica' is firmly rooted in the history of CSA. Only quite recently, during the second feministic wave in the last two decades of the 20ieth century it was acknowledged by academic psychology that CSA really occurs and that the effects can be traumatic enough to meet the criteria of PTSD (see Finkelhor & Browne, 1985; Albach & Everaerd, 1992; Albach, 1993; Zeitlin et al., 1993). However, the battle had not been won yet. In particular women with repressed memories of sexual abuse (those who experienced episodes of inability to recall the event) had a long history of being treated with great suspicion (Albach et al., 1996). The last revival of this skeptic tradition (the abuse did not really happen) evolved after 1990 and was based on the idea of false or implanted memories created under hypnosis in psychotherapy (Ceci & Loftus, 1994; Loftus, 1993, 1997). The foregoing on credibility illustrates well that war victims and CSA women have in common that both were accused of pretending or lying, however on different grounds. Soldiers were accused of lying about their illness; by malingering they tried to avoid being sent back to the deadly frontlines, while CSA women were accused of lying about what had happened to them, e.g. about the sexual abuse as an excuse or explanation for their current miserable psychological state (Crombach & Merkelbach, 1996).

Until recently studies on CSA were almost uniquely based on women. Empirical studies on the impact of CSA in male victims were beyond the scope of the feministic perspective. However the numerous recent reports of male CSA victims within the Roman Catholic Church in the media inevitably had to lead to a shift of focus in this female-only approach. Comparisons between female and male victims are a logical consequence. It is striking that in all female cases fantasy-proneness or high suggestibility is used as a personality trait causing women to report such lies or false memories, while in the recent cases of male sexual abuse, in the media hardly any doubts on the credibility of the reports of the male victims has been expressed. It might be that under enormous political pressure from the media, the already badly wounded Catholic Church had no other way-out than to stand in a white sheet, and the priests, some of whom are still alive, lost their status of inviolability and as a consequence had to confess their misconduct. Although it cannot be denied that in some cases women do lie about or simulate sexual abuse (see the literature on false memories, for instance Yapko, 1994), as by the way happens with many other events in court, it remains remarkable that *even the second feministic wave has not been robust enough to prevent women from being accused of hysteria, making up stories or lying about sexual abuse, while the credibility of men reporting being molested by priests apparently is not an issue of serious debate*. If this line of reasoning is true then, even in the 21st century the impact of sexual abuse for women is far greater than for men, as the credibility of women is even nowadays under debate. They are still considered to be liars, fantasy-prone, too emotional and therefore their credibility is dubious. The recent case of 'DSK' seems to confirm that 'pseudologia phantastica' still rules in court. This almost archetypal denigrated attitude towards women might also explain the negative self, commonly reported by victimized women (Russell, 1986).

3. Impact of CSA on alexithymia, dissociation, and self

3.1 Impact of CSA on alexithymia

Alexithymia has been introduced by Sifneos and literally means *'wordless affect'*, indicating the incapacity to recognize and express the emotional experience in verbal forms. Sifneos (1973) came up with this term after observing that a great amount of patients suffering from psychosomatic complaints were not able to verbally express and describe their affective experience and also distinguish it from bodily sensations; such difficulty constituted only a part of a wider cluster of cognitive and affective characteristics also including restricted imagination characterized by a marked paucity of fantasy and a literal, utilitarian cognitive style that is externally oriented. This cluster of characteristics constitutes a major obstacle in the process of treatment and contributes to the failure of response to therapy (Sifneos, 1975).

Krystal (1988) was probably the first to emphasize that alexithymia is one of the sequelae of traumatic experiences. From research data evidence exists for the idea that psycho-traumata can indeed induce alexithymia (Hyer et al., 1990; Thomas et al., 1992; Berenbaum & James, 1994; Zlotnick, et al., 2001; Frewen et al., 2008). Victims of both rape (Zeitlin et al., 1993) and CSA (Albach & Everaerd, 1992; Berenbaum, 1996; Cloitre et al., 1997; Moormann et al, 1997; Sher & Twaite, 1999; Bermond et al., 2008) are known to suffer from alexithymia. Milder forms of CSA are not always associated with alexithymia (Paivio & McCulloch, 2004; Kooiman et al., 2004; Modestine, Furrer, & Malti, 2005).

3.2 Impact of CSA on dissociation

Pierre Janet (1889) was the first to describe the concept of dissociation as a result of his extensive work with hysteric patients. He referred to dissociation as a process involving the breaking down of those structures of the mind that are interconnected within a single stream of consciousness. More specifically, the mind is constructed by separate compartments constituting from emotions, cognitions and actions; however as a consequence of trauma, stress or weakness the breakdown of this stream of consciousness may occur as a result of the splitting of one of those structures from the rest. Such alternations then in those structures inhibit the normal integration of information to the components that are involved and induce alternations in memory and identity, promoting in such way the development of different kinds of dissociative disorders, depending on the severity of the symptoms (Putnam, 1993).

Dissociation, one of the adverse effects of CSA (Chu & Dill, 1990; Ensink, 1992; Kirby et al., 1999; Kisiel & Lyons, 2001), is often studied together with alexithymia, and both constructs are considered to contribute to the enhancement of emotional disengagement from the traumatic event (Zlotnick et al., 1996; Irwin & Melbin-Helberg, 1997; Grabe, et al., 2000; Elzinga, et al. (2002); Moormann et al., 2004).

3.3 Impact of CSA on self

The first psychologist to develop a theory of self was William James (1890). According to his theory self consists of four integrated parts: the "spiritual self" (what we most truly seem to be), the "social self" (individuals and groups about whose opinion we care), the "material self" (material possession we see as part of us) and the "bodily self" (body image). These four selves combine to constitute each person's view of himself and his self-concept. Furthermore, James developed his theory as to the position a person holds in the world, which determines his self-esteem depending on his success or failure. Our perceptions of where we see ourselves standing in relation to others whose skills and abilities are similar to our own determine our inner feeling of self-worth.

Regarding self and CSA, Janoff-Bulman and Frieze (1983) argue that the trauma of victimization activates negative self-images. Victims see themselves as weak, helpless, needy, frightened and out of control. They are also apt to experience a sense of deviance. Therefore, effective coping with victimization requires not only coming to terms with a world in which bad experiences happen to one-self, but also restoring a damaged self-image. Low self-regard, commonly found among victims of repeated sexual abuse is emphasized by Russell (1986) as follows (p. 190):

"Women who place or find themselves in risky situations in the predatory world in which we live are quite likely to be raped. This does not, of course, mean they want to be raped, or that they don't mind it. It means that their self-esteem may be so damaged that they don't feel they deserve their own loving self-protection. This, in turn, can result in repeated victimizations, each one of which can undermine a women's self-esteem still further".

A survey done by Russell and co-workers (1986) shows that re-victimization is most of the time neither a one-time experience nor a rare occurrence, but more often extremely common. The kind of behavior displayed by the victim might be the reason why re-victimization in children happens so often. Clinical accounts indicate that sexual offenders who don't know about a child's previous victimization may be experts at picking up cues of vulnerability, such as low self-image or a strong but unsatisfied need for affection and attention. Finkelhor and Browne (1985) have developed a theoretical model for analyzing child sexual abuse in terms of four trauma-causing factors: traumatic sexualization (i.e., a child's sexuality is shaped in a developmentally inappropriate and interpersonally dysfunctional fashion as a result of sexual abuse), stigmatization (i.e., negative connotations - e.g., badness, shame, and guilt, that are communicated to the child around the experiences and that then become incorporated into the child's self-image), betrayal (i.e., children discover that someone on whom they were vitally dependent has caused them harm), and powerlessness (i.e. the child's will, desires, and sense of efficacy are continually contravened). Finkelhor and Browne refer to these factors as *traumagenic dynamics*, and suggest that these factors alter children's cognitive and emotional orientation to the world, and create trauma by distorting children's self-concept, world-view, and affective capacities.

3.4 Hypotheses

Victims of CSA will display:

a. A high prevalence of alexithymia.
b. High dissociation scores, indicative of Dissociative Identity Disorder (DID).
c. A negative self.

4. Explorative part: Gender differences

Gender differences in alexithymia, dissociation, and self have been published in populations other than CSA. The general picture reveals higher alexithymia scores for men on the BVAQ (Vorst & Bermond, 2001). However, reports using the TAS, failed to demonstrate such gender differences in alexithymia (Parker, Taylor & Bagby, 1989). While, in general men were found to be more alexithymic, women tended to be more vulnerable to dissociation (Coons, 1996; Ross, 1996). Many researchers though reported surpassing scores for males on the frequency of dissociative disorders in various populations including children, adolescents, criminal offenders and forensic patients are reported as well (Kluft, 1996; Putnam et al., 1996). These inconclusive findings can be attributed to methodological problems, such as comparing outcomes from classification systems with outcomes from questionnaires, different populations, and different instruments. For self gender outcomes are even more confusing because researchers have a tendency to make a distinction between an interdependent and an independent self-construal. The social, institutional, and cultural environment of the United States for instance promotes development of independence and autonomy in men and interdependence and relatedness in women (Bakan, 1966; Maccoby, 1990; Markus & Oyserman, 1989). Therefore the outcome of the comparison is dependent upon the self-construal chosen which hampers the making of absolute statements on gender differences.

The comparatively few studies that did investigate both male and female CSA victims seem to indicate that the variety of maladaptive psychological behaviours and psychiatric disorders associated with CSA are expressed differently in boys and girls (Walker et al., 2004). In general, girls manifest a tendency to *internalizing* behaviours (Butler & Nolen-Hoeksema, 1994). Boys on the other hand have been found to display a coping style in response to CSA characterized by more *externalizing* behaviours (Garnefski & Arends, 1998; Kuhn et al., 1998). The different expressions of the impact of CSA on gender may be partly explained by the influence of CSA on gender identity. Male victims seem to become more commonly confused about their sexual identity and orientation in heterosexual relationships (Tzeng & Schwarzin, 1990). Such confusion stems from any type of perceived responsiveness to the incident taking place from the same sex abuser and may lead to the assumption that the masculinity of the victim has been compromised (Moody, 1999). In such cases boys may be more prone to acting out aggression and engaging in delinquent activities in an effort to compensate for and re-establish their perceived loss of masculinity (Rogers & Terry, 1984). Girls on the other hand tend to display a more damaged self esteem and self blame, not only because of their tendency to ruminate, but also because in many cases they are often held responsible for the abuse by suggesting that girls seduced and encouraged the perpetrator (Carmen et al., 1984; Herman, 1981; Kohn 1987), with shame and guilt feelings as a consequence. Additionally, fear and distress enhance a maladaptive vulnerability that stems from their perception that the world is a dangerous and threatening place (Feiring et al., 1999). The above seems to be confirmed by case studies, where male victims of sexual abuse were found to have low self-esteem as well (Myers, 1989). Expressions were as being flawed, and shame and guilt for participating in the sexual activities were reported as well, which later may become personality traits. Hunter (1990) reports significantly lower self-esteem scores for male victims of sexual abuse as opposed to non-victims. Dhaliwal et al. (1996) report reduced sexual self-esteem as a consequence of sexual abuse.

In contrast with the above studies where gender comparisons are more relative than absolute, in the present research possible differences in symptom reporting between the sexes will be tested using the same constructs and the same instruments.

5. Method

5.1 Sample

Seventy-five subjects, reporting CSA volunteered in our research. The total group consisted of seventeen men and fifty-eight women, ranging from sixteen to sixty-one years of age (M age males = 37.31; M age females = 37.83).

5.2 Procedure

Respondents were recruited through newspaper announcements and through contact persons, working in CSA self-help groups supervised by clinical psychologists, where group members were encouraged to both share and cope with their traumatic past by receiving support and understanding from their fellow group members. It should be noted that it was much harder to find male than female subjects. Furthermore the data of the male subjects were collected at another location and time. Hence the sessions consisted of either males only or females only. Before entering the first session a test battery was administered to each gender group consisting of a Checklist for CSA Characteristics, the BVAQ, the DES, and the LSQ.

5.3 Instruments

Checklist for Childhood Sexual Abuse Characteristics, specially developed for this occasion, mainly based on the results and insights derived from in-depth interviews taken by Ensink (1992) and Albach (1993) for their PhD research.

The checklist contains 8 categories:

1) Perpetrator (a. father; b. brother or sister; c. other relative (grandfather, uncle, etc.); d. family friend; e. stranger; f. familiar persons other than relatives or family friends); *2) Onset before the age of 10; 3) Duration; 4) Frequency; 5) Assault* (a. sexual harassment; b. masturbation; c. attempted penetration; d. penetration; e. fellatio; f. anal penetration; 6) *Coercion* (a. position of power; b. misleading; c. presents; d. threatening; 7) *Enforcing secrecy* (a. shame on you; b. emotional pressure; c. physical violence); 8) *Memory recovery* (a. having experienced an episode of inability to recall the traumatic event; b. number of years)

If otherwise mentioned all items were coded in a yes/no format. In the category perpetrator for instance the number of perpetrators could be indicated in the subcategory strangers. Duration related to the numbers of years the abuse had lasted and frequency related to how many times a week the abuse had taken place. In the category coercion misleading meant that the child was told it was perfectly normal for children to be involved in the kind of sexual activities the perpetrator demanded. Giving presents to the victims supposedly was a strategy to consolidate the bond between perpetrator and child and thereby avoiding betrayal. Threatening meant that the child would no longer benefit from all kind of privileges if it refused to cooperate. Giving the child the idea that he/she was responsible for the abuse by seducing the perpetrator was applied to ensure the abuse was kept a secret. The child was bad and should be ashamed. Exerting emotional pressure happened when the perpetrator convinced the child that he acted out of love and that revealing "our secret" would make the perpetrator very sad and would ruin his life. Physical pressure was another way of preventing the child from revealing the abuse. Finally memory recovery was investigated by asking the subjects whether he/she had ever experienced an episode of inability to recall the traumatic events and if so how many years this period lasted.

Bermond-Vorst Alexithymia Questionnaire (BVAQ, Bermond & Vorst, 1993), consisting of five subscales (Vorst & Bermond, 2001) which relate to a reduced ability to: a) verbalize emotional experiences (Verbalizing), b) differentiate between emotional feelings (Identifying), c) reflect upon emotions (Analyzing), d) fantasize (Fantasizing), and e) experience emotional feelings (Emotionalizing).

Reliability and validity of the BVAQ are good (Vorst & Bermond, 2001; Bermond et al., 2007). Assessing the prevalence of alexithymia is based on impairment of the cognitive component (sum total of reduced Verbalizing, Identifying, and Analyzing), as an impaired cognitive component (belonging to Type I and Type II alexithymia) appeared to be related to a broad range of psychological disorders (Moormann et al., 2008; see also the 2007 publication of Bailey & Henry for the relation between Type I & II alexithymia and somatization), while an impaired affective component (sum total of reduced Emotionalizing & Fantasizing) primarily related to activities where expressive behaviour and creative imagination were hampered. For both alexithymia components scores ≥ percentile 70 were used as an indication of impairment while scores ≤ percentile 30 were used as an indication of unimpairement. In the Moormann et al. study of 2008 the cut-off scores for the alexithymia types (based on a student population of 354 subjects) were computed as follows: raw scores ≥54.0 related to an impaired cognitive component while raw scores ≤43.0 related to an unimpaired cognitive component. Regarding the affective component raw scores ≥42.0 related to an impaired affective, while raw scores ≤34.0 related to an unimpaired affective component. Using the above cut-off scores for an impaired cognitive BVAQ component as an indication of the prevalence of alexithymia resulted in an incidence of alexithymia of 20.4% in the Netherlands (Moormann et al., 2008) and of 18.2% in Australia (Bailey & Henry, 2007). On the basis of an albeit small clinical sample of 39, Taylor et al. (1997) suggest a cut-off value of 61 and above on the Toronto Alexithymia Scale (TAS-20). Despite the different instrument for alexithymia the statistics given in Finland (21.0%; Honkolampi et al., 2000), using these TAS-20 cut-off scores, are practically the same as the statistics obtained with the BVAQ in Australia and The Netherlands. Older studies using a cut-off on the earlier 26-item TAS have reported rates of 23% for a normal group in France (Loas et al., 1995) and 18.8% in Canada (Parker et al., 1989). Hence, the cut-off scores used in the present research seem a fair indication for the prevalence of alexithymia.

Dissociative Experiences Scale (DES - Bernstein & Putnam, 1986), a widely used self-report scale, containing 28 items, using a visual analogue scale (from 0-100). A Dutch adaptation was administered, consisting of the 3 subscales, as defined by Ross et al. (1995): a) Absorption-imaginative involvement ("So involved in fantasy that it seems real"), b) Activities of dissociated states ("Finding oneself in a place, but unaware how one got there"), and c) Depersonalization / Derealization ("Not recognizing one's reflection in a mirror; Other people and objects do not seem real")

Summing up all the scores and then dividing them by 28 results in the average DES score. The test retest reliability is good (0.84-0.96) and effectively differentiates patients with Dissociation from other psychiatric groups (Bernstein & Putnam, 1986). The DES can be used as a screening instrument for Dissociative Identity Disorder (DID). However semi-structured interviews are needed for a reliable diagnosis. Several cut-off values are used, ranging from 20 (Ross et al., 1991) to 31.3 (Bernstein & Putnam, 1986). In The Netherlands the DES cut-off scores were validated using the outcomes from clinical diagnostic interviews (Boon & Draijer, 1993), which resulted in an optimal cut-off score of 25 for the screening of DID. The mean DES scores in normal populations vary from 3.7 to 7.8, while scores of a group of a-select psychiatric patients vary from 14.6 to 17.0 (in Boon & Draijer, 1993).

Leiden Self Concept Questionnaire (LSQ ; Moormann & Duikers, 1984). The items relate to intellectual functioning, social functioning, physical appearance and self-efficacy. It consists of 27 items, first formulated in the present tense (present self), then in the past tense (past self), and finally in the future tense (future self). Only the present self will be discussed in our study. The Cronbach alphas are based on the 1989 publication by Moormann et al., and are given for the sexes separately (male: ⟨ = .89; female: ⟨ = .87). Scores ≤ percentile 30 is considered to be indicative of a low self (cut-off score of ≤ 103 for a student population (based on the data of the Moormann et al. study of 2008), cut-off score of ≤ 80 for male and ≤ 63 for female poly hard drug addicts (based on the data of the Moormann et al. study of 1989, and the Bauer et al. study of 1992), and cut-off scores ≤ 98 for the elderly (74-98 years of age), discussed in the data of the Moormann, et al. study of 1997.

5.4 Statistical analyses

First *Independent-Samples t Tests* will be run on all abuse characteristics (dependent variable) to identify whether the sexes (independent variable) differ on these variables. If so then in all analyses where means are compared it will be controlled for those abuse characteristics where sexes differ.

Regarding **Hypothesis 1** it was decided to use *cut-off scores* to identify the prevalence of alexithymia, dissociation and low self in the CSA group.

Gender differences will be tested by again performing *Independent-Samples t* Tests with gender as independent and alexithymia, dissociation and self as dependent variable.

6. Results

6.1 Gender differences in abuse characteristics and age

The results are given in Table 1 and demonstrate that the sexes didn't differ significantly neither on any of the abuse characteristics nor on age. However there was one trend on anal penetration that was more prominent in male than in female subjects.

Regarding the category perpetrator only t-tests where the father had been the perpetrator (29% for males, 40% for females) could be computed as in all other cases one of the groups contained empty cells: 18% of the males reported abuse by brother or sister, none of the females; No males reported abuse by other relatives (grandfather, uncle, etc.), while 24% of the females did; No males reported abuse by a family friend, while 6% of the females did; No males reported abuse by strangers, while the average numbers of abusive strangers was 1.12 for females; however 47% of the males reported abuse by people they knew other than relatives or a family friend, whereas none of the females did.

Abuse Characteristics	**MALE**			**FEMALE**				
	N	**M**	**SD**	**N**	**M**	**SD**	**t-test** (2-tailed)	**Sig**
1. FATHERperpetrator	17	0.29	0.47	50	0.40	0.50	t(1, 65) = -0.77	ns
2.ONSET< 10	17	0.71	0.47	49	0.78	0.42	t(1, 64) = -0.57	ns
3. DURATION	17	3.12	1.36	45	4.62	4.13	t(1, 60) = -1.47	ns
4. FREQUENCY	17	3.82	1.47	40	4.35	1.25	t(1, 55) = -1.38	ns
5. ASSAULT								
a. sexual harassment	17	0.94	0.24	47	1.00	0.00	t(1, 16) = -1.00	ns
b. masturbation	17	0.76	0.44	44	0.70	0.46	t(1, 59) = 0.46	ns
c. att. penetration	17	0.41	0.51	44	0.66	0.48	t(1, 59) = -1.78	ns
d. penetration	17	0.47	0.51	45	0.64	0.48	t(1, 60) = -1.24	ns
e. fellatio	17	0.65	0.49	45	0.47	0.50	t(1, 60) = 1.26	ns
f. anal penetration	17	0.41	0.51	45	0.16	0.37	t(1,22.61)=1.90	.07
6. COERCION								
a. position of power	17	0.76	0.44	49	0.92	0.28	t(1,20.62)=-1.4	ns
b. misleading	17	0.71	0.47	49	0.67	0.47	t(1, 64) = 0.24	ns
c. presents	17	0.53	0.51	49	0.51	0.51	t(1,64) = 0.13	ns
d. threatening	17	0.53	0.51	49	0.49	0.51	t(1, 64) = 0.28	ns
7. ENFOR. SECRECY								
a. shame	17	0.94	0.24	47	0.91	0.28	t(1, 62) = 0.34	ns
b. emotional pressure	17	0.71	0.47	47	0.72	0.45	t(1,62) = -0.14	ns
c. physical violence	17	0.35	0.49	48	0.35	0.48	t(1,63) = -0.01	ns
8. MEM RECOVERY	17	0.41	0.51	46	0.57	0.50	t(1, 61) = -1.08	ns
duration MEM REC	16	8.19	13.63	46	11.67	12.89	t(1, 60) = -.92	ns
AGE	16	37.31	11.36	52	37.83	9.73	t(1,66) = -0.18	ns

Table 1. Gender differences in abuse characteristics and age

Because of empty cells only the scores for the father were given in Table 1. None of the differences reached significance. The elevated percentages suggest a severe form of CSA.

The average abuse lasted 3-4 years (ranging from 1-30 years), and happened 3-4 times a week. Furthermore the prevalence of the various assaults (ranging from 16% to 100%) indicates severe abuse when considering:

a. The high incidence of coercion measures ranging from 51% to 92%,
b. The moderate to very high incidence of enforcing secrecy measures ranging from 35% to 94%, and
c. The considerable incidence of reported memory recovery, e.g. 41% for males and 57% for females with a mean duration of 8.19 years for males and 11.67 years for females. In one case a memory recovery had been reported after 46 years.

The finding that 71% of the males and 78% of the females reported that the abuse had started before the age of 10 suggests that we are really dealing with *childhood* sexual abuse.

Because neither on age nor on any abuse characteristic significant gender differences could be demonstrated, there was no further need for controlling for these variables in the upcoming statistical analyses where gender differences were tested on alexithymia, dissociation and self.

6.2 Impact of CSA on alexithymia, dissociation and self

Considerable evidence was found for **Hypothesis 1**, stating that CSA-victims display:

A *high prevalence of alexithymia* (e.g. scores ≥ 54.0 on the cognitive component of the BVAQ), as 40% of the CSA subjects (see Table 1 in the next chapter by Moormann, Albach & Bermond on alexithymia, dissociation and memory recovery) could be classified as either Type I (14%) or Type II (26%) alexithymia compared with the common guideline that about 1/5th of the normal population is alexithymic (see Instruments for prevalence statistics).

High dissociation scores (DES/28 > 25), as the average DES scores of both male (M = 25.79) and female (M = 38.23) CSA respondents exceeded the optimal cut-off value of 25 (see Table 2), indicative of Dissociative Identity Disorder (DID). Regarding the incidence of severe dissociation it was found that 47% of male and 78% of the females had average DES scores > 25

A *negative Self* as the average Self scores for male (M = 88.39) and female (M = 71.06) CSA respondents (see Table 2) were far below the cut-off value for students (N = 1061) corresponding to ≤ percentile 30 (Mean LSQ ≤ 103). Unfortunately norms for the normal population were not yet available. However compared with the elderly (N = 30; 74-98 years of age) the scores of both male and female CSA respondents were also far below the cut-off value of 98, corresponding to values lower than percentile 25. Compared with poly hard drug addicts, known for a negative self, the average mean self scores of both male and female CSA respondents fell in stanine 4 (for norm references see Instruments).

6.3 Explorative part: Gender differences

In Table 2 the statistics for this paragraph are given.

Dependent Variable	MALE			FEMALE			
	N	M	SD	N	M	SD	**t-tests** (2-tailed)
ALEX Total	17	109.71	24.98	43	123.98	19.23	t(1,58) = -2.38*
COG	17	65.53	18.95	45	77.44	16.67	t(1, 60) = -2.42*
a. Identifying	17	21.88	7.30	44	30.30	7.46	t(1, 59) = -3.97***
b. Verbalizing	17	24.47	8.23	45	29.91	7.53	t(1, 60) = -2.47*
c. Analyzing	17	19.18	7.59	44	18.32	6.40	t(1, 59) = 0.45
AFF	17	44.18	9.99	45	45.60	8.65	t(1, 60) = -0.55
a.Emotionalizing	17	21.24	5.62	45	19.71	6.98	t(1, 60) = 0.81
b. Fantasizing	17	22.94	5.58	45	25.89	8.03	t(1, 60) = - 1.39
DES/28	17	25.79	15.50	58	38.23	18.03	t(1, 73) = -2.58*
a. Absorption	17	418.90	201.10	58	546.01	225.62	t(1, 73) = -2.09*
b. Diss. Amnesia	17	123.82	116.76	58	175.06	143.11	t(1, 73) = -1.35
c. Deper & Derea	17	179.45	146.03	58	349.29	181.19	t(1, 73) = -3.54**
SELF	17	88.39	17.34	58	71.06	19.66	t(1, 73) = 3,27**

Table 2. Differences between male and female respondents on alexithymia, dissociation and self (*: p<0.05, **: p<0.01, ***: p<0.001)

Females scored significantly more alexithymic than men on the cognitive component, particularly on Identifying and Verbalizing emotions (on Analyzing the sexes did not differ significantly). Neither on the affective component nor on its subscales Emotionalizing and Fantasizing gender differences was significant. With the exception of the subscale 'Activities of Dissociated States', also called Dissociative amnesia, women scored significantly higher on all dissociation measures as well. Furthermore CSA women had a significantly lower self-concept. From the above it is concluded that that the impact of CSA is greater for women than for men.

7. Discussion

7.1 Impact of CSA on alexithymia, dissociation and self

Subjects in our sample have been victims of severe CSA and the results on alexithymia, dissociation, self and memory recovery confirm the notion that severe CSA has a devastating effect on psychological health in adulthood. The incidence of alexithymia (40%) was found to be substantially higher than the statistics published in non-abused populations in various different countries (around 20%; see the BVAQ description in the instruments part). Furthermore it was found that 47% of males and 78% of the females had average DES scores > 25, indicating DID. Finally CSA respondents reported a negative self. The outcomes above can be criticized on a common problem with prevalence indices for psychological disorders, e.g. where the exact cut off value should be located to ensure a valid diagnosis of alexithymia, dissociation or self. To some extent cut off scores always remain arbitrary and subjective. Even when sensitivity and specificity requirements are fulfilled the choice of the criterion remains an arbitrary decision. Furthermore the reliability on the reported abuse characteristics, a common problem in all retrospective studies using self-report questionnaires, can be questioned as well.

7.2 Gender specific outcomes

The impact for female victims was significantly stronger than for male victims (see Table 2). This result parallels the outcomes of gender differences in normal populations. Women generally have both stronger dissociative tendencies and a more negative self. However, in general men are more alexithymic and less emotional than women. Our results indicate the contrary, e.g. CSA women were found to be significantly more alexithymic than men, but only on the cognitive component (reduced Verbalizing and Identifying). The credibility issue, discussed in the introduction, and still associated with the feminine stereotype (hysterical, emotional, fantasy prone, liar, etc.) might be responsible for the highly impaired cognitive component in women, as not being taken seriously by expressing doubts on the credibility of their accounts, hampers the formation between the emotional experience and its cognitive labels. This invalidating environment where cries for help of the abused child are ignored or denied, often even by the mother, is described by Huber (1997) as one of the four factors associated with the development of DID. On the affective component (reduced Fantasizing and Emotionalizing) however, the sexes did not differ significantly from each other, which is remarkable as well because women usually are more emotional than men (Carpenter & Addis). The reported gender differences cannot be attributed to particular abuse characteristics because the sexes didn't differ significantly on any characteristic (see Table 1). It should be noted that in one category, e.g. 'perpetrator', only t-tests where the father had been the perpetrator (29% for males, 40% for females) could be performed, as in all other cases one of the groups contained empty cells. The data on perpetrators suggest, that adult relatives (grandfather, uncle) and strangers more often abused girls, while older siblings and adults they knew well, other than relatives (teachers, priests, coaches in sport clubs, etc.), more often abused boys. As it is extremely difficult to escape abuse in invalidating environments if an adult relative is the perpetrator it might be that threatening, physical violence and other coercions employed by the perpetrator to enforce secrecy (don't tell anybody about our secret otherwise ...) have led to the reported higher impairment of the cognitive alexithymia component in combination with higher dissociation scores in female victims.

7.3 Gender differences from a neurobiological perspective

An alternative way of discussing the results is looking for neurobiological substrates explaining behavioural gender differences. Larger prefrontal lobe CSF volumes and smaller midsaggital area of the corpus callosum subregion 7 (splenium) were seen in both boys and girls with maltreated-related PTSD (De Bellis & Keshavan, 2003). Subjects with PTSD did not show the normal age related increases in the area of the total corpus callosum and splenium. However this finding was more prominent in males with PTSD. Significant sex by group effects demonstrated smaller cerebral volumes and corpus callosum regions 1 (rostrum) and 6 (isthmus) in PTSD males and greater lateral ventricular volume increases in maltreated males with PTSD than maltreated females with PTSD. According to De Bellis and Keshavan their findings suggest that males are more vulnerable to the effects of severe stress in global brain structures than females. In the well-controlled, highly elegant study of De Bellis and Keshavan maltreated males with PTSD did show a trend towards reporting of more cluster C symptoms (e.g. avoidant and dissociative behaviors) than maltreated females with PTSD. The associated behavior includes efforts to avoid traumatic reminders, diminished interest in others, feelings of detachment, a restricted range of affect, and dissociation. Emotional numbing and diminished interest in others, particularly during development, may result in lack of empathy and an increased risk for anti-social behaviors and externalizing behaviors.

7.4 Incongruence between what is expected from the neurobiological substrate on gender differences in symptomatology and its behavioral manifestation

However, our results on gender differences are the opposite of what would be expected from a neurobiological perspective. How can this be explained? De Bellis and Keshavan note that their cross-sectional investigation does not imply causation. Neither does our investigation. It is not possible to disentangle whether observed sex differences are the consequence of the stress and trauma or a preexisting risk factor for the development of a disorder. It might well be that the male subjects in our sample did not have a preexisting risk factor but instead a preexisting protective buffer (low levels of neuroticism) against the development of a specific disorder. In this context it should be noted that only seventeen male respondents were willing to volunteer in our research. They were hard to find. There is still a 'taboo' on talking about male sexual abuse, in particular because it concerned same-sex relationships, which could make others think the victim consented to the abuse and is homosexual. It might well be that the male respondents who were willing to share their experiences with others were the stronger ones with more healthy personality profiles (lack of neuroticism), who were better equipped to cope with the adverse effects of CSA.

Even though our findings are not in agreement with what could be expected from a neurobiological point of view they do correspond to the general notion that women display a higher level of symptom reporting than men (Wool & Barsky, 1994; Kroenke & Spitzer, 1998). However it should be noted as well that one of the more controversial issues in terms of mental disorder diagnoses has been their differential sex prevalence (Hartung & Widiger, 1998). The point to be made is that it cannot be denied that what is suggested by neurobiological studies, e.g. that males are more vulnerable to the effects of severe stress in global brain structures than females, does not always correspond to what has been reported on the behavioral level in symptomatology. Hence, it remains striking that women who on the neurobiological level are assumed to be less vulnerable to stress (the stronger sex) have on the behavioral level both a reputation for and do show the symptoms of vulnerability to stress in a wide array of activities (the weaker sex). It might well be that the immensely popular brain model in contemporary academic science also has its flaws and does not account yet for the more phenomenological (how people experience events and impressions) aspects of human existence. Anyway we sincerely hope that our research with all its weaknesses and limitations is challenging enough to stimulate future research on the virgin territory of gender differences in CSA.

8. Conclusions

CSA-victims display: 1) a high prevalence of alexithymia (40% as opposed to 20%, reported in general populations), 2) high dissociation scores (> 25 on the average DES), indicative of Dissociative Identity Disorder, and 3) a negative self.

The impact of CSA on alexithymia, dissociation and self is significantly stronger for women than for men, and cannot be attributed to differences in abuse characteristics and age.

9. References

Albach, F. & Everaerd, W. (1992). Posttraumatic stress symptoms in victims of childhood incest. *Psychotherapy and Psychosomatics,* Vol.57, pp. 143-151

Albach, F. (1993). *Freud's Verleidingstheorie: Incest, trauma en hysterie* [Freud's seduction theory: Incest, trauma and hysteria]. PhD thesis, University of Amsterdam, Stichting Petra, ISBN 90-74214-04-5, Middelburg, The Netherlands

Albach, F.; Moormann, P.P. & Bermond, B. (1996). Memory recovery of childhood sexual abuse. *Dissociation,* Vol.9, pp. 258-269

Bakan, D. (1966). *The duality of human existence,* Beacon Press, Boston, MA

Bauer, H.; Moormann, P.P. & Hagtvet, K. (1992). Anxiety and perceived development of self at different stages of poly-hard-drug addicts, In: *Advances in in Tests Anxiety Research* (Vol. 7), K.A. Hagtvet (Ed.), 189-205, Swets & Zeitlinger, Lisse

Bailey, P.E. & Henry J.D. (2007). Alexithymia, somatisation and negative affect in a community sample. *Psychiatry Research,* Vol.150, pp. 13-20

Berenbaum, H. (1996). Childhood abuse, alexithymia and personality disorder. *Journal of Psychosomatic Research,* Vol.41, pp. 585-595

Berenbaum, H. & James, T. (1994). Correlates and retrospectively reported antecedents of alexithymia. *Psychosomatic Medicine,* Vol.56, pp. 353-359

Bermond, B. & Vorst, H. (1993). *The Bermond Vorst Alexithymia Questionnaire.* Unpublished internal report, Deparment of Psychology, University of Amsterdam.

Bermond, B.; Clayton, K.; Liberova, A.; Luminet, O.; Maruszewski, T.; Ricci Bitti, P. E.; Rime, B.; Vorst, H.; Wagner, H. & Wicherts, J. (2007). A cognitive and an affective dimension of alexithymia in six languages and seven populations. *Cognitions and Emotions,* Vol.21, Nr.5, pp. 1125-1136

Bermond, B.; Moormann, P.P.; Albach, F. & Dijke, A. van (2008). Impact of severe childhood sexual abuse on the development of alexithymia in adulthood. *Psychotherapy and Psychosomatics,* Vol.77, *260-261*

Bernstein, E.M. & Putnam, F.W. (1986). Development, reliability, and validity of a dissociation scale. *Journal of Nervous and Mental Disease*, Vol.174, pp. 727-735

Birnbaum, B. (1915). *Die sexuellen Falschanschuldigungen der Hysterischen. [The false sexual accusations of the hysterics].* Gross-Archiv, Band 64

Boon, S. & Draijer, N. (1993). *Multiple personality disorder in the Netherlands: A study on reliability and validity of the diagnosis*, Zwets & Zeitlinger, Lisse

Butler, L. D. & Nolen-Hoeksema, S. (1994). Gender differences in responses to depressed mood in a college sample. *Sex Roles*, Vol.30, pp. 5-6

Carmen, E. H.; Rieker, P. P. & Mills, T. (1984). Victims of violence and psychiatric illness. *American Journal of Psychiatry*, Vol.141, pp. 378-383

Carpenter, K.M. & Addis, M.E. (2000). Alexithymia, gender, and responses to depressive symptoms. *Sex Roles*, Vol.43, pp. 629-644

Ceci, S.J. & Loftus, E.F. (1994). 'Memory work': A royal road to false memories? *Applied Cognitive Psychology,* Vol.8, pp. 351-364

Chu, J.A. & Dill, L.D. (1990). Dissociative symptoms in relation to childhood physical and sexual abuse. *American Journal of Psychiatry, Vol.147,* pp. 887-892

Cloitre, M.; Scarvalone, P. & Difede, J. (1997). Posttraumatic stress disorder, self- and interpersonal dysfunction among sexually retraumatized women. *Journal of Traumatic Stress,* Vol.10, pp. 437-442

Coons, P. M. (1996): The dissociative disorders. Rarely considered and underdiagnosed. *Psychiatric Clinics of North America,* Vol.21, pp. 637-648

Crombag, H.F.M. & Merckelbach, H.L.G.J. (1996). *Hervonden herinneringen en andere misverstanden [Recovered memories and other misapprehensions],* Contact, Amsterdam

De Bellis M.D. & Keshavan, M.S. (2003). Sex differences in brain maturation in maltreatment-related pediatric posttraumatic stress disorder. *Neuroscience and Biobehavioral Reviews,* Vol.27, pp. 103-117

Dhaliwal, G.K.; Gauzas, L.; Antonowicz, D.H. & Ross, R.R. (1996). Adult male survivors of child sexual abuse: Prevalence, sexual abuse characteristics and long term effects. *Clinical Psychology Review,* Vol.16, pp. 619-639

Eliot, D.M. & Briere, J. (1992). Sexual abuse trauma among professional women: Validating the Symptom Trauma Checklist-40 (TSC 40). *Child abuse and Neglect,* Vol.16, pp. 391-398

Elzinga, B.; Bermond, B. & Van Dyck, R. (2002). The relationship between dissociative proneness and alexithymia. *Psychotherapy and Psychosomatics,* Vol.71, pp. 104-111

Ensink, B.J. (1992). *Confusing realities: A study on child sexual abuse and psychiatric symptoms,* Ph.D. thesis, VU University Press, Amsterdam

Feiring, C.; Taska L. & Lewis, M. (1999). Age and gender differences in children's and adolescent's adaptation to sexual abuse. *Child abuse and Neglect,* Vol.23, pp. 115-128

Finkelhor, D. & Browne, A. (1985). The traumatic impact of child sexual abuse: A conceptualization. *American Journal of Orthopsychiatry,* Vol.55, 530-541

Frewen, P.A.; Dozois, D.J.A.; Neufeld, R.W. & Lanius., R.A. (2008). Meta-analysis of alexithymia in Post Traumatic Stress Disorder. *Journal of Traumatic Stress,* Vol.21, pp. 243-246

Garnefski, N. & Arends, E. (1998). Sexual abuse and adolescent maladjustment: Differences between male and female victims. *Journal of Adolescence,* Vol.21, pp. 99-107

Garnier, P. (1903). Les hystériques accusatrices [The accusing hysterics]. *Annales d'hygiène publique et de médicine légale, troisième série, tome L.,* J-B Ballière et fils, Paris

Grabe, H. J.; Rainermann, S.; Spitzer, C.; Gansicke, M. & Freyberger, H.J. (2000). The relationship between dimensions of alexithymia and dissociation. *Psychotherapy and Psychosomatics,* Vol.69, pp. 128-131

Gold, S.N.; Hill, E.L.; Swingle, J.M. & Elfant, S. A. (1999). Relationship between childhood abuse characteristics and dissociation among women in therapy. *Journal of Family Violence,* Vol.14, pp. 157-17

Hartung, C.M. & Widiger, T.A. (1998). Gender differences in the diagnosis of mental disorders: Conclusions and controversies of the DSM-IV. *Psychological Bulletin,* Vol.123, Nr.30, pp. 260-278

Honkalampi, K,; Hintikka, J.; Taskanen, A.; Lehtonen, J. & Viinamki, H. (2000). Depression is strongly associated with alexithymia in the general population. *Journal of Psychosomatic Research,* Vol.48, pp. 99-104

Herman, J.L. (1981). *Father-daughter incest,* Harvard University Press, Cambridge

Horowitz, M.J. (1976). *Stress response syndromes* (2nd. Ed.), Jason Aronson, Northvale, NJ

Huber, M. (1997). *Meervoudige persoonlijkheden: Een handboek voor overlevenden van extreme geweld* [Multiple personalities: A manual for survivors of extreme violence, translated from German, first published in 1995 by Fischer Tachenbuch Verlag GmbH, Frankfurt am Main], Wereldbibliotheek, Amsterdam

Hunter, M. (1990). *Abused boys: The neglected victims of sexual abuse,* Lexington Books & D. C. Health and Company, Lexington

Hyer, L.; Woods, G.; Summers, M.N.; Boudewyns, P. & Harrison, W.R. (1990). Alexithymia among Vietnam veterans with Post Traumatic Stress Disorder. *Journal of Clinical Psychiatry,* Vol.51, pp. 243-246

Irwin, H.J. & Melbin-Helberg, E.B. (1997). Alexithymia and dissociative tendencies. *Journal of Clinical Psychology,* Vol.53, pp. 159-166

James, W. (1890). *Principles of Psychology,* Holt, New York

Janet, P. (1889). *L'automatisme psychologique* [The psychological automatism], Félix Alcan, Paris

Janoff-Bulman, B. & Frieze, I. H. (1983). A theoretical perspective for understanding reactions to victimization. *Journal of Social Issues,* Vol.39, pp. 1-17

Kirby, J.S.; Chu, J.A. & Dill, D.L. (1993). Correlates of dissociative symptomatology in patients with physical and sexual abuse histories. *Comprehensive Psychiatry,* Vol.34, pp. 258-263

Kisiel, C.L.L. & Lyons, S.J. (2001). Dissociation as a mediator of psychopathology among sexually abused children and adolescents. *American Journal of Psychiatry,* Vol.158, pp. 1034-1039

Kluft, R.P. (1996). Dissociative Identity Disorder, In: *Handbook of Dissociation: Theoretical, empirical and clinical perspectives,* L.K. Michelson & W.J. Ray (Eds.), 337-366, Plenum Press, New York

Kohn, A. (1987). Shattered innocence. *Psychology Today,* Vol.21, 54-58

Kooiman, C.G.; Rees Vellinga, S van; Spinhoven, P., Draijer, N.; Trijsburg, R.W & Rooijmans, H.G.M. (2004). Childhood adversities as risk factors for alexithymia and other aspects of affect dysregulation in adulthood. *Psychotherapy & Psychosomatics,* Vol.73, pp. 107-116

Kroenke, K. & Spitzer, R.L. (1998). Gender differences in reporting of physical and somatoform symptoms. *Psychosomatic Medicine,* Vol.60, pp. 150-155

Krystal, H. (1988). *Integration and self-healing: Affect, trauma and alexithymia,* Analytic Press, Hillsdale, NY

Kuhn, J.A.; Arellano, C.M. & Chavez, E.L. (1998). Correlates of sexual assault in Mexican-American and White non-Hispanic adolescent males. *Violence and Victims,* Vol.13, pp. 11-20

Loas, G.; Fremaux, D.; Otmani, O. & Verrier, A. (1995). Prevalence of alexithymia in a general population. Study in 183 "normal" subjects and in 263 students. *Annales médico-psychologiques,* Vol.153, Nr.5, pp. 355-357

Loftus, E.F. (1993). The reality of repressed memories. *American Psychologist,* Vol.48, pp. 518-537

Loftus, E.F. (1997). Creating false memories: Researchers are showing how suggestion and imagination can create "memories" of events that did not actually occur. *Scientific American,* September, pp. 50-55

Maccoby, E. (1990). Gender and relationships: A developmental account. *American Psychologist,* Vol. 45, pp. 513-520

Markus, H. & Oyserman, D. (1989). Gender and thought: The role of the self-concept, In: *Gender and thought,* M. Crawford & M. Hamilton (Ed.), 100-127, Springer-Verlag, New York

Myers, M. F. (1989). Men sexually assaulted as adults and sexually abused as boys. *Archives of Sexual Behaviour,* Vol.18, pp. 203-215

Modestine, J. ; Furrer, R. & Malti, T. (2005). Different traumatic experiences are associated with different pathologies. *Psychiatry Quaterly,* Vol.76, pp. 19-32

Moody, W.C. (1999). Male child sexual abuse. *Journal of Pediatric Health Care,* Vol.13, Nr.3, pp. 112-119

Moormann, P.P. & Duijkers, T.J. (1984). *Het psychologische moeras van drugverslaving* [The psychological morass of drug addiction], Internal report LPR-PP: 84-061, Department of Psychology, Leiden University, The Netherlands

Moormann, P.P., Cocq van Delwijnen, H. de, Wessel, K. van, & Bauer, H. (1989). *Personality characteristics of drug addicts in the Netherlands,* Internal report LPR-PP: 02-89, Department of Psychology, Leiden University, The Netherlands

Moormann, P.P.; Bermond, B.; Albach, F. & Dorp, I. van (1997). The etiology of alexithymia from the perspective of childhood sexual abuse, In: *The (non)expression of emotions in health and disease,* Ad Vingerhoets, Frans van Bussel, & Jan Boelhouwer (Eds.), 139-153, Tilburg University Press, Tilburg

Moormann, P.P.; Bermond, B. & Albach, F. (2004). The Reality Escape Model: The intricate relation between alexithymia, dissociation, and anesthesia in victims of child sexual abuse, In: *Emotional Expression and Health,* Ivan Nyklicek, Ad Vingerhoets, & Lydia Temoshok (Eds), 82-98, Brunner Routledge, Hove

Moormann, P.P.; Bermond, B.; Vorst, H.C.M.; Bloemendaal, A.; Teijn, S. & Rood, L. (2008). New avenues in alexithymia research: The creation of alexithymia types. In: *Emotion Regulation: Conceptual and Clinical Issues,* Johan Denollet, Ivan Nyklicek, & Adrianus Vingerhoets (Eds.), 27-42, Springer, New York

Paivio, S.C. & McCulloch, C.R. (2004). Alexithymia as a mediator between childhood trauma and self-injurious behaviors. *Child Abuse and Neglect,* Vol.28, pp. 339-354

Parker, J.D.A.; Taylor, G.J. & Bagby, M. (1989). The alexithymia construct: Relationship with sociodemographic variables and intelligence. *Comprehensive Psychiatry,* Vol.30, pp. 434-444.

Putnam, F.W. (1993). Dissociative disorders in children: behavioural profiles and problems. *Child abuse and Neglect,* Vol.17, pp. 39-45

Putnam F.W.; Carlson E.B.; Ross, C.A.; Anderson, G.; Clark P.; Torem; M., Bowman, E.S.; Coons, P.; Chu, J.A.; Dill, D.L.; Loewenstein, R.J. & Braun, B.G. (1996). Patterns of dissociation in clinical and non clinical samples. *Journal of Nervous and Mental Disorders,* Vol.184, pp. 673-679

Rogers, C.N. & Terry, T. (1984). Clinical interventions with boy victims of sexual abuse, In: *Victims of sexual aggression: Treatment of children, women, and men,* I.R. Stuart & J.G. Greer (Eds.), 91-104, Van Nostrand Reinhold, New York

Ross, C.A. (1996). History, phenomenology and epidemiology of dissociative disorders, In: *Handbook of dissociation,* L.K. Michelson & W.J. Ray (Eds), 3-24, Plenum Press, New York

Ross, C.A.; Ellason, J.W. & Anderson, G. (1995). A factor analysis of the Dissociative Experience Scale (DES) in dissociative identity disorder. *Dissociation, Vol.8,* pp. 229-235

Russell, D.E.H. (1986). *The secret trauma: Incest in the lives of girls and women.* Basic Books, New York

Sher, D. & Twaite, J.A. (1999). The relationship between child sexual abuse and alexithymic symptoms in a population of recovering adult substance abusers. *Journal of Child Sexual Abuse,* Vol.8, pp. 25-40

Sifneos, P.E. (1973). The prevalence of alexithymic characteristics in psychosomatic patients. *Psychotherapy and Psychosomatics,* Vol.22, pp. 250-262.

Sifneos, P.E. (1975). Problems of psychotherapy of patients with alexithymic characteristics and physical disease. *Psychotherapy and Psychosomatics,* Vol.26, pp. 65-70

Taylor, G.J.; Bagby, R.M. & Parker, D.A. (1997). *Disorders of affect regulation: Alexithymia in medical and psychiatric illness,* Cambridge University Press, Cambridge

Thomas, R.K.; Krystal, J.H.; Giller, E.L.; Frank, J. & Dan., E. (1992). Alexithymia as a predictor response in post traumatic stress disorder. *Journal of traumatic stress,* Vol.5, pp. 563- 573

Tzeng, O.C.S. & Schwarzin, H.I. (1990). Gender and race differences in child sexual abuse correlates. *International Journal of Intercultural Relations,* Vol.14, pp. 135-161

Vorst, H.C.M. & Bermond, B. (2001). Validity and reliability of the Bermond-Vorst Alexithymia Questionnaire. *Personality and Individual Differences,* Vol.30, pp. 413-434

Walker, J.L.; Carey, P.D.; Mohr; N.; Stein, D.J. & Seedat, S. (2004). Gender differences in the prevalence of child sexual abuse and in the development of pediatric PTSD. *Archive of women's mental health,* Vol.7, Nr.2, pp. 111-121.

Wool, C.A. & Barsky, A.J. (1994). Do women somatize more than men? Gender differences in somatization. *Psychosomatics,* Vol.35, pp. 445-452

Yapko, M.D. (1994). *Suggestions of abuse: True and false memories of childhood sexual trauma,* Simon & Schuster, New York

Zeitlin, S.B.; McNally, R.J. & Cassiday, K.L. (1993). Alexithymia in victims of sexual assault: An effect of repeated traumatization? *American Journal of Psychiatry,* Vol.150, pp. 661-663

Zlotnick, C.; Shea, M.T.; Pearlstein, T.; Simpson, E.; Costello, E. & Begin, A. (1996). The relationship between dissociative symptoms, alexithymia, impulsivity, sexual abuse, and self-mutulation. *Comprehensive Psychiatry,* Vol.37, pp. 12-16

Zlotnick, C.; Mattia, J. I. & Zimmermann, M. (2001). The relationship between post traumatic stress disorder, childhood trauma and alexithymia in an outpatient sample. *Journal of Traumatic Stress,* Vol.14, pp. 177-187

Part 2

The Physiological Impact of Sexual Assault

6

Psychobiological Effects of Sexual Abuse

Dorie A. Glover, John K. Williams and Kimberly A. Kisler
UCLA Semel Institute for Neuroscience and Human Behavior
USA

1. Introduction

Sexual abuse represents a stressor that challenges psychobiological homeostasis. Basic survival requires an ability to maintain internal equilibrium by adjusting physiological processes to match the demands of the external and internal environment. "Stress" is a broad term representing any physical or psychological demand that challenges equilibrium. When outside temperatures rise, physiological systems respond with multiple changes so as to keep internal temperatures from rising to a dangerous level. As nourishment is depleted, hunger is an internal cue that prompts food seeking. If ignored, energy resources will be shut down to non-critical bodily functions and shunted to those most critical for continued survival (e.g., the brain). Threat of physical or psychological harm activates biological systems that facilitate an appropriate response, including aggressive defensive actions ("fight") or avoidance behavior ("flight"). Unfortunately, a protective response is often unavailable or ineffective in the context of sexual abuse. Alternatively, a psychobiological response may prove effective in the short-term, but ultimately lead to a chain of processes that set the stage for long-term mental and physical health risk.

In this chapter, we will: a) describe the biological systems most closely involved in regulating stress responses; b) review existing literature on the psychobiological consequences of child and adult sexual abuse; c) discuss limitations of existing data; and d) introduce a conceptual framework for understanding sexual abuse as it relates to future mental and physical health.

2. The biological response to threat

Stressful experiences bring about a complex and counterbalancing set of hormonal responses in the sympathetic-adrenomedulary (SAM) and the hypothalamic-pituitary-adrenal axis (HPAA) systems, as well as the immune system. The basic components of these systems have been mapped out through animal studies, which allow for scientific control over the timing, frequency, type, and severity of the stress. Widely examined in animal and human research, the HPAA is best known as the regulator of the "fight-flight" response to threat, diverting energy resources needed for protective actions and promoting a subsequent return to homeostasis when the threat is no longer present. Such a system exists in all vertebrates (Lovejoy, 2005). Thus, the HPAA has been a central focus of basic animal research on fear conditioning, general effects of environmental stress, the developing brain, "learned helplessness" models of depression, as well as human studies of anxiety and mood disorders more generally (Friedman, Charney, & Deutch, 1995). More recently, it has been proposed that stimuli perceived as significant may not only elicit aggressive or avoidance behavior (i.e., fight/flight), but also approach and affiliation behaviors, referred to as "tend and befriend" (Taylor et al., 2000). These behaviors are suggested to be controlled primarily by the neurosubstances of oxytocin and arginine vasopressin (AVP) (known alternatively as vasopressin, argipressin, or antidiuretic hormone (ADH). When triggered by threat, the hypothalamus releases corticotrophin-releasing hormone (CRH/alternatively "factor" or CRF) to the anterior pituitary. CRH, oxytocin, and AVP are all secreted in the paraventricular nucleus (PVN) and the arcuate nucleus (AN) of the hypothalamus. Mutual origination from the PVN and excitatory and inhibitory cross-talk between CRH, OXY, and AVP suggest these may be more interrelated than previously thought (van den Burg & Neumann, 2011). Nonetheless, biological assessment of oxytocin or AVP following sexual abuse has not yet been examined. Thus, we restrict our discussion here to the better known sequelae of the SAM and HPAA.

In humans, the perception and interpretation of stimuli occurs within the limbic system, consisting mainly of the hippocampal formation, amygdala, and entorhinal cortex. When stimuli are identified as potential perturbations to the basic state of equilibrium (i.e., physical or psychological "stressors"), the SAM system immediately (within seconds) releases the catecholamines epinephrine (adrenaline) and norepinephrine (noradrenaline, or NE). The catecholamines facilitate subsequent processes that increase the heart rate, blood pressure, and blood glucose levels in muscles and vital organs in order to allow the body to adapt to the increased demand. Stressors also trigger the HPAA to begin a slower process occurring over minutes. This response begins with the hypothalamus, a cone-shaped brain structure that sits below the thalamus, projecting downward into the pituitary (infundibular) stalk which ends at the roundish-shaped pituitary gland (Afifi & Bergman, 1998). Once triggered, the hypothalamus releases corticotrophin-releasing hormone (CRH/alternatively "factor" or CRF) to the anterior pituitary. The pituitary response to CRH is to release adrenocorticotropic hormone (ACTH). In turn, ACTH stimulates release of glucocorticoids (in humans, "cortisol") and dehydroepiandrosterone (DHEA) from the adrenal glands located above the kidneys. Cortisol and the catecholamines further act on the immune system, which results in changes in the levels and activity of cytokines that are especially relevant for host protection against viral infections like HIV (i.e., CD4 and CD8 T-cells) (Coe & Laudenslager, 2007; Glaser & Kiecolt-Glaser, 2005).

Under normal circumstances, specialized feedback systems are designed to ensure a return to homeostasis once the threat is gone. Once released, cortisol has an important role in shutting down the sympathetic activation of the SAM system and suppressing further release of CRH by a negative feedback mechanism on the pituitary, hippocampus, hypothalamus, and amygdala. The anti-glucocorticoid properties of DHEA are also believed to contribute to an up-regulation of HPAA responses, as well as mitigate possible deleterious effects of high cortisol levels on the brain (Rasmusson, Vythilingam, & Morgan, 2003). Once the perception of threat recedes, the negative feedback mechanisms help restore neurosubstance levels to resting states (allostasis). Thus, the HPAA represents a "negative feedback" loop by which cortisol release is triggered *and* subsequently inhibited.

However, when stress exposure is very intense, frequent, or chronic, the effects of the SAM, HPA axis, and immune system on target cells and organs may be prolonged. The interaction of the stress hormones (cortisol and the catecholamines) with cell receptors produce both short-term changes in cell processes, as well as changes in gene expression that have long-lasting consequences for cell function. Over time, these effects can lead to tissue damage, and changes in cell functioning and the brain (structural atrophy, suppressed neurogenesis, and synaptic and dendritic remodeling). Such central neurobiological changes may lead to HPAA dysregulation that is opposite to expected patterns. A counter-intuitive *low* level of urinary cortisol was first reported in men diagnosed with Posttraumatic Stress Disorder (PTSD) (Yehuda et al., 1990). PTSD is, by definition, a fear-based psychiatric condition. Diagnostic requirements include: a) exposure to a traumatic event involving perceived threat of death or harm to physical integrity of the self or another person; and b) an acute emotional reaction of fear, helplessness, or horror. Brain imaging studies confirm distinct neurological areas are activated in PTSD patients who show heightened peripheral SAM system reactivity (e.g., increased heart rate) versus those showing blunted reactivity (Lanius et al., 2010) with an explanatory proposal that there are two forms of PTSD. These and subsequent studies in other psychiatric populations (e.g., Major Depressive Disorder: Ahrens et al., 2008; Panic Disorder: Petrowski, Herold, Joraschky, Wittchen, & Kirschbaum, 2010) and otherwise healthy individuals experiencing chronic stress (Juster et al., 2011) demonstrate the bi-directional nature of HPAA output at rest and/or in response to new threat. The general direction of HPAA dysregulation (hyper vs. hypo responsive) is thought to depend upon characteristics of the threat (e.g., the intensity, frequency, and chronicity), the timing of assessment relative to the threat (immediate or minutes/hours versus days or months), or the developmental stage in which the threat occurs (McEwen, 2010; McEwen & Gianaros, 2011). Also, the directional impact of cortisol on other neurotransmitters and systems appears to depend upon the perceived anticipatory immediacy of new and recurring threat (Sapolsky, Romero, & Munck, 2000). Of note, these are environmental, not genetic factors. A study of monozygotic twins discordant for bullying (one with and one without a victimization history) supports the experiential nature of threat effects on HPAA reactivity (Ouellet-Morin et al., 2011). Bullied twins showed a blunted cortisol response to a psychosocial stress test, whereas their non-bullied siblings had a normal cortisol rise. There was no evidence that these group differences were due to genetic makeup, family environment, pre-existing or concomitant individual factors, and the perception of stress or the level of subjective emotional responding to the stress test.

Ultimately, stress effects are associated with poor health outcomes across multiple systems, including cardiovascular, metabolic, and immune systems (McEwen, 2008; McEwen & Gianaros, 2011). Emerging data on telomeres, which are deoxyribonucleic acid (DNA)/protein repeats at the end of chromosomes that regulate cellular replicative life span, indicate stress prematurely shortens telomere length (Epel et al., 2004) and thus may hasten all-cause mortality. Telomere length is receiving widespread attention as a potential biomarker proxy for cumulative stress burden, accelerated aging processes, and expected lifespan for a given individual (Epel et al., 2009).

Sexual abuse, either as a single or re-occurring event, represents a significant threat to the physical and psychological integrity of the individual and thus acts to "perturb" homeostasis. The ability to successfully adapt to this challenge, both immediately and in the long term, is key to psychological and physical health and perhaps even how long one can expect to live.

3. Assessment of biological dysregulation in sexually abused children and adults

In preclinical studies of rodents and primates, neurotransmitters and their effects can be measured centrally in a temporal sequence concurrent with presentation and removal of stress. In humans, we are rarely able to assess immediate post-trauma biology. Sexual abuse remains a terrible and stigmatized secret for many victims who often do not disclose the abuse (London, Bruck, Ceci, & Shuman, 2005; Sorsoli, Kia-Keating, & Grossman, 2008). If they do, they may not receive the emotional support and protection that is needed to avoid further victimization. Childhood sexual abuse (CSA) is particularly unlikely to be revealed until long after it has occurred. It may be revealed to others only as an adult survivor, or may never be revealed. Non-disclosure of adult sexual abuse (ASA) is also common. Thus, treatment seeking in any form (from a psychologist, counselor, religious leader, or other supportive professional) is low, particularly among low-income racial/ethnic minorities.

Widespread under-reporting is likely to result in inaccurate prevalence rates (Pereda, Guilera, Forns, & Gomez-Benito, 2009). As a result, the full effects of sexual abuse on development and long-term physical health across the lifespan are not well known. Studies of biological functioning in sexual abuse victims soon after an incident are limited, with most sequelae being reported retrospectively in adulthood (Burns-Loeb et al., 2002; Glover, Garcia-Aracena, Lester, Rice, & Rothram-Borus, 2010). Thus, most biological data on CSA survivors come from retrospective studies among adult women with self-reported histories of CSA. Studies among sexually abused women are also rarely conducted near the time of an ASA incident. Very little research exists on biological effects of sexual abuse among males, including assessment of CSA effects among boys or adult men reporting retrospectively, or among adult men soon after ASA (Burns-Loeb et al., 2002).

3.1 Biological functioning after CSA among children

CSA victims are often exposed to multiple types of maltreatment (including physical abuse, neglect, and psychological maltreatment) and adversity factors (including variables reflecting interpersonal loss, parental dysfunction, family violence, economic adversity, and life-threatening illness) (Higgins, 2004). Nonetheless, research generally limits investigations to a single type (Kendler et al., 2000), combines different types of adverse exposure into a single group, does not include measures of severity and developmental timing, and rarely includes non-English-speaking participants (Green et al., 2010; McLaughlin et al., 2010; Scott, Smith, & Ellis, 2010). These factors do not have equal effects on outcomes and their joint effects are not additive nor specific to a particular outcome (Green et al., 2010).

Of the few studies reporting biological outcomes in sexually and/or physically abused children, it is clear that physiological disturbances may be widespread. The effects of even a single severe traumatic event involving threat of or actual physical harm to the victim may permanently alter functioning of neurotransmitters from the HPAA and SAM systems. These abnormalities may be detected at rest or only in response to new stressors. Examples of affected systems include autonomic activity, cortisol and catecholamines, and immune system indicators, although findings are not consistent in direction or pattern (Cicchetti & Rogosch, 2001; Gunnar & Quevedo, 2007; McEwen & Gianaros, 2011; McEwen & Wingfield, 2003; Nemeroff, 2004; Putnam, 2003; Turner-Cobb, 2005). Biological studies have largely examined the HPAA, although acute stress is known to affect the limbic system and have potential effects on gene expression of widespread neurohormonal receptors (DeBellis et al., 1994; DeBellis, Lefter, Trickett, & Putnam, 1994; Heim et al., 2000; Heim & Nemeroff, 2001; Penza, Heim, & Nemeroff, 2003; Wise, Palmer, Rothman, & Rosenberg, 2009).

A recent review of the literature on neuroendocrine dysregulation after CSA showed that of 127 publications from 1990 to January 2007, only 7 studies with biological data soon after a CSA event could be found (Bicanic, Meijer, Sinnema, van de Putte, & Olff, 2008). Of these, several did not report the time since abuse and so are not discussed here. King, Mandansky, King, Fletcher, and Brewer (2001) identified 10 girls who had experienced CSA in the past month (as reported by parents and/or social service agencies). The group was mostly white (70%), and 5 to 7 years of age. Although study eligibility required one CSA incident within the past 2 months, most (80%) also reported multiple incidents occurring over as many as 12 months before study entry. Salivary cortisol was collected on the morning of a physician-scheduled exam designed to identify "physical or emotional" signs to support sexual abuse" (p 72). Morning salivary cortisol was then also collected from non-abused controls matched on age, ethnicity, sex, and socio-economic status. CSA survivors showed significantly lower morning salivary cortisol relative to controls, suggesting HPAA dysregulation can be detected within months of CSA.

In another study reporting assessment soon after CSA, a cohort of sexually abused girls were identified within 6 months of their disclosure of the abuse. In the first assessment, morning plasma cortisol levels were found to be significantly elevated as compared to controls matched for demographics (Putnam, Trickett, Helmers, Dorn, & Everett, 1991). The next assessment of a subsample of this cohort (6 or more months later) collected 24-hour urinary free cortisol and also involved administration of exogenous (ovine) CRH in order to measure plasma ACTH and cortisol reactivity (DeBellis et al., 1994). On this occasion, cortisol secretion detected from urine and plasma following CRH did not differ across abused and non-abused groups, but CSA girls showed reduced ACTH reactivity to the CRH infusion. Results indicate that dysregulation is detectable months and years after the initial abuse and may change over time. Unfortunately, such dysregulation cannot be attributed to the abuse itself because new trauma and/or adverse conditions could have occurred in the period between the initial abuse and the biological assessment.

The findings on ACTH reactivity in CSA (DeBellis, Lefter, Trickett, & Putnam, 1994) preceded a large number of subsequent studies among traumatized adults with PTSD focusing on mechanisms of HPAA dysregulation (for recent updates on mechanisms see Friedman & Pitman, 2007). This focus is reflected in one other study of biomarkers found among CSA survivors during childhood. Duval and colleagues (2004) examined hospitalized adolescents (aged 10 to 14) with PTSD who reported sexual abuse years earlier (mean 5.6 +/- 4 years). ACTH and cortisol levels were measured following administration of an HPAA stimulating hormone, dexamethasone. Compared to controls, these CSA survivors showed ACTH hypersuppression to dexamethasone. Whether dysregulation among these teens was due to PTSD, exposure to child sexual abuse, or both was not possible to determine.

Brain imaging of abused children indicates changes in the size or symmetry of key brain structures (hippocampus, corpus collosum, prefrontal cortex) as well as neuronal quality (density and integrity) of certain brain regions (Bremner et al., 1997; Teicher, Tomoda, & Andersen, 2006). Carrion, Weems, and Reiss (2007) reported brain changes associated with cortisol and PTSD symptoms in 15 children exposed to at least one traumatic event. Most had experienced multiple traumatic events, including sexual, physical, and emotional abuse as well as witnessing violence. The sample included 6 boys and 9 girls ages 8 to 14 (mean=10.4), and a mixed ethnic composition of primarily whites (n=7) or African Americans (n=6). The children were assessed twice, with assessments separated by 12-18 months. Brain imaging techniques were used to evaluate changes in hippocampal size over time in relation to PTSD symptoms and home-collected cortisol levels across the day. Results showed that participants with the highest severity of PTSD symptoms at Time 1 showed the greatest reductions in the right hippocampus from the first to the second assessment. Elevated evening (pre-bed) salivary cortisol at Time 1 was also related to reductions in hippocampal size at the next assessment.

3.2 Biological functioning among adult survivors of sexual abuse

Most sexual abuse (SA) data relevant for biological functioning come from retrospective studies among adult women who were abused as children. For example, Leserman (2005) reviewed studies of physical health among sexually abused samples, indicating higher than expected associations between SA and headache, gastrointestinal, gynecologic, and panic-related symptoms. Retrospective biomarker assessments with control groups indicate CSA exposure is associated with differences in 24-hour urinary cortisol excretion (e.g., Lemieux & Coe, 1995) and smaller hippocampal volume (e.g., Stein, Walker, Hazen, & Forde, 1997). Retrospective studies of adult women with a history of CSA *or* other types of abuse (e.g., neglect and physical abuse) have shown changes in autonomic activity and ACTH responses to laboratory stress (Heim et al., 2000; Heim & Nemeroff, 2001; Heim & Nemeroff, 2002) as well as smaller hippocampus volume (Bremner et al., 1997; Vythilingam et al., 2002). One study indicated brain volume differences in specific regions were found for women abused at ages 3-5 years (hippocampus) versus ages 9-10 years (corpus callosum), ages 11-13 years (hippocampus), or 14-16 years (frontal cortex) (Andersen et al., 2008). Studies of CSA survivors categorized as having PTSD or not sometimes indicate biological dysregulation occurs only among CSA survivors with current PTSD (e.g., T cell activation of the immune system) (Lemieux, Coe, & Carnes, 2008). Functional brain imaging of CSA exposed adults with PTSD demonstrate changes in activation patterns (Lanius, Bluhm, Lanius, & Pain, 2006). The direction of neuroendocrine differences (higher vs. lower cortisol or ACTH response) has been inconsistent. Trickett, Noll, Susman, Shenk, and Putnam (2010) report data indicating discrepancies may be due to changes in neuroendocrine functioning in the initial period after abuse (associated with elevated cortisol) versus after many years have passed (associated with attenuated cortisol).

Only one study is known to have conducted biological assessments soon after adult sexual abuse. Resnick, Yehuda, Pitman, and Foy (1995) collected plasma cortisol levels from female rape victims within hours of the SA. Those who reported a history of prior assault showed significantly lower cortisol levels in the acute aftermath than those who reported no prior assault histories. Other biological assessment studies among abused adults typically combine SA with other forms of physical and psychological abuse (e.g., Garcia-Linares, Sanchez, Lorente, Coe, & Martinez, 2004; Sanchez-Lorete, Blasco-Ros, Coe, & Martinez, 2010).

4. Problems of interpretation

In the absence of assessment soon after an initial incident of sexual abuse, and periodically thereafter (i.e., longitudinal studies), it is difficult to interpret biological findings in relation to past events. Numerous intervening events can affect outcomes and the longer the period between CSA and assessment, the less likely scientists can be confident in proper interpretation of findings.

There are two related intervening factors that make interpretation of retrospective studies especially difficult. First, CSA has been linked to a greater likelihood of sexual revictimization both later in childhood and in adulthood (Classen, Palesh, & Aggarwal, 2005; Messman-Moore & Long, 2000; Messman-Moore & Long, 2003). There have been numerous studies conducted with diverse samples of women who were sexually abuse as children and then subsequently revictimized (Messman-Moore & Long, 2003). Studies have included college students (Gidycz, Hanson, & Layman, 1995; Mayall & Gold, 1995; Messman-Moore & Long, 2000; Messman-Moore, Long, & Siegfried, 2000), clinical samples (Briere & Runtz, 1987; Bryer, Nelson, Miller, & Krol, 1987; Shields & Hanneke, 1988), military samples (Merrill et al., 1999), community samples (Fergusson, Horwood, & Lynskey, 1997; Messman-Moore & Long, 2000; Wyatt, Guthrie, & Notgrass, 1992), and lesbian and bisexual female samples (Morris, Balsam, & Rothblum, 2002). Research on sexual revictimization with men, specifically gay and bisexual men is an emerging field (Heidt, Marx, & Gold, 2005; Kalichman et al., 2001). Experiences of CSA have been correlated with negative contributions to mental, physical, and sexual health (Burns-Loeb et al., 2002; Whiffen & MacIntosh, 2005). However, it is not clear why some victims of sexual abuse are at greater risk of revictimization or how singular versus multiple experiences affect mental and physical health outcomes. For example, evidence exists supporting that sexual abuse during certain stages of development, severity of CSA, and additive forms of trauma such as sexual and physical abuse may be important factors in distinguishing survivors of CSA who are revictimized from those who are not (Classen, Palesh, & Aggarwal, 2005). Most of the research on CSA and revictimization is derived from cross-sectional and retrospective studies. As a consequence, it is difficult to distinguish between correlational and causal relationships.

The second related intervening factor that complicates interpretation of retrospective studies is the common comorbidity of mental health disorders, multiple non-sexual trauma types, and concurrent child and adult adversities. Exposure to CSA, as with other childhood trauma and adversities, is associated with increased prevalence of adult DSM-IV mood disorders, anxiety disorders, and substance use disorders in numerous large epidemiological studies (Green et al., 2010; McLaughlin et al., 2010; Scott, Smith, & Ellis, 2010). Abnormal biological assessment profiles in adulthood may be due to: a) child sexual abuse; b) other trauma or adversity occurring in childhood or as an adult; c) the current (adult) presence of a psychological disorder; or d) some combination of these factors.

A landmark longitudinal study by Koenen, Moffitt, Poulton, and Caspi (2007) illustrates this issue. Records for a New Zealand birth cohort (N=1037) were reviewed for childhood neurodevelopment, temperament, behavioral, and family environment characteristics and in-person follow-up assessments at ages 26 and 32 were conducted. Data revealed a cumulative negative effect of exposure to both acute trauma and adversity in childhood (before the age of 11). One set of factors (low IQ and chronic environmental adversity, including poverty) increased risk for PTSD at age 26, but not the number of lifetime trauma exposures. A second set of factors (childhood externalizing characteristics, maternal depression, and loss of a parent) not only increased risk for having a PTSD diagnosis at age 26, but also increased risk for exposure to more lifetime acute traumas even in the absence of PTSD symptoms. Subsequent victimization could be due to increased risk-taking behaviors, poor cognitive functioning that would normally allow escape from risky situations, the negative impact of early trauma on subsequent educational and vocational achievement, or the impairments associated with PTSD symptoms. If subsequent trauma exposure in adulthood occurred between age 26 and 32, those with the greatest childhood burden of trauma and adversity were also more likely to develop PTSD even if they had not experienced such psychological symptoms before. Thus, a host of developmental factors, including exposure to CSA, contribute to vulnerability for increased trauma exposure and for mental health sequelae.

Among CSA survivors, additional sexual abuse (revictimization), exposure to other trauma and adversities, and the development of mental health disorders are common co-occurrences. Unless a careful history is obtained and these factors systematically controlled (e.g., through research study design or statistical covariance), reliable interpretation of biological outcomes in adulthood is limited.

Studies designed to address these limitations exist. For example, Heim, Mletzko, Purselle, Musselman, and Nemeroff (2008) examined HPAA functioning among healthy men (aged 18-60) recruited into four study groups, including: 1) normal subjects with no childhood abuse history or psychiatric disorder (*n* =14); 2) men with childhood abuse histories without current major depressive disorder (MDD) (*n*=14); 3) men with childhood abuse histories with current MDD (*n* =15); and 4) men with current MDD and no childhood abuse history (*n*=6). HPAA functioning was examined using the dexamethasone/corticotropin-releasing factor (CRF) test, which is a sensitive measure of HPAA hyperactivity and has been demonstrated to be altered in patients with MDD. Men with childhood trauma histories exhibited increases in ACTH and cortisol responses to dexamethasone/CRF relative to non-abused men with and without depression. Increased response was associated with the severity, duration, and earlier onset of the child abuse. Statistical analyses indicated effects were not due to concurrent PTSD symptoms (Heim et al., 2008).

5. Discussion of limitations of existing studies

Well-designed psychobiological research that includes appropriate comparison groups is surprisingly limited. Timely disclosure of an event is clearly a prerequisite for immediate assessment, but even when reporting has occurred (e.g., to social service agencies or police), psychobiological data are rarely collected. Even when data is collected, researchers now know that the specific form of biological dysregulation after acute or chronic stress is highly variable. As noted earlier, both very high and very low cortisol levels have been found in adults with PTSD (Glover & Poland, 2002) and among physically and sexually abused children (Gunnar & Quevedo, 2007). Bi-directional heart rate and functional magnetic imaging responses in adults with PTSD have also been documented (Lanius, Bluhm, Lanius, & Pain, 2006). Lanius and colleagues (2010) propose there are two types of PTSD based on the pattern of reactivity to new stressors. Some individuals exposed to trauma subsequently fail to react to new stress, showing blunting of the normal cardiovascular and neuroendocrine increases. This pattern is referred to as a "dissociative" type of PTSD and may be related to behavioral tendencies for dissociative amnesia, fantasy proneness, and depersonalization used to cope with extreme stress. Others may react normally, but fail to recover within the expected time frame for a given biomarker. These data are in keeping with emerging awareness of the fluid and counterbalancing nature of biological systems and their primary output. For example, recent findings show norepinephrine's capacity as both an anxiogenic and anxiolytic (Nemeroff, 2004) and cortisol effects not only reduce immune system activity, but also heighten it depending upon the stress context (i.e., type, duration, imminence of threat) (Sapolsky, 2000). Future research on the psychobiology of sexual abuse must begin to use updated methods, including examining individual biomarkers bi-directionally and multiple biomarkers across systems known to counterbalance each other.

It is now clear that the form of bio-dysregulation may change as a function of the amount of time that has elapsed since the last sexual abuse event or the last traumatic event, if numerous types of traumas are concurrently being experienced (Weems & Carrion, 2007). In a study of mothers of children with life-threatening illness, Glover, Garcia-Aracena, and Mohlman (2008) found that maternal hippocampal volume, known in animal studies to shrink after exposure to stress-related high cortisol, showed a significant positive association with the time elapsed since the child's illness diagnosis. That is, the more time that had passed since the onset of the child's illness, the larger the hippocampus size (after controlling for age of the mother). This cross-sectional study indicates plasticity of the hippocampus, with the greatest negative effect close in time to the stressor and a gradual recovery. The timing of sexual abuse exposure in relation to developmental stage (e.g., child vs. adult, pre- vs. post-puberty, during women's child-rearing vs. post-menopausal years) is also quite likely to influence the psychobiological sequelae of abuse (Heim, Plotsky, & Nemeroff, 2004).

Peri-traumatic factors at the time of sexual abuse may influence mental and physical health effects, including severity (e.g., penetration vs. fondling) and the victim's relationship to the perpetrator (e.g., immediate family member or intimate partner vs. distant acquaintance or stranger) (Glover et al., 2010). The absence of information on specific characteristics of trauma and the socio-cultural context in which trauma occurs is a recognized limitation of large scale epidemiological studies of trauma and adversities (Green et al., 2010). This may be particularly relevant for sexual abuse in the context of racial/ethnic minority cultures that are associated with strong gender roles and expectations (Sciolla et al., 2011).

Finally, perhaps as a result of outside agendas from potential funding providers (e.g., pharmaceutical companies) many existing studies recruit only a narrow band of sexually abused study participants who do or do not meet criteria for a specific mental health disorder (e.g., PTSD or MDD) or physical health problem (e.g., gynecological abnormalities). Ideally, studies should include sexual abuse exposed individuals with and without mental and physical health symptoms and control groups who also vary on abuse and health histories. Although not based on sexual abuse trauma, a series of studies examining multiple biomarkers of health risk (BHR) in highly stressed women with and without PTSD or MDD is informative (Glover, Steele, Stuber, & Fahey, 2005; Glover, Stuber,& Poland, 2006; Glover et al., 2010). Whereas BHR was highest among those with current mental health symptoms, neither PTSD or depression symptoms were a necessary prerequisite for elevations in BHR relative to controls (Glover, Stuber, & Poland, 2006). Furthermore, elevated BHR was linked to lower volume of the hippocampus (Glover, Garcia-Aracena, & Mohlman,2008), independent of any mental health symptoms as determined by clinical interview. Together, these data suggest that psychobiological dysregulation following sexual abuse may be detected even when mental health symptoms as assessed via self-report are absent. Nonetheless, self-reported mental health symptoms, even at sub-clinical levels as measured by conventional psychological assessments, may exacerbate dysregulation and ultimately, pose a risk for health problems.

6. A framework for understanding psychobiological consequences of sexual abuse

Challenges for understanding psychobiological sequelae of sexual abuse include complex, bi-directional, and counterbalancing biological systems, a paucity of studies among child and adult victims, and research design and omission limitations in existing research. As biological investigations of sexual abuse sequelae become more sophisticated, these must also connect with the growing knowledge of personal, interpersonal, and community level moderating and mediating variables, particularly for revictimization (Breitenbecher, 2001; Classen, Palesh, & Aggarwal, 2005; Messman-Moore, & Long, 2003).

6.1 Personal and interpersonal level factors

Age, gender, and race/ethnicity are likely to have significant effects for long term biological outcomes following SA. Research among boys and men is greatly lacking and may show outcome differences than those from females. Sexual abuse during adolescence has been shown to place a woman at greater risk for revictimization in adulthood than that occurring at earlier times (Gidycz, Coble, Latham, & Layman, 1993; Humphrey & White, 2000). Developmental stage of occurrence not only during childhood but also critical stages during the lifespan (e.g., during pregnancy or SA as the mother of young children) may have profound effects on biological health outcomes. The racial/ethnic background of the victim is now understood to be a major influence on the meaning and interpretation of SA for the individual as well as the response from others if/when abuse is revealed (Behl, Crouch, May, & Valente, 2001; Bohn, 2003; Urquiza & Goodlin-Jones, 1994; Wyatt, Guthrie, & Notgrass, 1992). A detailed **sexual history**, including severity, duration, frequency, use of force, number of perpetrators, and relationship to perpetrators are all variables critical to health outcomes and risks for sexual revictimization (Arata, 2000; Bifulco, Brown, & Adler, 1991; Collins, 1998; Kessler & Bieschke, 1999; Koverola, Proulx, Battle, & Hanna, 1996; West, Williams, & Siegel, 2000; Wyatt, Loeb, Solis, Carmona, & Romero, 1999). Recency of abuse in relation to the assessment appears important; the more recent the abuse, the greater the likelihood that it will predict revictimization (Himelein, 1995). A detailed history of **other forms of trauma** including child physical abuse and family adversity have also been linked to negative sequelae (Molnar, Buka, & Kessler, 2001) and sexual revictimization (Arata & Lindman, 2002; Desai, Arias, Thompson, & Basile, 2002; Heidt, Marx, & Gold, 2005; Jankowski, Leitenberg, Henning, & Coffey, 2002). **Family structure and dynamics and interpersonal relationships** should be assessed including the composition of the family unit and of primary social groups, the use of alcohol and drugs by members in these groups, and the methods for resolution of conflict are also relevant issues (Hamilton & Browne, 1999; Kellogg & Hoffman, 1997; Koverola et al., 1996; Long & Jackson, 1991; Nash, Hulsey, Sexton, Harralson, & Lambert, 1993; Nelson et al., 2002; Swanston et al., 2002). **Psychiatric disorders** (e.g., depression and anxiety or substance abuse) as well as **psychological factors** (e.g., shame, self-blame, and resiliency) are critical variables to explore (Neumann, Houskamp, Pollock, & Briere, 1996). **Medical illnesses** prior to, during, or after sexual abuse need to be assessed as they may be associated with and/or sequelae of sexual abuse (Wegman & Stetler, 2009).

6.2 Community level factors

Social Support including relationships with extended family, friends, church, etc., is especially important as it relates to sexual abuse sequelae. Social support has been shown to have an impact on disclosure and on moderating the psychological impact of sexual abuse (Borja, Callahan, & Long, 2006; Feiring, Taska, & Lewis, 1998). However, very little research has been conducted examining whether such support protects against the biological sequelae of sexual abuse. **Cultural, community and religious norms** need to be evaluated as these may provide scripts which influence how individuals appraise and respond to stress. Sparse research exists on examining how norms influence the way in which individuals interpret and define experiences such as sexual abuse. Also, little is known regarding how appraisal based upon these cultural, community, and religious norms subsequently impact or contribute to psychological or biological/physical manifestations. These factors need to be explored as they may influence health outcomes.

7. Conclusion

There is still much to examine with respect to the psychobiology of sexual abuse. The understanding of moderating and mediating variables for sexual abuse itself is increasing, but these have largely been studied independent of biological assessments. A more holistic model that considers biopsychosocial mediating and moderating variables as complex predictors for and consequential effects of sexual abuse is needed to enhance and accelerate the development of effective prevention and intervention efforts.

8. Acknowledgements

Funding to support this research and to write this chapter was provided from the National Institute of Mental Health (The ES-HIM Project [1 R34 MH077550] and the Center for Culture, Trauma, and Mental Health Disparities [5P50MH073453]).

9. References

Afifi, A. K., & Bergman, R. A. (1998). *Functional Neuroanatomy*. United States: McGraw-Hill.

Ahrens, T., Deuschle, M., Krumm, B., van der Pompe, G., den Boer, J. A., & Lederbogen, F. (2008). Pituitary-adrenal and sympathetic nervous system responses to stress in women remitted from recurrent major depression. *Psychosomatic Medicine*, 70(4), 461-467.

Andersen, S. L., Tomada, A., Vincow, E. S., Valente, E., Polcari, A., & Teicher, M. H. (2008). Preliminary evidence for sensitive periods in the effects of childhood sexual abuse on regional brain development. *Journal of Neuropsychiatry and Clinical Neurosciences*, 20(3), 292-301.

Arata, C. M. (2000). From child victim to adult victim: A model for predicting sexual revictimization. *Child Maltreatment*, 5, 28-38.

Arata, C. M., & Lindman, L. (2002). Marriage, child abuse, and sexual revictimization. *Journal of Interpersonal Violence*, 17, 953-971.

Behl, L. E., Crouch, J. L., May, P. F., & Valente, A. L. (2001). Ethnicity in child maltreatment research: A content analysis. *Child Maltreatment*, 6, 143-147.

Bicanic, I. A., Meijer, M., Sinnema, G., van de Putte, E. M., & Olff, M. (2008). Neuroendocrine dysregulations in sexually abused children and adolescents: A systematic review. *Progress in Brain Research*, 167, 303-306.

Bifulco, A., Brown, G. W., & Adler, Z. (1991). Early sexual abuse and clinical depression in adult life. *The British Journal of Psychiatry*, 159, 115-122.

Bohn, D. K. (2003). Lifetime physical and sexual abuse, substance abuse, depression, and suicide attempts among native american women. *Issues in Mental Health Nursing*, 2(4), 333-352.

Borja, S. E., Callahan, J. L., & Long, P. J. (2006). Positive and negative adjustment and social support of sexual assault survivors. *Journal of Traumatic Stress*, 19(6), 905-914.

Breitenbecher, K. H. (2001). Sexual revictimization among women: A review of the literature focusing on empirical investigations. *Aggression and Violent Behavior*, 6, 415-432.

Bremner, J. D., Randall, P., Vermetten, E., Staib, L., Bronen, R. A., Mazure, C., … Charney, D. S. (1997). Magnetic resonance imaging-based measurement of hippocampal volume in posttraumatic stress disorder related to childhood physical and sexual abuse- A preliminary report. *Society of Biological Psychiatry*, 41(1), 23-32.

Briere, J., & Runtz, M. A. (1987). Post sexual abuse trauma: Data and implications for clinical practice. *Journal of Interpersonal Violence*, 2, 367–379.

Bryer, J. B., Nelson, B. A., Miller, J. B., & Krol, P. A. (1987). Childhood sexual and physical abuse as factors in adult psychiatric illness. *American Journal of Psychiatry*, 144, 1426–1430.

Burns-Loeb, T., Williams, J. K., Rivkin, I., Vargas-Carmona, J., Wyatt, G., Chin, D., & Asuan-O'Brien, A. (2002). The effects of child sexual abuse on adolescent and adult sexual functioning. In J. R. Heiman & C. M. Davis (Eds.), *Annual Review of Sex Research: An Integrative and Interdisciplinary Review* (307-345). Allentown, PA: The Society for the Scientific Study of Sexuality.

Carrion, V. G., Weems, C. F., & Reiss, A. L. (2007). Stress predicts brain changes in children: A pilot longitudinal study on youth stress, posttraumatic stress disorder, and the hippocampus. *Pediatrics*, 119(3), 509-516.

Cicchetti, D., & Rogosch, F. A. (2001). The impact of child maltreatment and psychopathology on neuroendocrine functioning. *Development and Psychopathology*, 13(4), 783-804.

Classen, C. C., Palesh, O. G., & Aggarwal, R. (2005). Sexual revictimization: A review of the empirical literature. *Trauma, Violence, & Abuse*, 6(2), 103-129.

Coe, C. L., & Laudenslager, M. L. (2007). Psychosocial influences on immunity, including effects on immune maturation and senescence. *Brain, Behavior, and Immunity*, 2(8), 1000-1008.

Collins, M. E. (1998). Factors influencing sexual victimization and revictimization in a sample of adolescent mothers. *Journal of Interpersonal Violence*, 13, 3-24.

DeBellis, M. D., Chrousos, G. P., Dorn, L. D., Burke, L., Helmers, K., Kling, M. A., … Putnam, F. W. (1994). Hypothalamic-pituitary-adrenal axis dysregulation in sexually abused girls. *Journal of Clinical Endocrinology & Metabolism*, 78(2), 249-255.

DeBellis, M. D., Lefter, L., Trickett, P. K., & Putnam, F. W. (1994). Urinary catecholamine excretion in sexually abused girls. *Journal of the American Academy of Child & Adolescent Psychiatry*, 33, 320-327.

Desai, S., Arias, I., Thompson, M. P., & Basile, K. C. (2002). Childhood victimization and subsequent adult revictimization assessed in a nationally representative sample of women and men. *Violence and Victims*, 17, 639-653.

Duval, F., Crocq, M. A., Guillon, M. S., Mokrani, M. C., Monreal, .J, Bailey, P., & Macher, J. P. (2004). Increased adrenocorticotropin suppression after dexamethasone administration in sexually abused adolescents with posttraumatic stress disorder. *Annals of the New York Academy of Sciences*, 1032, 273-275.

Epel, E. S., Blackburn, E. H., Lin, J., Dhabhar, F. S., Adler, N. E., Morrow, J. D., & Cawthon, R. M. (2004). Accelerated telomere shortening in response to life stress. *Proceedings of the National Academy of Sciences USA*, 101(49), 17312-17315.

Epel, E. S., Merkin, S. S., Cawthon, R., Blackburn, E. H., Adler, N. E., Pletcher, M. J., & Seeman, T. E. (2009). The rate of leukocyte telomere shortening predicts mortality from cardiovascular disease in elderly men. *Aging*, 1(1), 81-88.

Feiring, C., Taska, L. S., & Lewis, M. (1998). Social support and childrens' and adolescents' adaptation to sexual abuse. *Journal of Interpersonal Violence*, 13, 240-260.

Fergusson, D. M., Horwood, L. J., & Lynskey, M. T. (1997). Childhood sexual abuse, adolescent sexual behaviors and sexual revictimization. *Child Abuse and Neglect*, 21(8), 789–802.

Friedman, M. J., Charney, D. S., & Deutch, A. Y. (Eds.). (1995). *Neurobiological and clinical consequences of stress: From normal adaptation to post-traumatic stress disorder*. Philadelphia, PA: Lippincott Williams & Wilkins Publishers.

Friedman, M. J., & Pitman, R. K. (2007). New findings on the neurobiology of posttraumatic stress disorder. *Journal of Traumatic Stress*, 20(5), 653-655.

Garcia-Linares, M. I., Sanchez-Lorente, S., Coe, C. L., & Martinez, M. (2004). Intimate male partner violence impairs immune control over herpes simplex virus type 1 in physically and psychologically abused women. *Psychosomatic Medicine*, 66(6), 965-972.

Gidycz, C. A., Coble, C. N., Latham, L., & Layman, M. J. (1993). Sexual assault experience in adulthood and prior victimization experiences: A prospective analysis. *Psychology of Women Quarterly*, 17, 151-168.

Gidycz, C. A., Hanson, K., & Layman, M. J. (1995). A prospective analysis of the relationships among sexual assault experiences. *Psychology of Women Quarterly*, 19, 5-29.

Glaser, R., & Kiecolt-Glaser, J. K. (2005). Stress-induced immune dysfunction: Implications for health. *Nature Reviews Immunology*, 5(3), 243-251.

Glover, D. A., Garcia-Aracena, E. F., Lester, P., Rice, E., & Rothram-Borus, M. J. (2010). Stress biomarkers as outcomes for HIV+ prevention: Participation, feasibility and findings among HIV+ latina and arican american mothers. *AIDS and Behavior*, 14(2), 339-350.

Glover, D. A., Garcia-Aracena, E. F., & Mohlman, J. (2008). Peripheral biomarker composite associated with smaller hippocampal volume. *NeuroReport*, 19(13), 1313-1316.

Glover, D. A., Loeb, T. B., Carmona, J. V., Sciolla, A., Zhang, M., Myers, H. F., & Wyatt, G. E. (2010). Childhood sexual abuse severity and disclosure predict posttraumatic stress symptoms and biomarkers in ethnic minority women. *Journal of Trauma & Dissociation*, 11(2), 152-173.

Glover, D. A., & Poland, R. E. (2002). Urinary cortisol and catecholamines in mothers of child cancer survivors with and without PTSD. *Psychoneuroendocrinology*, 27(7), 805-819.

Glover, D. A., Steele, A. C., Stuber, M. L., & Fahey, J. L. (2005). Preliminary evidence for lymphocyte distribution differences at rest and after acute psychological stress in PTSD-symptomatic women. *Brain Behavior and Immunity*, 19(3), 243-251.

Glover, D. A., Stuber, M., & Poland, R. E. (2006). Allostatic load in PTSD-symptomatic middle-aged mothers of child cancer survivors. *Psychiatry: Biological and Interpersonal Processes*, 69(3), 191–203.

Green, J. G., McLaughlin, K. A., Berglund, P. A., Gruber, M. J., Sampson, N. A., Zaslavsky, A. M., & Kessler, R. C. (2010). Childhood adversities and adult psychiatric disorders in the national comorbidity survey replication I: Associations with first onset of DSM-IV disorders. *Archives of General Psychiatry*, 67(2), 113-123.

Gunnar, M., & Quevedo, K. (2007). The neurobiology of stress and development. *Annual Review of Psychology*, 58, 145-173.

Hamilton, C. E., & Browne, K. D. (1999). Recurrent maltreatment during childhood: A survey of referrals to police child protection units in England. *Child Maltreatment, 4*, 275-286.

Heidt, J. M., Marx, B. P., & Gold, S. D. (2005). Sexual revictimization among sexual minorities: A preliminary study. *Journal of Traumatic Stress*, 18, 533-540.

Heim, C., Mletzko, T., Purselle, D., Musselman, D. L., & Nemeroff, C. B. (2008). The dexamethasone/corticotropin-releasing factor test in men with major depression: Role of childhood trauma. *Biological Psychiatry*, 63(4), 398-405.

Heim, C., & Nemeroff, C. B. (2001). The role of childhood trauma in the neurobiology of mood and anxiety disorders: Preclinical and clinical studies. *Biological Psychiatry*, 49, 1023-1039.

Heim, C., & Nemeroff, C. B. (2002). Neurobiology of early life stress: Clinical studies. *Seminars in Clinical Neuropsychiatry*, 7(2), 147–159.

Heim, C., Newport, D. J., Heit, S., Graham, Y. P., Wilcox, M., Bonsall, R., Miller, A. H., & Nemeroff, C. B. (2000). Pituitary-adrenal and autonomic responses to stress in women after sexual and physical abuse in childhood. *Journal of the American Medical Association*, 284(5), 592-597.

Heim, C., Plotsky, P. M., & Nemeroff, C. B. (2004). Importance of studying the contributions of early adverse experience to neurobiological findings in depression. *Neuropsychopharmacology*, 29(4), 641-648.

Higgins, D. J. (2004). The importance of degree versus type of maltreatment: A cluster analysis of child abuse types. *Journal of Psychology*, 138(4), 303-324.

Himelein, M. J. (1995). Risk factors for sexual victimization in dating: A longitudinal study of college women. *Psychology of Women Quarterly*, 19, 31-48.

Humphrey, J. A., & White, J. W. (2000). Women's vulnerability to sexual assault from adolescence to young adulthood. *Journal of Adolescent Health*, 27, 419-424.

Jankowski, M. K., Leitenberg, H., Henning, K., & Coffey, P. (2002). Parental caring as a possible buffer against sexual revictimization in young adult survivors of child sexual abuse. *Journal of Traumatic Stress, 15*, 235-244.

Juster, R. P., Marin, M. F., Sindi, S., Nair, N. P., Ng. Y. K., Pruessner, J. C., & Lupien, S. J. (2011). A clinical allostatic load index is associated with burnout symptoms and hypocortisolemic profiles in healthy workers. *Psychoneuroendocrinology*, 36(6), 797-805.

Kalichman, S. C., Benotsch, E., Rompa, D., Gore-Felton, C., Austin, J., Luke, W., … Simpson, D. (2001). Unwanted sexual experiences and sexual risks in gay and bisexual men: Associations among revictimization, substance abuse, and psychiatric symptoms. *Journal of Sex Research*, 38(1), 1-9.

Kellogg, N. D., & Hoffman, T. J. (1997). Child sexual revictimization by multiple perpetrators. *Child Abuse and Neglect*, 21, 953-964.

Kendler, K. S., Bulik, C., Silberg, J., Hettema, J. M., Myers, J., & Prescott, C. A. (2000). Childhood sexual abuse and adult psychiatric and substance use disorders in women. *Archives of General Psychiatry*, 57, 953-959.

Kessler, B. L., & Bieschke, K. J. (1999). A retrospective analysis of shame, dissociation, and adult victimization in survivors of childhood sexual abuse. *Journal of Counseling Psychology*, 46, 335-341.

King, J. A., Mandansky, D., King, S., Fletcher, K. E., & Brewer, J. (2001). Early sexual abuse and low cortisol. *Psychiatry and Clinical Neurosciences*, 55, 71-74.

Koenen, K. C., Moffitt, T. E., Poulton, J. M., & Caspi, A. (2007). Early childhood factors associated with the development of post-traumatic stress disorder: Results from a longitudinal birth cohort. *Psychological Medicine*, 37, 181-192.

Koverola, C., Proulx, J., Battle, P., & Hanna, C. (1996). Family functioning as predictors of distress in revictimized sexual abuse survivors. *Journal of Interpersonal Violence*, 11, 263-280.

Lanius, R., Bluhm, R., Lanius, U., & Pain, C. (2006). A review of neuroimaging studies in PTSD: Heterogeneity of response to symptom provocation. *Journal of Psychiatric Research*, 40(8), 709-729.

Lanius, R. A., Vermetten, E., Loewenstein, R. J., Brand, B., Schmahl, C., Bremner, D., & Spiegel, D. (2010). Emotion modulation in PTSD: Clinical and neurobiological evidence for a dissociative subtype. *American Journal of Psychiatry*, 167(6), 640-647.

Lemieux, A. M., & Coe, C. L. (1995). Abuse-related post-traumatic stress disorder: Evidence for chronic neuroendocrine activation in women. *Psychosomatic Medicine*, 57(2), 105-115.

Lemieux, A. M., Coe, C. L., & Carnes, M. (2008). Symptom severity predicts degree of T cell activation in adult women following childhood maltreatment. *Brain, Behavior, & Immunity*, 22(6), 994-1003.

Leserman, J. (2005). Sexual abuse history: Prevalence, health effects, mediators, and psychological treatment. *Psychosomatic Medicine*, 67(6), 906-915.

London, K., Bruck, M., Ceci, S. J, & Shuman, D. W. (2005). Disclosure of child sexual abuse. What does the research tell us about the ways that children tell? *Psychology, Public Policy and Law*, 11(1), 194-226.

Long, P. J., & Jackson, J. L. (1991). Children sexually abused by multiple perpetrators: Familial risk factors and abuse characteristics. *Journal of Interpersonal Violence*, 6, 147-159.

Lovejoy, D. A. (2005). *Neuroendocrinology: An Integrated Approach*. England: John Wiley & Sons, Ltd.

Mayall, A., & Gold, S. R. (1995). Definitional issues and mediating variables in the sexual revictimization of women sexually abused as children. *Journal of Interpersonal Violence*, 10(1), 26–42.

McEwen, B. S. (2008). Central effects of stress hormones in health and disease: Understanding the protective and damaging effects of stress and stress mediators. *European Journal of Pharmacology*, 583(2-3), 174-185.

McEwen, B. S. (2010). Stress, sex, and neural adaptation to a changing environment: Mechanisms of neuronal remodeling. *Annals of the New York Academy of Sciences*, 1204 Suppl, E38-59.

McEwen, B. S., & Gianaros, P. J. (2011). Stress and allostasis-induced brain plasticity. *Annual Review of Medicine*, 62, 431-445.

McEwen, B. S., & Wingfield, J. C. (2003). The concept of allostasis in biology and biomedicine. *Hormones and Behavior*, 43(1), 2-15.

McLaughlin, K. A., Green, J. G., Gruber, M. J., Sampson, N. A., Zaslavsky, A. M., & Kessler, R. C. (2010). Childhood adversities and adult psychiatric disorders in the national comorbidity survey replication II. *Archives of General Psychiatry*, 67(2), 124-132.

Merrill, L. L., Newell, C. E., Thomsen, C. J., Gold, S. R., Milner, J. S., Koss, M. P., & Rosswork, S. G. (1999). Childhood abuse and sexual revictimization in a female Navy recruit sample. *Journal of Traumatic Stress*, 12(2), 211–225.

Messman-Moore, T. L., & Long, P. J. (2000). Child sexual abuse and revictimization in the form of adult sexual abuse, adult physical abuse and adult psychological maltreatment. *Journal of Interpersonal Violence*, 15(5), 489-502.

Messman-Moore, T. L., & Long, P. J. (2003). The role of childhood sexual abuse sequelae in the sexual revictimization of women: An empirical review and theoretical reformulation. *Clinical Psychology Review*, 23(4), 537-571.

Messman-Moore, T. L., Long, P. J., & Siegfried, N. J. (2000). The revictimization of child sexual abuse survivors: An examination of the adjustment of college women with child sexual abuse, adult sexual assault, and adult physical abuse. *Child Maltreatment: Journal of the American Professional Society on the Abuse of Children*, 5(1), 18–27.

Molnar, B. E., Buka, S. L., & Kessler, R. C. (2001). Child sexual abuse and subsequent psychopathology: Results from the national comorbidity survey. *American Journal of Public Health*, 91, 753-760.

Morris, J. F., Balsam, K. F., & Rothblum, E. D. (2002). Lesbian and bisexual mothers and nonmothers: Demographics and the coming-out process. *Journal of Family Psychology*, 16(2), 144-156.

Nash, M. R., Hulsey, T. L., Sexton, M. C., Harralson, T. L., & Lambert, W. (1993). Long-term sequelae of childhood sexual abuse: Perceived family environment, psychopathology and dissociation. *Journal of Consulting & Clinical Psychology*, 61(2), 276-283.

Nelson, E. C., Heath, A. C., Madden, P. A. F., Cooper, M. L., Dinwiddie, S. H., Bucholz, K. K., ... Martin, N. G. (2002). Associations between childhood sexual abuse and adverse psychosocial outcomes: Results from a twin study. *Archives of General Psychiatry*, 59(2), 139-145.

Nemeroff, C. B. (2004). Neurobiological consequences of childhood trauma. *Journal of Clinical Psychiatry*, 65(Suppl 1), 18-28.

Neumann, D. A., Houskamp, B. M., Pollock, V. E., & Briere, J. (1996). The long-term sequelae of childhood sexual abuse in women: A meta-analytic review. *Child Maltreatment*, 1(6), 6-16.

Ouellet-Morin, I., Danese, A., Bowes, L., Shakoor, S., Ambler, A., Pariante, C. M., ... Arseneault, L. A. (2011). Discordant monozygotic twin design shows blunted cortisol reactivity among bullied children. *Journal of the American Academy of Child and Adolescent Psychiatry*, 50(6), 574-582.

Penza, K. M., Heim, C., & Nemeroff, C. B. (2003). Neurobiological effects of childhood abuse: Implications for the pathophysiology of depression and anxiety. *Archives of Women's Mental Health*, 6(1), 15-22.

Pereda, N., Guilera, G., Forns, M., & Gomez-Benito, J. (2009). The prevalence of child sexual abuse in community and student samples: A meta-analysis. *Clinical Psychology Review*, 29(4), 328-338.

Petrowski, K., Herold, U., Joraschky, P., Wittchen, H. U., & Kirschbaum, C. (2010). A striking pattern of cortisol non-responsiveness to psychosocial stress in patients with panic disorder with concurrent normal cortisol awakening responses. *Psychoneuroendocrinology*, 35(3), 414-421.

Putnam, F. W. (2003). Ten-year research update review: Child sexual abuse. *Journal of the American Academy of Child & Adolescent Psychiatry*, 42(3), 269-278.

Putnam, F. W., Trickett, P., Helmers, K., Dorn, L., & Everett, B. (1991). Cortisol abnormalities in sexually abused girls. Poster presented at the Annual Meeting of the American Psychiatric Association: Washington, D.C.

Rasmusson, A. M., Vythilingam, M., & Morgan, C. A. (2003). The Neuroendocrinology of posttraumatic stress disorder: New directions. *CNS spectrums*, 8(9), 651-667.

Resnick, H. S., Yehuda, R., Pitman, R. K., & Foy, D. W. (1995). Effect of previous trauma on acute plasma cortisol level following rape. *American Journal of Psychiatry*, 152, 1675-1677.

Sanchez-Lorente, S., Blasco-Ros, C., Coe, C. L., & Martinez, M. (2010). Recovery of immune control over herpes simplex virus type 1 in female victims of intimate partner violence. *Psychosomatic Medicine*, 72(1), 97-106.

Sapolsky, R. M. (2000). Stress hormones: Good and bad. *Neurobiology of Disease*, 7(5), 540-542.

Sapolsky, R. M., Romero, L. M., & Munck, A. U. (2000). How do glucocorticoids influence stress responses? Integrating permissive, suppressive, stimulatory and preparative actions. *Endocrine Reviews*, 21(1), 55-89.

Sciolla, A., Glover, D. A., Loeb, T. B., Zhang, M., Myers, H. F., & Wyatt, G. E. (2011). Childhood sexual abuse severity and disclosure as predictors of depression among adult african-american and latina women. *Journal of Nervous and Mental Disease*, 199(7), 471-477.

Scott, K. M., Smith, D. R., & Ellis, P. M. (2010). Prospectively ascertained child maltreatment and its association with DSM-IV mental disorders in young adults. *Archives of General Psychiatry*, 67(7), 712-719.

Shields, N. M., & Hanneke, C. R. (1988). Multiple sexual victimization: The case of incest and marital rape. In G. T. Hotaling, D. Finkelhor, J. T. Kirkpatrick, & M. A. Straus (Eds.), *Family Abuse and Its Consequences: New Directions in Research* (255–269). Newbury Park, CA: Sage Publications.

Sorsoli, L., Kia-Keating, M., & Grossman, F.K. (2008). "I keep that hush-hush": Male survivors of sexual abuse and the challenges of disclosure. *Journal of Counseling Psychology*, 55(3), 333-345.

Stein, M. B., Walker, J. R., Hazen, A. L., & Forde, D. R. (1997). Full and partial posttraumatic stress disorder: Findings from a community survey. *American Journal of Psychiatry*, 154, 1114-1119.

Swanston, H. Y., Parkinson, P. N., Oates, R. K., O'Toole, B. I., Plunkett, A. M., & Shrimpton, S. (2002). Further abuse of sexually abused children. *Child Abuse and Neglect*, 26, 115-127.

Taylor, S. E., Klein, L.C., Lewis, B. P., Gruenewald, T. L., Gurung, R. A., & Updegraff, J. A. (2000). Biobehavioral responses to stress in females: Tend-and-befriend, not fight-or-flight. *Psychological Review*, 107, 411-429.

Teicher, M. H., Tomoda, A., & Andersen, S. L. (2006). Neurobiological consequences of early stress and childhood maltreatment: Are results from human and animal studies comparable? *Annals of the New York Academy of Sciences*, 1071(1), 313-323.

Trickett, P. K., Noll, J. G., Susman, E. J., Shenk, C. E., & Putnam, F. W. (2010). Attenuation of cortisol across development for victims of sexual abuse. *Development & Psychopathology*, 22(1), 165-175.

Turner-Cobb, J. M. (2005). Psychological and stress hormone correlates in early life: A key to HPA-axis dysregulation and normalisation. *Stress: The International Journal on the Biology of Stress*, 8(1), 47-57.

Urquiza, A. J., & Goodlin-Jones, B. L. (1994). Child sexual abuse and adult revictimization with women of color. *Violence and Victims*, 9, 223-232.

van den Burg, E. H., & Neumann, I. D. (2011). Bridging the gap between GPCR activation and behaviour: Oxytocin and prolactin signalling in the hypothalamus. *Journal of Molecular Neuroscience*, 43, 200–208.

Vythilingam, M., Heim, C., Newport, J., Miller, A. H., Anderson, E., Bronen, R., ... Bremner, J. D. (2002). Childhood trauma associated with smaller hippocampal volume in women with major depression. *American Journal of Psychiatry*, 159(12), 2072-2080.

Weems, C. F., & Carrion, V. G. (2007). The association between PTSD symptoms and salivary cortisol in youth: The role of time since the trauma. *Journal of Traumatic Stress*, 20(5), 903-907.

Wegman, H. L., & Stetler, C. (2009). Meta-analytic review of the effects of childhood abuse on medical outcomes in adulthood. *Psychosomatic Medicine*, 71, 805-812.

West, C. M., Williams, L. M., & Siegel, J. A. (2000). Adult sexual revictimization among Black women sexually abused in childhood: A prospective examination of serious consequences of abuse. *Child Maltreatment*, 5, 49-57.

Whiffen, V. E., & MacIntosh, H. B. (2005). Mediators of the link between childhood sexual abuse and emotional distress. *Trauma, Violence, & Abuse*, 6(1), 24-39.

Wise, L. A., Palmer, J. R., Rothman, E. F., & Rosenberg, L. (2009). Childhood abuse and early menarche: Findings from the Black Women's Health Study. *American Journal of Public Health*, 99(S2), S460-466.

Wyatt, G. E., Guthrie, D., & Notgrass, C. M. (1992). Differential effects of women's child sexual abuse and subsequent sexual revictimization. *Journal of Consulting and Clinical Psychology*, 60, 167–173.

Wyatt, G. E., Loeb, T. B., Solis, B., Carmona, J. V., & Romero, G. (1999). The prevalence and circumstances of child sexual abuse: Changes across a decade. *Child Abuse & Neglect*, 23(1), 45-60.

Yehuda, R., Southwick, S. M., Nussbaum, G., Waahby, V., Giller, E. L., & Mason, J. W. (1990). Low urinary cortisol excretion in patients with post-traumatic stress disorder. *Journal of Nervous and Mental Disorders*, 178, 366-369.

7

Risk Factors in Sexually Abused Children Reporting to the One Stop Centre at University Teaching Hospital in Zambia

Elwyn Chomba
University of Zambia, University Teaching Hospital
Zambia

1. Introduction

1.1 Definition of Child Sexual Abuse

Child sexual abuse (CSA) is the involvement of a child in sexual activity that he or she does not fully comprehend, is unable to give informed consent to, or for which the child is not developmentally prepared and cannot give consent, or that violate the laws or social taboos of society (Faller 1988,Kempe 1978, Sedlak & Broadhurst 1996, Sgroi 1988).

CSA is evidenced by an activity between a child and an adult or another child who by age or development is in a relationship of responsibility, trust or power, the activity being intended to gratify or satisfy the needs of the other person(Kempe 1978, Sgroi 1988). The sexual act can be divided into penetrative and non-penetrative and this may include but is not limited to the following;

Child sexual abuse includes:

- Actual or attempted penetrative sexual intercourse or oral sex with a child.
- Non-penetrative sexual activity, e.g. rubbing the penis between the child's thighs or genitals;
- Fondling of a child's sexual parts, i.e. genitals, breasts, buttocks, etc.;
- Masturbation between adult and child;
- Displaying or exposing a person's genitals to a child (exhibitionism);
- The exploitative use of a child in prostitution or any other unlawful sexual practice;
- The exploitative use of children in pornography;
- Forced early marriages;
- Peeping on a child when he or she is bathing or undressed for the purpose of sexual gratification;
- The inducement or coercion of a child to engage in any unlawful sexual activity
- The exploitative use of a child in prostitution or other unlawful sexual practices
- The exploitative use of children in pornograpghic performances and materials (WHO 1999)

1.2 Other definition of sexual abuse

- RAPE happens when a person has sex that he or she did not agree to. It includes intercourse in the vagina, anus or mouth. Sometimes it happens when aone person forces another to have sex. Rape can happen to men and women.
- STATUTORY RAPE is sexual intercourse with a girl under the age set down by the law (16 years for girls and 14 for boys in Zambia) with his/her consent.
- INCEST means the performance of any sexual act between persons who are forbidden by law to marry because they are family members. It applies not only to biological family members, but also to sexual acts between stepparents and stepchildren or adopted children and their parents.
- FELATIO is penal satisfaction by licking or sucking with the mouth and tongue (oral sex).
- SODOMY is anal sexual intercourse
- INDECENT ASSAULT is assault involving the sexual organs. It includes such actions as forced oral or anal sex, fondling, and attempted rape such actions as forced oral or anal sex, fondling, and attempted rape.

1.3 Risk factors in Child Sexual Abuse

CSA has been in existence since time immemorial. CSA occurs in all societies as well as all social structures. It has been difficult to quantify the magnitude of CSA grobally including Zambia as most cases go unreported. There are a number of factors that make children vulnerable to sexual abuse. The key determinants are:

- Increased number of orphans has a big impact on the increase of CSA.
    - Zambia has one of the largest numbers of AIDS orphans in the world. This is estimated to be a total of 1,100,000 orphan of which two thirds of these orphans are AIDS orphans (Central Statistics Office - Lusaka)
    - Orphans are taken into foster home or orphanages where it is not uncommon to be sexually abused. Some may be taken in by relatives or find themselves in child-headed homes and are often forced to trade sex for money, food or abused by their caretakers
- Female sex - The most common cases of CSA in Zambia are that of a girl child by an adult man or with a few between an adult woman with an under aged boy
- HIV pandemic resulting in loss of parent has children into prostitution
- Broken homes have been well documented in the United States as an important risk factor for child sexual victimization. In Zambia, loss of one parent has resulted in increase of repoted cases of CSA.
- Children whose parents suffer from mental illness or drug dependency have an increased risk of being sexually abused.
- War/ armed conflicts: Sexual abuse has been reported to be rampant communities engaged in wars and armed conflicts. Zambia is surrounded by neighbours who have had armed conflicts and resulting in setting up of these camps within the Zambian borders.
- Children who are mentally impaired are more likely to be sexually and the abuse not be detected until the child presents with pregnancy.

CSA is not limited to the categories itemized above. It happens in any forum or society. It exists amongst the rich and the poor, the highly educated people and the illiterates.

1.4 Definition of a child

There are multiple definitions of a child in the Zambian laws and these create disparities in interpretation. In the context of One Stop Centre (OSC) children are defined as those aged 16 years and below in keeping with the medical definition at the University Teaching Hospital (UTH).

1.5 Prevalence of Child Sexual Abuse in Zambia

Zambia is a country in sub-Saharan Africa where the problem of CSA is compounded by HIV prevalence of 19.7 % in urban adults compared 10.3% in rural adults ($p<0.00001$)(ZHDS 2007). There are no studies on the prevalence of CSA in Zambia. The OSC was established specifically to offer post exposure HIV prophylaxis to children sexually abused.

Lusaka is the capital of Zambia with a population of close to 2 million (ZHDS 2007).

UTH houses the only medical school in the country and the schools of Registered Nurses and Midwifery. The paediatric department is the busiest deparment within the UTH catering mainly for management of the aqcutely ill. Most of the children before the establishment of the OSC were cared for at the department of obsterics and gynaecology. Though there is significant emphasis on prevention of mother to child HIV transmission in Zambia, HIV transmission through CSA had been a neglected issue. The contribution of CSA to the HIV pandemic remains unknown. However, the impact of HIV on children has been evaluated.

Children have been much affected by the HIV/AIDS epidemic in Zambia, where over 30,000 children are HIV positive (UNAIDS Report 2007). Perinatal transmission accounts for the majority of pediatric HIV infections where HIV prevalence is high. However, sexual exposure remains an important risk factor in children in the post-weaning period. While HIV transmission rates attributable to sexual abuse are unknown, pediatric victims of sexual abuse are at a higher risk of HIV transmission due to physical trauma and due to the fact that multiple exposures often occur prior to discovery of the abuse (Lindegren ML et al 1998).

In a pilot study conducted at the UTH in 2003, 99% of sexually abused children reporting to the gynecology ward were female, which also placed them at a higher risk for HIV acquisition (Chomba et al 2006).

Although epidemiologic data for the prevalence of child sexual abuse (CSA) in Zambia is not available (Collings 2002), recent establishment of one stop centres will help in providing some information on factors associated with child sexual abuse thus help to unravel the extent of the problem.

Literature from countries surrounding Zambia documents the existence of a CSA epidemic in the region. Prevalence studies rely on cross-sectional study design, most often surveying school children about their experiences of sexual abuse. In a review article of child sexual abuse in sub-Saharan Africa, Lalor et.al. report that between 3.2 and 7.1% of all respondents report unwanted or forced sexual intercourse before the age of 18 years (Lalor 2004). Jewkes et al. surveyed 11, 735 South African women between the ages of 15 and 49 years about their history of rape during childhood. Overall, 1.6% reported unwanted sexual intercourse before the age of 15 years of age. 85% of child rape occurred between the age of 10 and 14 years and 15% between the ages of 5 and 9 years (Jewkes, Levin et al. 2002). In a study in Zimbabwe, Birdthistle reports that among unmarried, sexual active adolescents, 52.2% had experienced forced intercourse at least one time. 37.4% of first sexual intercourse acts were forced (Birdthistle IJ 2008). In a study of 487 university students in Tanzania, 11.2% of women and 8.2% of men reported unwanted sexual intercourse. The average age at the time of abuse was 13.6 years (McCrann D 2006). Collings et al (Collings 2002) surveyed a sample of 640 female university students in South Africa and found that 34.8% had experienced contact sexual abuse before the age of 18 years. Another study among high school students in South Africa (Nadu 2002), found that almost 20% were victims of parental or guardian sexual abuse. Additional research suggests that the prevalence of child sexual abuse in sub-Saharan Africa is similar to other countries across the world (Lalor 2004).

2. Rationale

In the era of HIV infection with the highest mortalities in the sub-Saharan region documenting the characteristics of children who are at risk of being sexually abused is an important strategy to reduce horizontal transmission of HIV in children.

The current preventative strategies for children from acquiring HIV are enveloped in the Prevention of Mother to Child Transmission (PMTCT) and there are no studies in Zambia to characterise risk factors on children who may be sexually abused nor strategies to prevent HIV acquisition in these vulnerable children as far as we are aware.

In a survey by Mathews et al (Mathews et al, 2011) of girls aged between 13 -24 years, respondents who lived in a rural environment were significantly less likely than those in an urban environment to report having experienced sexual violence before the age of 18. Compared with respondents who had been close to their biological mothers as children, those who had not been close to her had higher odds of having experienced sexual violence, as did those who had had no relationship with her at all.

In the second quarter of 2003, Zambian police handled 300 cases of child rape and some experts believe that for every case reported another 10 go unreported. (Agence France-Presse 2003). The number of reported cases and the realization that these cases were likely to be the tip of iceberg, in combination with high HIV prevalence led to the identification of the need to establish a comprehensive multidisciplinary centre to train health workers in the recognition of CSA, to increase public awareness of CSA, to improve management of sexually abused children with an emphasis on preventing HIV acquisition and document the characteristics and risk factors of sexually abused children.

3. Objective

The aim is to identify risk factors of child sexual abuse in children reporting to the OSC and propose possible interventions. Currently the OSC is offering PEP to children who are at risk of contracting HIV through sexual abuse. Other services offered include;

- psychosocial counseling,
- treatment of sexually transmitted infections (STIs.)
- Emergency contraceptives
- Evaluation of Post Traumatic Stress Disorders
- Referral to HIV Clinic for HIV positive children (PTSD)

4. Methodology

In most western countries Child Advocacy Centers (CACs) are not located within medical institutions and offer a more comprehensive package to include physical abuse as well as child neglect (Downing 2002, Hansen 1998). We chose to establish the multidisciplinary centre within the pediatric department because most the sexually abused children came to the attention of the health workers because of medical complications (Chomba,Kasese-Bota Haworth, Fuller, Amaya, 2006) and in order to offer PEP to abused children, which was only available at the UTH. The centre would not provide services for isolated physical abuse cases nor neglected children.

The One Stop Centre was established in the pediatric department on 26th April 2006. A location was selected where there was minimal foot traffic, and there are no conspicuous notices indicating its function to help preserve the confidentiality of the children and their guardians attending the center. The Centre included a physical examination room and several interview rooms including one with a two way mirror, microphone and speakers which allows one person to interview (usually a medical person) whilst the police officers and counsellors take notes from another room. The centre is equipped with comfortable child-friendly waiting facilities (TV set, toys and educational materials).

The Centre has employed one medical doctor who oversees medical examinations and attends to court cases, one clinical officer who performs physical examinations; one police officer who documents on police medical forms and ensures that they are delivered to the prosecutors; one social worker who follows up children in the community and advises on rehabilitation; and three nurses who assist the physician and the clinical officer.

Intake interviews are conducted with the caregiver and child separately (if the child is able). Information on demographic characteristics and abuse history is collected. A medical/laboratory form includes the following tests: HIV, RPR, pregnancy, Hepatitis B and forensic specimens (High vaginal swab for wet prep, gram stain and culture to identify gonorrhoea, trichomonas, and spermatozoa).

Mental health assessments for the youth include the Post-traumatic stress disorder - Reaction Index, the Strengths and Difficulties Questionnaire, and My Feelings About the Abuse. This last measure specifically examines the construct of shame, which is considered to be critical in the Zambian culture. The mental health assessment administered to the caregivers about the abused child is the Child Behaviour Checklist.

A systematic flow has been designed to promote excellence in the care of sexually abused youth.

1. Family register at UTH main desk and receives a treatment form
2. Once the family has both forms, they are directed to the centre where they are greeted by the social worker and/or nurses. Youth and their care-givers are immediately asked if the abuse happened within the last 72 hours.

a. If abuse occurred within 72 hours, the child is immediately brought to a nurse to take the necessary blood tests, and administer PEP if appropriate. After blood tests and PEP administration, the intake forms and the questionnaire for assessment of level of trauma are completed by the nurse or social worker. A physical exam is completed and the UTH treatment form and police medical forms are completed.
b. If abuse did NOT occur within 72 hours, the child/care-giver is interviewed by one of the staff , blood tests are performed, a physical exam of the child is conducted and the forms are completed as well as the police medical form are completed (The police officer stationed at the centre completes the relevant potion of the form.
c. If a child is HIV positive, they are referred to the Paediatric Antiretroviral Therapy (ART) Clinic for further management and follow up.
d. If a child is found to be pregnant, she is referred to the Antenatal and/or Prevention of Mother to Child HIV Transmission (PMTCT) clinic.
e. If abuse did NOT occur within 72 hours, the child/care-giver is interviewed by one of the staff, blood tests are performed.

Drugs used for PEP were Zidovudine 240mgs/m^2 in combination with Lamivudine 4mg/kg (Combivir) twice daily for 28 days. No syrups were available initially leaving the very young children without any PEP options until later when syrup formulations were made available. Initially, a two drug regimen was recommended as effective (WHO, Geneva Report 2006) though currently a 3 drug regimen is in place in accordance with current guidelines

5. Results

For the purposes of this chapter, data for 2010 was analysed. A total of 1068 children were seen during this period.

Of the total 1068 children , most of the abused children were girls 1042 (97.6%),boys 46 (2.4%) were boys. Those most likely to be abused were aged between 0-5 years 246 (23%), 6-10 years 223 (20.9%) and 11 and 16 599 (56.1%) (Table 1).

	Frequency	Percent
Age		
0-5 Years	246	23.0
6-10 Years	223	20.9
11-16 Years	599	56.1
Total	1068	100.0
Sex		
F	1042	97.6
M	26	2.4
	1068	100.0

Table 1. Age and Sex Distribution

Of the 1068 children who reported to the centre only 628 (59%) had complete data consistent with the analysis.

Most of the abusers are non relative adults known to the child (66.4%). Strangers accounted for only 7% (Table 2) (Figure 1)

	Frequency	Percent
Father	18	2.9
Known Adult (Neighbor, teacher)	417	66.4
Stranger	44	7.0
Multiple people at the same time	5	.8
Grandfather	4	.6
Auntie	1	.2
Uncle	33	5.3
Cousin	13	2.1
Sibling	11	1.8
Don't know	82	13.1
Total	628	100.0

Table 2. Who is the Abuser?

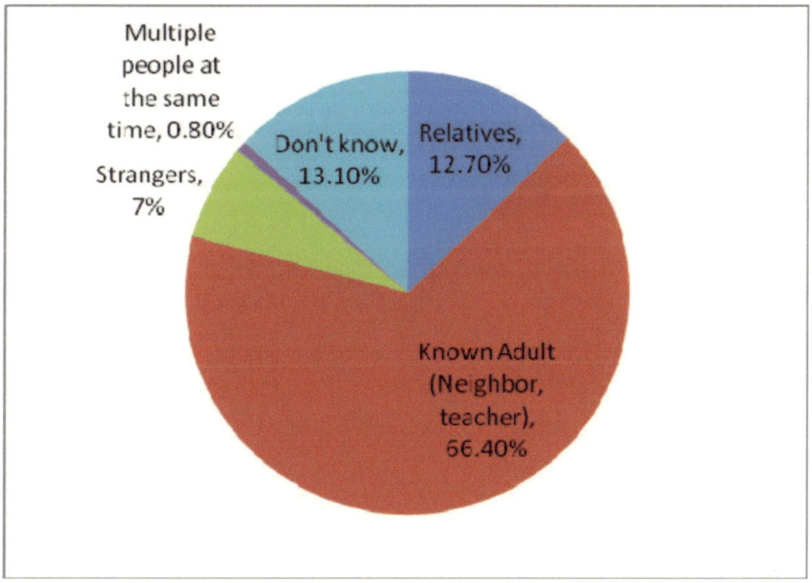

Fig. 1. Summary of Abuser Information

26.6% of these children were reported to be orphans (Table 3)

Is this child an Orphan	Frequency	Percent
No	461	73.4
Yes	167	26.6
Total	628	100

Table 3. Number of Orphans

15.6% reported that the were living in the same household as the abuser during the time of the abuse. About 24% of the children in contact with the abuser (Table 4).

	FREQUENCY	PERCENT
Did abuser live in the child's household during the abuse?		
No	508	80.9
Yes	98	15.6
Don't Know	22	3.5
Total	628	100.0
Since the abuse had been disclosed, does the child has any contact with the abuser?		
No	480	76.4
Yes, seen around	140	22.3
Yes, unsupervised contact	3	.5
Yes, in court, VSU,police	4	.6
Total	627	99.8
999	1	.2
Total	628	100.0

Table 4. Abuser location and Contact with child

Of the 628 children reporting to the centre 86% were referred by the police. Most of the children reporting within 72hrs of abuse at the OSC were given PEP (Table 5).

	Frequency	Percent
Who referred you to the clinic?		
Medical facility/doctor	55	8.8
Police	540	86.0
Parent/caregiver/relative	20	3.2
Friend	3	.5
VSU	7	1.1
Total	625	99.5
Other	3	.5
Abuse Reporting Time		
No	245	39.0
Yes	353	56.2
Don't know	30	4.8
Total	628	100.0
PEP Administration		
No	6	1.7
Yes	347	98.3
Total	353	100.0

Table 5. Refferal, Reporting Time and PEP Adminstration of CSA victims

At the OSC physical force was used in about 20% of the victims of CSA, 23.7% playful/gentle coaxing was applied. 52% had no presenting complaints and 28.2% had genital pain. (Table 6)

	Frequency	Percent
How Did The Abuser Engage The Child?		
Don't know	122	19.4
Playful/gentle coaxing	149	23.7
Bribes	91	14.5
Commands/instructions	8	1.3
Verbal threats	21	3.3
Physical threats	98	15.6
Physical force	125	19.9
offering alcohol	4	.6
Other	10	1.6
What is the presenting complaint?		
None	329	52.4
Genital Pain	177	28.2
Abdominal Pain	48	7.6
Discharge	9	1.4
Bleeding	5	.8
Genital itching	5	.8
Bruising	1	.2
Behavior change	8	1.3
Other	46	7.3

Table 6. Methods used to engage the child and presenting signs and symptoms

6. Discussion

Child sexual abuse in the sub-saharan region is a risk factor to the acquisition of HIV infection (Dunkle 2006, UNICEF 2001, WHO 2006). Risk factors to child sexual abuse are evaluated in this chapter to help guide health workers, psychosocial counsellors, organisations and other professionals tasked in the protection of children to help manage sexually abused children. Planning strategies to mitigate against child sexual abuse requires understanding risk factors associated with CSA.

The female child was by far more likely to be abused. Other studies in the sub-Saharan region have reported similar findings (Birdthistle et al2009, Mathew et al 2011). Zambia has one of the highest HIV prevalence rates 14% (Zambia NAC 2009) and females aged between 15-19 are more likely to be HIV infected 16% as compared to their male counterparts 10%

(Zambia NAC 2009). These high rates amongst females may suggest that CSA may be putting females at higher risk of HIV acquisition.

There is a high proportion of children aged below 10 reporting to the OSC and 23% of these are aged below 5 years. In Zambia, the school enrolment is between 6 to 7 years for the first grade suggesting that about 20% of the children are being abused right in the home. The statistics also show that 66% of the abusers were non-relative adults (neighbours, teachers, etc). Only 7% was attributed to strangers. This finding explains the absence of clinical presenting complaints and lack of pathological findings on examination inspite of the history of physical force having been used in 20% of those who were sexually abused. This could be attributed to delayed in reporting to the OSC allowing for healing which occurs rapidly in children. However in a review of CSA literature done by Pitche (Pitche 2005), though 30-60% abusers were known to the child, 97% of cases had penetrative sex resulting in injuries. However this study was retrospective.

Among the 628 children seen, 56.2% reported within the 72hrs required leaving a large number of children who did not qualify for PEP. This also has been shown in several studies (Birdthistle et al, Bablet al 2000, Chesshyre et al 2009,Speight et al 2006) that PEP as a strategy for preventing HIV acquisition has not been very successful. This may be due to the fact that the very nature of the abuse being committed by some trusted adult or on who the child depends on for upkeep becomes the abuser. This may lead to delays in reporting to health authorities as opposed to when the abuser is a stranger.

In Zambia a large number of children are orphans. One estimate is that 1.656 million children, or more than one-third of those under the age of 15, are orphans who have lost one or both parents (Kelly 2000). Of the 628 children who had complete data 26.6% were orphans.In another study (Birdthistle 2009) 30.1% reporting to a the facility were orphans. This puts this group of children at high risk of sexual abuse.They more likely to be greatly economically disadvanted and lack adult protection from abuse.

Though the OSC set-out to screen for syphilis which is known to increase HIV aquisition (Dunkle et al 2006, Pitche 2005) most children did not have this labortatory test done due to the shortage of re-agents. Hepatitis B similarly was not performed consistently for us to evaluate the prevalence of this in these children.

7. Conclusion

Child sexual abuse is prevalent in Lusaka.The female child is by far the most vulnerable and there needs to urgent policy and support for prevention of CSA for this vulnerable group. Communities need to be sensitised on the dangers of CSA as numbers reporting to the OSC are the tip of the iceberg. The 23% of children abused aged 0-5 years pose a great challenge as this is a helpless vulnerable group when abuse is occurring within the home.Understanding family dynamic should be part of the prevention strategy of CSA. There needs to be more resources and better tools for collection of data to better unravel risk factors associated with sexual abuse.

8. Limitations

The data was not obtained in a research setting but in a clinic setting where the workers are busy with managing acute cases. Lack of adequate human and material resources led to incomplete data collection. The results cannot be extrapolated to the rest country as they were collected from children living in Lusaka an urban area where about 20% of the population lives.

9. Acknowledgment

We acknowledge the courage of the young children and their caregivers who came to University Teaching Hospital One Stop Centre.

I would like to thank the Centre for Disease Control and Prevention (CDC) Zambia for funding the establishment of the One Stop Centre at UTH. Also I would like to thank the following people for their efforts in the collection and gathering of information that was used for this chapter:

Mr. Elson Chama
Mr. Katai Chola
Ms. Mafunase Mako

Special thanks are also extended to:

Dr. Lackson Kasonka Managing Director UTH, Dr. Chipepo Kankasa Director Paediatric Centre of Excellence, Dr. Jonathan Mwansa Paediatrician, Mr. Kabanda Sampa OSC Clinic Coordinator and all the OSC Staff.

10. References

Agence France-Press 2003, Sexual Abuse of young girls rife in Zambia 29th September 2003

Babl FE, Cooper ER, Damon B, Louie T, Kharasch S, Harris JA. HIV postexposure prophylaxis for children and adolecents. Am J Emerg Med. 2000 May;18 (3) 282-7

Birdthistle IJ, F. S., Machingura A, Mudziwapasi N, Gregson S, Glynn JR. (2008). "From affected to infected? Orphanhood and HIV risk among female adolescents in urban Zimbabwe." AIDS 22: 750-766.

Birdthistle I.J. , Floyd S., Mwanasa S., Nyagadza A., Gwiza E, Glynn J. Child sexual abuse and links to HIV and orphanhood in urban Zimbabwe. J Epidemiol Community Health *doi:10.1136/jech.2009.094359*

Chesshyre EL, Molyneux EM. Presentation of child sexual abuse cases to Queen Elizabeth Central Hospital following the establishment of an HIV post-exposure prophylaxis programme. Malawi Med J. 2009 Jun;21(2):54-8.

Chomba E, Kasese Bota M, Haworth A, Fuller B, Amaya M. Circumstances of child abuse in a cohort of children eligible to receive post-exposure prophylaxis at the University of Zambia Teaching Hospital: a descriptive study. International AIDS Conference August 2006 http://www.futuredirections.org/Abstracts/A2197011.aspx retrieved on 19th July 2011

Collings, S. J. 2002. The prevalence and characteristics of child sexual abuse among South African University Students: Comments on S. N. Madu. South African Journal of Psycology, 32(3), 62-63

Downing M, Once is Enough; A Unique Sex Abuse Centre Ensures that Tender Young Lives Aren't Torn Apart by the System, Huston Press March 16, 2000.

Dunkle KL, Jewkes RK, Nduna M, *et al* Perpetration of partner violence and HIV risk behaviour among young men in the rural Eastern Cape, South Africa. AIDS2006;20:2107–14.

Faller,K. C. (1988). *Child Sexual Abuse: An interdisciplinary manual for diagnosis, case management and treatment*. New York : Columbia Univeristy Press

Government Republic of Zambia (2010,April) Zambia Country Report: Monitoring the Declaration of Commitment on HIV and AIDs and the Universal Access Biennial Report http://www.unaids.org/en/CountryResponses/Countries/zambia.asp Website Retrieved on 15th May 2010

Jewkes, R., J. Levin, et al. (2002). "Rape of girls in South Africa." Lancet 359(9303): 319-20.

Kelly M.J., S.J. School of Education University of Zambia, The Orphan Crisis in Zambia, http://www.jctr.org.zm/bulletins/orphan_crisis.htm Accessed on 19th July 2011

Kempe, C. H. (1978). Sexual abuse, another hidden paediatric problem. The 1977 C. Anderson Aldrich Lecture. Peadiatircs,62,382-389

Lalor, K. Child Sexual Abuse in sub-Saharan Africa: a literature review. Child Abuse and Neglect 28 (2004); 439-460

Lindegren ML, Hanson IC, Hammett TA, et al. Sexual Abuse of Children: Intersection with the HIV Epidemic. Pediatrics 1998: 102: e46).

Matthew J Breiding , Avid Reza , Jama Gulaid , Curtis Blanton , James A Mercy , Linda L Dahlberg, Nonhlanhla Dlamini & Sapna Bamrah. Risk factors associated with sexual violence towards girls in Swaziland Bulletin of the World Health Organization 2011;89:203-210. doi: 10.2471/BLT.10.079608

McCrann D, L. K., Katabaro JK. (2006). "Childhood sexual abuse among university students in Tanzania." Child Abuse Negl 30: 1343-1351.

Nadu S.M. (2002). The relationship between perceived parental physical availability and child sexual, physical and emotional abuse among highschool students in the Northern Province, South Africa. Social Science Journal, 39 (4), 639-745.

National HIV/AIDS/STI/TB Council. Zambia HIV Prevention Response and Modes of Transmission Analysis Report June 2009

Pitche P. Child sexual abuse and sexually transmitted infections in sub-saharan Africa. Med Trop (Mars). 2005 Nov;65(6):570-4

Sedlak, A. J. & Broadhurst D. D. (1996). Third National Incidence oStudy of Child Abuse and Neglect (NIS-3 final report, Contract#105-94-1840) Washington DC : US Department of Health and Human Services

Sgroi, S. M. (1982) Handbook of clinical intervention in child sexual abuse. Lexington MA : Lexington Books

Speight CG, Klufio A, Kilonzo SN, Mbugua C, Kuria E, Bunn JE, Taegtmeyer MPiloting post-exposure prophylaxis in Kenya raises specific concerns for the management of childhood rape. Trans R Soc Trop Med Hyg. 2006 Jan;100(1):14-8. Epub 2005 Oct 12.

UNICEF Analysis of the situation of sexual exploitation of children in the Eastern and Southern Africa region. 2001.

WHO. Clinical Management of Sexual Abuse Survivors By World Health Organization, Geneva. Reproductive Health and Research UNHCR- Health and Community Development Section 1999 www.The-ecentre.net/toolkit/Health/HTP-8pdf retrived on 19th July 2011

WHO. Preventing child maltreatment: a guide to taking action and generating evidence. In: *WHO-ISPCAN*, ed. Geneva, 2006
Zambia Health Demographics Survey 2007

8

How Do We Recognize Recent Sexual Abuse in Children Less than 10 Years of Age? What Is the Role of Paediatric Wards? Experience in a French Paediatric Hospital

G. Picherot, N. Vabres, J. Fleury, E. Launay and C. Gras-Leguen
Clinique Médicale Pédiatrique, UAED,
CHU Nantes,
France

1. Introduction

A diagnosis of sexual abuse in children is being made increasingly in France and in all Western countries. Sexual abuses in France represent a third of all cases of maltreatment [1]. In children less than 10 years of age, discovery of the circumstances varies according to the situations experienced by the adolescents. Stories can involve silence or a revelation by indirect signs or consequences of abuses. To approach this diagnosis, we will successively address three aspects: the usual circumstances of the revelation or evocation of this diagnosis, a speech and behavioral side, and a clinical examination and its difficulties.

2. Circumstances

Generally, children under the age of 10 years are brought by their parents, and come more rarely with a social worker or forensic expertise.

A child's speech or a sudden change in behavior could disturb the relatives [2]. The diagnosis can be done in an environmental context of sexual assault: the revelation of a sibling or the child himself. It sometimes involves an investigation around an abuser or abnormal behavior of parents [2-3-4-5].

The evocation in less than three years old chidren may revolve around a child-minder, represented by doubt concerning behavioral or clinical abnormalities after returning home following a child-minding period, or more frequently, a situation evoking suspicion in the context of parental separation [6].

The diagnosis can be sought in circumstances of clinical abnormalities discovered by the parents or physician, as represented by suspicious perineal lesions or the consequences of sexual assault such as sexually transmitted disease atypical for the child's age [5].

The American Academy of Pediatrics established several factors which may lead to suspicion of sexual assault in children [7]:

1. Declaration of the victim or witness (sibling, friend)
2. Questions for the family who suspects abuse
3. Discovery of direct or indirect suspect signs during a routine examination
4. Review requested by judicial authorities

In all cases, the evocation depends on the vigilance of the physician who receives the child [1]. Process of protection is possible if the child can be "heard" in those circumstances [7].

3. The words and silent stories

The interpretation of a word depends on the development and age of the child. The language of a child is structured between the ages of 4 and 6 years [8].

However, it is informative and based on cognitive and language development despite the age. "A young child of two years may report sexual abuse directly and clearly" [9]. The words are simple and correlated to the possibilities of the child. They sometimes refer to the act of aggression, and sometimes to the pain and consequent anxiety. They are called in special circumstances of personal hygiene, diaper or clothes changing, and sometimes during a clinical examination for instance when the child shows the assaulted area.

It is often a story without words, indirect consequences on the child's behavior may suggest the diagnosis. The subjective perception of one parent or the environment will lead to a discussion on recent changes. Many signs have been described as true indices [6], and often reflect the impact of recent trauma [9]:

- Fear: restlessness, irritability, insomnia, nightmares, screaming in front of a similar situation, feeling insecure
- regressive signs: refusal of parental separation, loss of developmental acquisitions
- painful reminders: refusal to change, to review
- somatic expressions: abdominal pain, anorexia, difficulty in swallowing
- indirect expressions of genital and perineal trauma: regression of cleanliness, appearance, constipation or faecal incontinence, voiding dysfunction revealed by urinary tract infections, sometimes up to Hinman syndrome or severe bladder dysfunction. [10]
- sexually transmitted diseases in spite of age will be discussed in terms of a clinical examination
- sexualized behavior: compulsive masturbation, precocious sex play or sexualized gestures of the child on the adult or another child
- unusual or even aggressive behavior with people nearby

If the child speaks or if its behavioral consequences reveals an history of abuse, its interpretation requests a rigorous approach [2-12-7].

The first adult who received the confidence should look for an experienced professional within 2-3 days after the revelation.

There is no way for the physician to bring together suspected children and adults, even to observe the reactions of the child.

The collection of the child's speech must be done with consideration to avoid leading questions at any age as the predictive value of words is not related to age [12].

Professionals must link the interpretation of a child's speech with its emotional and cognitive development and remember that memory for detail is unstable. The perception of time is more revealing than a chronological relation of facts as many temporal expressions have no meaning for younger children [11]. Emotional factors are also significant: the child's fear related to unsuitable for any age experiences may inhibit expression.

Early sexualized behaviors of children are not in themselves proof of aggression. Within three years there may be "periods of intense masturbation" without a past sexual assault as sexual curiosity in young children is widespread [5].

Strategies for assessing the validity of the statements described by Yuille are hardly applicable in younger children [13].

At this age, repeted situations of interrogation lead to an even greater possibility for misinterpretation and this is an important argument for filmed audition strategies [5]. None of these signs as a consequence of trauma is *a priori* indicative of sexual assault, and only their association to the context will lead to the diagnosis.

The circumstances of abuse would lead to a discernment of different disorders of the child by its family. Extrafamilial abuse may lead to earlier recognition of changes in the child.

Situations of alleged sexual assault in connection with parental separation are increasingly frequent. The interpretation of anxious behavior after a weekend at the ex-spouse's home, or confusion with necessary care and intimate assaults may lead to repeated investigations and traumatic experiences. This is also the case in the same situations of actual sexual assault [1-5-7].

There is no way to support an instrumental evaluation.[14] The use of sexed dolls is very controversial: the method is not recommended in the assessment of Yuille [13], and is to be used with great caution and interpretation by experts as reported by August [15]. The child can use ordinary toys (Bear, Figurines) to stage events or to describe the assaulted body parts. Older children may use drawings to express themselves. Among younger girls (less than 5 years of age), this method rarely leads to get a direct word or a specific behavioral sign, but "gives the child to see and hear something of grave concern," [16] and we must therefore raise the possibility of sexual assault.

4. Clinical examination

Clinical examination of a child in circumstances of sexual abuse is difficult for a child of any age. Its interpretation requires a skill that will avoid repetition of intolerable procedures [17]. Misinterpretations are common, particularly in young children.

The legal and social services eagerly await objective evidence of sexual assault. **However, this rarely leads to a review of the findings of abnormalities.**

The work of Heger et al. and their analysis with a rigorous methodology of 2384 records shows that an abused child and clinical abnormalities are found in only 4% of cases [3]. In 96% of cases, the diagnosis is based on the child's words and on the circumstances. Without denying the importance of a clinical examination, it must be considered in the course of the child's assessment as an important and sometimes significant element specific to this age, but rarely as a contributing factor.

Consultation, even on the basis of a court application, must be part of the caring process. The complete pediatric examination should resemble, as closely as possible, the usual consultations. Apart from the objective forensic aspect, it is also designed to detect a sexually transmitted disease and reassure the child and its family of the normality of the body as this participates in the repair process [1-2]. The review is integrated into the comprehensive pediatric examination and requires no sedation beyond exceptional cases of lesions requiring surgery.

The examination may be experienced by the child as a second attack if not conducted in a supportive manner: explanations are allways required. We must use language appropriate to the age of the child, and must ask the parents for the words they usually use to name the genitals [6].

The examination is performed at this age in the presence of a parent that is not suspected and another person (from the nursing team). In our experience, the physician should never examine the child alone. This fits into the general reception which will be discussed.

Instrumental help with a genital examination is discussed at this age: using a pediatric colposcope to improve the performance of the examination or consideration for some simple situations, including systematic use of a video colposcope for the discussion of lesions. The use of a catheter with balloon inflation for a better visualization of the hymen is unnecessary and traumatic at this age. Instrumental help requires expertise [3-18], and should be reserved for pubescent patients [20].

The urgency of the review is still under discussion. It is indisputable if the abuse was less than 72 hours ago. Between three and 15 days after the abuse, the examination must be made quickly. Beyond 15 days, the examination may be delayed [6-21].

J.A. Adams gives further indications of an emergency medical examination [20]:

- genital or anal pain or bleeding
- need for medical care or urgent intervention
- the child's particular concern about possible damage

The physical examination cannot be separated from the history of the child. The verbal responses or attitudes of the child during the examination must be carefully noted. Children sometimes give additional information during the examination of the genitals [1-2-20].

In practice, it is recommended that this review include apart from genital and anal examinations "a complete physical examination with emphasis on growth parameters and sexual development of children examined mucocutaneous rigorous, searching for traces of violence throughout the body and especially at the inner thighs and chest, as well as areas of support and restraint (neck, wrists, ankles) a review of the oral cavity in search of lesions dental and mucous membranes, as well as the tongue-an observation of child behavior during clinical examination" [1].

The clinical findings can be of three types:

- General clinical abnormalities
- Abnormal perineal genital or anal
- Sexually transmitted infections despite age or suspicious vulvitis (rarely specific apart from sexually transmitted infections)

General clinical abnormalities are traumatic signs in non genital areas reflecting physical abuse (hematoma shoulders, trace of restraint on the limbs, oral mucosa lesion, etc.).

Genital anomalies are looked at in a **girl** of that age in a supine position in the attitude of the so-called "frog" [6-20-22]. Children less than three years of age can also be considered sitting or lying on the lap of an accompanying individual [6]. There is no need to touch and it should be painless. The examiner should have precise notions about normal anatomical variations [6-20] as the large variations of aspects of the hymen before puberty to avoid errors [22].

Adams classifies the aspect of girls' genital into 4 categories [20-23]:

- variants of normal
- damage caused by other medical conditions
- injury uncertain
- more specific lesions

Fifty lesions or situations are thus classified.

Among the specific lesions, we find direct acute injury (laceration, bruises) or injuries related to the penetration (bruises, cuts, lacerations, and even destruction of the hymen). Scarring may have a high specificity (scarring of the posterior fourchette).

Good knowledge of the circumstances and clinical aspects of genital trauma of a girl can distinguish sexual assaults [24].

The genitals of **boys** are examined by simple inspection.

Anal anomalies are sought by examination in the supine or sometimes prone position [1-6-20]. They can be distinguished by examining the simple assault suspect fissure cracks associated with frequent constipation, and are always sagittal. The interpretation of anal dilatation is difficult. Instances of anal dilatation isolated to a degree greater than or equal to two centimeters are regarded by Adams as unspecific [20]. Warts also have a low specificity [1]. The practice of rectal examination or anuscopy is not recommended as routine. Anuscopy under suitable conditions can allow a rare staging of lesions.

Sexually transmitted infections must be sought and treated. They sometimes reveal elements of sexual abuse. Vaginal swabs and blood tests are sometimes informative, particularly if the abuse was less than 72 hours ago or if there is a local sign (flow). They are regarded under the same conditions as for other ages. The preparation of the child is necessary. The use of local analgesia for blood sampling is required.

The analysis of sexually transmitted infections depends on the age of the child.

The transmission of certain germs may be perinatal.

The presence of gonorrhea in the genital, anal, or oral region should be considered suspect after the neonatal period according to Adams [20]. Non-sexual transmission has been demonstrated beyond this period by other authors [6-25].

The diagnosis of syphilis should suggest sexual abuse outside of a maternal-fetal transmission.

The presence of *Trichomonas vaginalis* (6 months) or *Chlamydia trachomatis* (after three years) is also very suspicious [1-6-20].

HIV transmission is theoretically possible, but exceptional with the waning of sexual abuse at that age. Maternal serology will eliminate maternal-fetal transmission [20].

Other transmissions are available: Papillomavirus, Herpes Hepatitis B, Hepatitis C, etc., but few are specific and are therefore of uncertain significance.

The sampling for forensic investigation involving the search for sperm, DNA identification, and a toxic syndrome (abuse under drug) is the subject of specific protocols for identification, storage, and transmission. Each country has determined these conditions, and hence they have a legal value.

Samples used to research sexually transmitted infections do not represent a consensus before puberty, and must be adapted to the circumstances:

- research of gonorrhea, *Chlamydia trachomatis, Trichomonas vaginalis* by culture and bacteriological examination
- indirect research techniques for chlamydia and gonorrhea by PCR have no forensic value and must be confirmed by bacteriological cultures [21]
- serology HIV, Syphilis, Hepatitis B, Hepatitis C, according to circumstances [20-21].(Figure 1)

Highly suggestive signs	Uncertain signs
Sexual contact shown by the presence of semen	Injury acute or scarring of the vulva does not reach the hymen
Hymen injury Acute: tear, bruise, abrasion Scarring: Total posterior tear (between 4 and 8 hours) Partial or total absence of hymen posterior notch or partial thinning of the posterior hymen	Notch or partial thinning of the posterior hymen
Lesion of the fourchette acute or healed	Anal dilatation
Important anal acute lesion or scar	Warts
STI Trichomonas after 6 month Chlamydiae after 3 years Syphilis (outside maternofoetal contamination) HIV (if seronegative mother)	Herpes simplex I and II

Fig. 1. Signs and those suggestive of uncertain significance [1-20-22]

Preventive treatment (Post Exposure Prophylaxis, PEP) is discussed at this age (pre-pubertal). There is no systematic chlamydia, trichomonas or syphilis, and assessment is based on laboratory diagnosis. HIV preventive treatment is evaluated according to the circumstances of the assault, and must be weighed against the disadvantages of treatment at this age. Serological surveillance in post-exposure is also tailored to the assessed risks [1-20-21].

The conditions of reception of the child victim of sexual assault are important.

They must be appropriate for the child's age during the entire process. The interview and examination should not repeat the trauma, and the permanent presence of a third adult caregiver is essential. Repeated examinations are unacceptable [1]. The review cannot be limited to the technical expertise of forensic aspects. The pediatric home team must be competent to collect details of history, examine the child, make a differential diagnosis with other causes of behavioral or clinical features, request additional tests, and send the certificates to ensure the appropriate care of the children [1-20].

In France, the passing of a law on 17 June, 1998 recognized the status of the victimized minor with enhanced rights, including assistance at hearings, filmed bond hearings, and the interests of health care professionals being represented at hearings. The association "Voice of Children" offered care to children affected by sexual abuse, and led to the assistance for "permanence and home units Multidisciplinary forensic child sexual assault victims" [26]. This "permanence" must improve the reception of minors. For the entire process of an initial investigation, the child is supported in one place suitable for children and is located in a pediatric hospital structure. In this structure, the child can be heard, admitted in cases of emergency if necessary, can receive treatment for pain if samples are needed under suitable conditions, and receive assessment on a psychological level. Psychological and social support of the child may be arranged with the relevant partner agencies. Management of these hotlines is conducted jointly by Social Services, the judicial services of Inquiry, Hospital Trust and the Regional Agency of Hospitalization, and advocacy groups for child victims (The Voice of the Child).

In Nantes, following the Prosecutor of the Republic's request, minors meet at first a pediatric nurse who explains the steps and accompanies the children and their families. Judicial investigators are invited to the hospital for a hearing filmed session under suitable and specific conditions. The medical team (pediatricians, gynecologists, psychiatrists and psychologists, including a social worker), conducts the initial medical and psychological assessments as requested. These reviews and assessments can be deferred after evaluation of the emergency level and safety of the child.

The nurse and social worker with the medical team organize an assessment of the psychological and social development of the child even if no judicial action results.

This new organization, dating back more than a decade, now covers more than 40 French hospitals. It has been, and remains, controversial. The main criticism is the concept of proximity Clinical (Pediatric ward) and Forensic (Justice) which could lead to a mixture of roles.

Our experience is very close to that of the CAC (Child Advocacy Center). The studies of Edinburgh [27] and Smith [28] focused on young adolescents, but included children of these structures as incorporated into pediatric hospitals. Their experience showed better results not only for the assessment of speech in a clinical approach, but also in relation to the advice given to children and their families. The organization of monitoring is also facilitated by this approach [27]. In accordance with the recommendation of Edinburgh, we incorporated a role for pediatric nurses with a long experience in childcare.

Tishelman confirms the value of an integrative model and justice for the pediatric care of affected children by setting 6 goals in these structures [29]:

- Evaluate specific forensic aspects
- Assess the overall health and psychological trauma of child victims
- Assess risk factors of abuse to prevent recurrence
- Evaluate opportunities for protection, therefore need to protect children by hospitalization
- Provide the child and its family psychological and social care
- Make recommendations to the social and legal services concerning the needs of the child and family

All this confirms the value of an integrated pediatric and forensic approach. This attitude is reinforced by the importance of physical and psychological consequences observed in adults who have suffered sexual assault in their childhood. Early care of the child within a pediatric approach should help to avoid such troubling developments [30]. Tishelman also speaks of a particular population of children whose judicial evaluation has not confirmed the sexual assault. Those children who leave without a judicial conclusion after a grueling investigation should also receive monitoring and care [29].

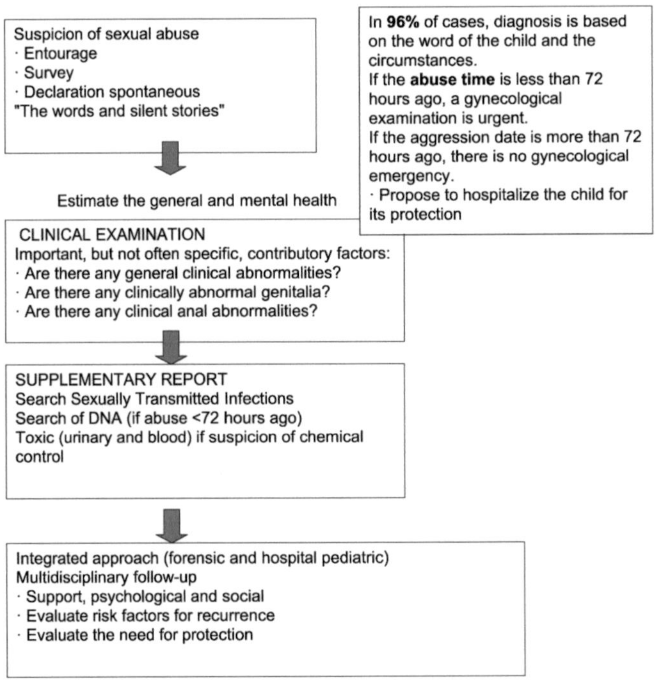

In conclusion, recognition of sexual abuse in children less than 10 years of age is based on the word of the child associated with indirect signs of a nonspecific nature. Clinical examination is essential, but it is difficult and rarely contributory. The forensic approach must be combined with an approach incorporating pediatric care and protection. The development of integrated units in forensic pediatric service for the reception of the whole child seems to us an essential change that will improve the entire process and prevent sequelae.

5. References

[1] Repérage et signalement de l'inceste par les médecins :reconnaître les maltraitances sexuelles intrafamiliales chez le mineur Haute Autorité de Santé France (HAS) 2011 www.has-sante.fr

[2] American Academy of Pediatrics Guidelines for the evaluation of sexual abuse of children: subject review. Pediatrics 1999;103:186-191

[3] Heger A, Ticson L, Velasquez O, Bernier R. Children referred for possible sexual abuse: medical finding in 2384 children. Child Abuse & Neglect 2002;26:645-59

[4] Nathanson M., Muller MH., Belasco C., Dieu-Osika S., Camard O. Gaudelus J. Les enfants et adolescents victimes d'abus sexuels. Diagnostic et prise en charge. Arch Pédiatr 1998;5:84-9

[5] Van Gisenghem H - L'enfant mis à nu: L'allégation d'abus sexuel: la recherche de la vérité. Montréal Ed. 1999

[6] Frappier JY., Haley N., Allard-Dansereau Cl. Abus sexuels Ed. Les presses de l'université. Montréal 1990

[7] Kellog N. American Academy of Pediatrics Committee on Child Abuse and Neglect. The Evaluation of Sexual Abuse in Children Pediatrics. 2005;116:506-12

[8] Messerschmitt P. La vérité sort elle de la bouche des enfants? Arch Pediatr 2011;18:55-6

[9] De Becker E, Hayez JY. L'enfant en dessous de 3 ans maltraité sexuellement: comment les tout petits parlent d'un abus et comment y faire face? Neuropsychiatrie de l'enfant et de l'adolescence. 2003;51:105-10

[10] Garignon C., Mure PY, Parapel P, Chiche D, Mouriquand P. Dysfonctionnement vésicaux graves chez l'enfant victime de maltraitance: Le syndrome d'Hinman Press Med 2001;30:1912-23

[11] Roussey M, Balençon M. La valeur de la parole de l'enfant dans les situations d'abus sexuels. Rev Int Ped 1999;9-14

[12] Ceci SJ, Ross DF, Toglia MP. Age differences in suggestibility; psychological implications. J Exp Psychol Gen 1987;117:38-49

[13] Yuille JC. L'entrevue de l'enfant dans un contexte d'investigation et l'évaluation systématique de sa déclaration in L'enfant mis à nu Ed. Méridien Psychologie Montréal 1996

[14] Jodoin Cl. L'expert et ses outils in Us et abus de la mise en mots en matière d'abus sexuel Van Gijsegehm H Ed. Méridien Psychologie Montréal 1999

[15] August RL, Forman BD. A comparison of sexually abused and non sexually abused children's behavioural responses to anatomically correct dolls. Child Psychiatry Human Dev 1989;20:39-47

[16] Hayez JY. Sexual abuse of underage children: incest and extra-familial abuse. Psychiat Enfant. 1992;35:197-271

[17] Makoroff K, Brauley J, Brandner A, Myers P, Shapiro R. Genital examinations for alleged sexual abuse of prepubertal girls: finding by pediatric emergency medicine physicians compared with child abuse trained physicians. Child Abuse & Neglect 2002;26:1235–42

[18] Balençon M, Roussey M. Examen et conduite à tenir chez le jeune enfant victime d'abus sexuels. J Pédiatr Puericulture 2000;13:36-42

[19] Palusci VJ, Cyrus TA. Reaction to video colposcopy in the assesment of child sexual abuse. Child Abuse & Neglect 2001;25:1535–46

[20] Adams JA, Kaplan RA, Starling SP, Mehta NH, Finkel MA, Botash AS, Kellog ND, Shapiro SA. Guidelines for medical care of children who may have been sexually abused. J Pediatr Adolesce Gynecol 2007;20:163–72

[21] Bernard D, Peters M, Makoroff K. The evaluation of suspected pediatric sexual abuse. Clin Ped Emerg Med 2006;7:161–9

[22] Myhre AK, Mykelstad K, Adams JA. Changes in genital anatomy and microbiology in girls between age 6 and age 12 years: a longitudinal study. J Pediatr Adolesc Gynecol 2010;23:77–85

[23] Adams JA. Medical evaluation of suspected child sexual abuse. APSAC Advisor 2010;22:2–7

[24] Benjamins LJ. Genital trauma in pediatric and adolescent females. J Pediatr Adolesc Gynecol 2009;22:129–33

[25] Goodyear-Smith F. What is the evidence for non-sexual transmission of gonorrhea in children after the neonatal period? A systematic review. Journal of Forensic and Legal Medicine 2007;14:489–502

[26] La Voix de L'Enfant: Permanences et unités d'accueil médico-légales pour les enfants victimes de Violences Sexuelles France 2002 www.lavoixdelenfant.org

[27] Edinburgh L, Saewy E, Levitt C. Caring for young adolescent sexual abuse victims in a hospital-based children's advocacy center. Child Abuse & Neglect 2008;32:119–26

[28] Smith DW, Witte TH, Fricker-Elhai AE. Service outcomes in physical and sexual abuse cases: a comparison of child advocacy center-based and standard services. Child Maltreat. 2006;11:354–60

[29] Tishelman AC, Meyer SK, Haney P, McLeod SK. The clinical-forensic dichotomy in sexual abuse evaluations: moving toward an integrative model. J Child Sex Abus. 2010;19:590–608.

[30] Bouchard EM, Tourigny M, Joly J, Hébert M, Cyr M. Les conséquences à long terme de la violence sexuelle, physique et psychologique vécue dans l'enfance. Revue d'épidémiologie et de santé publique 2008;56:333–44

9

Childhood Sexual Abuse and Adult Physical and Dental Health Outcomes

Kathleen Monahan[1] and Carol Forgash[2]
Stony Brook University, Stony Brook, N. Y.,
Private Practice, Smithtown, N.Y.,
USA

1. Introduction

This chapter addresses the negative health outcomes for adult childhood sexual abuse (CSA) survivors. It is now well established that CSA survivors have a myriad of long- term physical health related disorders and disease processes (Boscarino, 2004; Irish, Kobayashi, & Delahanty, 2010; Monahan & Forgash, 2000) mental health difficulties, (Briere & Scott, 2006; Briere & Weathers, 2005; Brown, 2009) and dental health issues (Teram; Leeners, Stiller, Block, Görres, Imthurn, Rath, 2007). Many of these individuals will exhibit health risk behaviors as well (Felitti, Anda, Nordenberg et al, 1998; Owens & Chard, 2001; Chartier, Walker, Naimark, 2008; Liebshutz et al., 2000; Meade, Kershaw, Hansen, Sikkema, 2009). Additionally, oral and dental health has been recognized as a strong predictor of physical health problems. Recently, the dental health of CSA survivors has been an area of investigation.

The trauma field has long recognized the association between childhood trauma, PTSD symptomatology and health issues (Schnurr, 1996). One of the most recognized studies to date is the Adverse Childhood Experiences (ACE) study which gathered information from 17, 337 adults 50 years and older (Felitti, Anda, Nordenberg et al, 1998). Information on current health status and childhood adverse experiences such as vitriolic divorce, abuse and neglect, a parent dying, and witnessing one's mother being beaten, were collected. The study found that 30.1% of the respondents reported being physically abused, 19.9% reported sexual abuse, and 11% reported being emotionally abused (Felitti, Anda, Nordenberg, et al, 1998). Moreover, the study found that childhood stressors are strongly related to the development and prevalence of risks factors for disease and health and social well-being throughout the life span (Felitti, Anda, Nordenberg et al, 1998). The authors state,

> The ACE study reveals a powerful relationship between our emotional experiences as children and our physical and mental health as adults, as well as the major cause of adult mortality in the United States. It documents the conversion of traumatic emotional experiences in childhood into organic disease later in life (p. 245).

In addition, the more adverse experiences one reported, the more likely one was to develop severe, life-threatening health outcomes such as heart disease, skeletal fractures, stroke, diabetes, and cancer (Filetti, Anda, Nordenberg et al, 1998; van der Kolk, 2005). The ACE study points out that childhood abuse has life-long impact on the health and well being of the victim. Filetti (2001) questions, "How does one perform reverse alchemy, going from a normal newborn with almost unlimited potential to a diseased, depressed adult? How does one turn gold into lead?" (p. 1).

2. Factors that contribute to deleterious outcome

There are several significant factors that contribute to the deleterious outcome from childhood sexual abuse. These factors, age at time of abuse, frequency of abuse, duration and severity of the abuse, originally identified by David Finkelhor (1984), formulates the "how and why" children can be so harmed by sexual abuse.

The age of the child when the abuse occurs signifies the interruption of a normal developmental trajectory. The traumatic sexualization occurs at a time when the child is not developmentally capable of understanding and processing sexual behavior and subsequently robs the child of childhood innocence.

Frequency and duration are two issues that create anticipatory fear and hyperarousal in a child. Frequency is how often the abuse occurs during a given time period. Duration is the ongoing nature of the abuse, (e.g., months, years) and can create a sense of futility in the child in that the abuse appears to be never ending. The longer-term consequences of frequency and duration are that they contribute to the socialization of trauma, creating a sense of victimhood.

The severity of the abuse creates fear, negative feelings regarding sex, (Sprei & Courtois, 1988; Jehu, 1989) and a general physiological hyperaroused state for the child (Teicher, Andersen, Polcari, Anderson, Navalta, 2002; van der Kolk, 2011). In cases where there was extreme, on-going abuse, the child may have been physically and genitally harmed.

While Finkelhor (1984) discusses the traumatic sexualization of the child as the core issue creating negative outcomes it is not, in and of itself, the primary contributing factor. The closer the relationship of the offender to the child, the stronger the level of betrayal, feelings of mistrust, and a damaged world-view and belief system. Courtois (2005) states, "Abuse by a stranger does not generate the divided loyalty and resultant denial or dismissal of abuse disclosure that is the case when abuse is intrafamilial, especially when it occurs in the nuclear family (involving parent and/or siblings)" (p. 95).

The presence or absence of familial support when disclosing abuse (Paine & Hansen, 2002) is another significant factor in the recovery process. There is significant literature that addresses the notion that when one is supported and believed by family members, the ability to heal and begin the recovery process has a better prognosis (London, Bruck, Ceci, & Shuman, 2005; Priebe & Svedin, 2008). The manner in which the family responds to disclosure is also important. Families who respond with demonstrations of aggressive anger and threats to the perpetrator in front of the victim only serve to instill fear and regret about disclosing, due to the nature of the adults seemingly "out of control" behavior.

Resilience and the interplay of genetics combined with risk and protective factors have been examined with children in high-risk environments for over 15 years. Cicchetti and Blender (2004) define resilience as, "… comprehending the factors contributing to positive outcomes despite the presence of significant adversity…" (p. 17325).

Previous anecdotal information relied on the conceptualization that social support alone (a significant family member, a teacher, etc.) could provide the at-risk child with the required coping mechanisms to mediate adversity. Social support combined with the child's innate capacity to ward off the negative aspects of adversity are thought to be the primary predictors of the child's ability to deal with and successfully survive maltreatment, and thus considered resilience.

Cicchetti and Blender (2004) point out that predictive factors have been narrowly focused. They state, "...adequate prediction of either disturbance or resilience requires considering multiple risks and protective factors and their interplay" (p. 17325).

3. Attachment

Bowlby (1980) presented the significance of early caregiving experiences on the ability of a neonate to attach to its caregivers, and thus internalize "working models" or representations of positive caregiving experiences. Van der Kolk (2005) states, "A child's internal working models are defined by the internalization of the affective and cognitive characteristics of their primary relationships" (p. 402).

For humans, brain development is optimally done in a social context, that is with primary caregivers providing not only sustenance but nurturance as well. When the caregiving relationship is less than optimal or in fact abusive, such as in the cases of neglect or physical and sexual child abuse, the child will experience deleterious outcomes.

For the CSA survivor's health, neglect may have reverberations on many levels throughout his or her life. Psychological and physical health, interpersonal functioning, and overall well-being are impacted by levels of neglect. A significant consideration is that the CSA survivor may lack the primary belief that he/she is an individual of worth, deserving to take care of her physical health. Therefore, her ability to be an educated health consumer, to ask questions during medical exams, and her ability to follow-up with annual visits, required immunizations, and diagnostic testing, etc., may all be compromised.

The CSA survivor may not have experienced good role models and thus may not have learned that brushing ones teeth every day is a necessary component of good health care. He or she may not have learned about the necessity of hygiene, immunizations, and annual check-ups and treatment for childhood illnesses, such as ear infections. Not having a good role model may have taught her that these types of behaviors are not a necessary part of life and certainly not a consideration for good health.

Posttraumatic Stress Disorder (PTSD), chronic PTSD, and Developmental Trauma Disorder

CSA survivors can suffer with posttraumatic stress symptomatology and PTSD. PTSD is defined as exposure to a traumatic event in which the threat of death or serious injury or witnessing threat or serious injury or the threat to physical integrity has occurred. In addition, intense fear, helplessness, or horror responses to a traumatic event may have occurred (DSM IV, TR p. 428). Symptomatology include avoidance of the initial traumatizing event or environment, frequent dreams or nightmares of the event, intrusive thoughts and images, flashbacks - feeling as if the event is occurring again - which is generally triggered by sensory stimuli, and physiological reactivity, e.g. a heightened state of agitation, motor activity, or physical reactions.

Chronic PTSD generally occurs when there is more than one traumatic event and/or if the initial ongoing traumatic event was severe and ongoing, e.g., combat situations. The CSA survivor may have been abused by a family member as a child, experienced dating violence, married an abusive spouse, and/or may have been sexually abused again by a stranger and/or another family member. Very often, these types of lifelong traumatic experiences involve the notion that many survivors carry; that life usually entails traumatic events that one cannot escape. CSA survivors with chronic PTSD often experience hyperarousal and hypervigilience that are continuous physiological states. Chronic PTSD frequently includes the inability to self-soothe and emotionally regulate. Health risk behaviors such as alcohol and substance abuse, cigarette smoking, eating disorders, and self-injurious behavior (cutting) are correlated with childhood sexual abuse. These health risk behaviors can be considered attempts by the CSA survivor, albeit poor ones, in the adaptive struggle in which self-medicating is necessary for survival. They may also be attempts to avoid intrusive memories.

The sexual abuse field has struggled with the inadequacy of the PTSD diagnosis for child victims of sexual abuse. Because the nature of sexual abuse is chronic, usually perpetrated by a caregiver, and occurs during childhood, it impacts critical periods of neurobiological development (van der Kolk, 2011). When caregivers are abusive, absent or neglectful, and/or helpless in the face of trauma, children cannot develop a sense of safety and stability that emanates from the caregiver nor can they rely on that caregiver to restore a sense of calm and reliability. The child's responses to stress become diffuse and inadequate. The ability to self-soothe and emotionally regulate - managing stress, impulsivity, and anxiety - are markedly impaired. A significant issue is that the child experiences a sense of betrayal and perceives the world as a hostile and attacking environment.

Mental health practitioners and researchers have examined the concept of complex PTSD (Herman, 1992a, 1992b) and the tentative diagnosis of Developmental Trauma Disorder (Cook et al, 2005; van der Kolk, 2005). Cook et al (2005) state, "A comprehensive review of the literature on complex trauma suggest seven primary domains of impairment observed in (traumatically) exposed children: attachment, biology, affect regulation, dissociation, (e.g., alterations in consciousness), behavioral regulation, cognition, and self-concept" (p. 392). Included in these domains are the child's worldview and functional impairments such as academic, interpersonal, legal interactions, and vocation (van der Kolk, 2005). This tentative diagnosis, yet to be wholly accepted by the trauma field, appears to encompass the chronic and devastating nature of trauma to the developing child.

4. How does trauma change your health?

Traumatic events are now known to change not only psychological well-being but also the basic structure of how the body perceives painful events, processes them and produces physical reactions. But how does this happen? How do traumatic events in childhood such as sexual abuse change health status? It is important to note that not all individuals exposed to traumatic events will experience noxious outcomes, therefore genetic predisposition/vulnerability (Neigh, Gillespie, Nemeroff, 2009) and environmental factors are suspected when examining etiology. Stern's oft quoted metaphor (Kazaks & Stern, 2005) "Genetics load the gun, and environment pulls the trigger," appears apropos.

Humans have the capacity to react to stressful events in ways that will protect them. Many people have heard of the fight/flight/freeze reaction to threatening events. This is the body's stress reaction alerting the individual to either stay and fight, run away from the stressful event, or sometimes freeze in place. Each reaction is designed to assist the individual to survive and is directly attributable to the autonomic nervous system and the endocrine system working together to deal with the stressful event.

The hypothalamic-pituitary-adrenal (HPA) axis is a mediating pathway of the stress response (Neigh, Gillespie, Nemeroff, 2009, van der Kolk, 2011) and it's the function of the HPA to modulate hormones that address stressful events. To promote survival, a chain reaction of powerful hormones and neurochemicals are produced to assist the individual in dealing with the immediate stressful event (Neigh, Gillespie, Nemeroff, 2009). Deactivation of these hormones occurs through a "negative feedback loop" alerting the individual that danger is no longer present. Neigh, Gillespie, and Nemeroff (2009) state,

However, if the stress response becomes chronic due to repeated exposure to stressors, defects at different levels of the negative feedback system, or both, the result is a sustained increase in the level of stress hormones and the initiation of pathological changes across multiple physiological systems, resulting in stress related diseases (p. 391; also see McEwen, 2008).

The sympathetic nervous system (SNS) is dominant over the parasympathetic nervous system (PNS), and will not yield to the PNS until some form of resolution takes place. Resolution can take the form of fighting, jogging, meditating (Howard, 2006). The adrenal glands release enough adrenaline to get your attention at the first sign of stress. Adrenaline also helps to "imprint" an emotional or traumatizing event. If the stress continues, the hypothalamus secretes corticotropin-releasing factor. In this process cortisol is also released.

Cortisol is a steroid hormone that is produced naturally in the body to assist in the adaptive struggle when an individual is facing acute traumatic situations. When the stress or the traumatic situation is chronic, high levels of cortisol become toxic. Prolonged cortisol production impairs the immune system and thus, healing. Vulnerability to stress-related disorders and diseases, such as gastrointestinal disorders (ulcers) and heart disease commences. Chronic trauma and stress induces lower cortisol production and this decrease creates an enhanced autoimmune system. In the absence of any other illnesses, the autoimmune system will attack various systems within the body and create illnesses such as Fibromyalgia, Chronic Fatigue Syndrome, thyroid diseases, and Krohn's disease (Bergmann, 2011). Howard (2006) states,

> Minor results of this stress-related impairment include colds, flu, backaches, tight chest, migraine headaches, tension headaches, allergy outbreaks, and skin ailments. More chronic and life-threatening results can include hypertension, ulcers, accident-proneness, addictions, asthma, infertility, colon or bowel disorders, diabetes, kidney disease, rheumatoid arthritis, and mental illness. Killers that can result include heart disease, stroke, cancer, and suicide (p. 816).

Chronic trauma, coupled with the severity of the abuse itself, has long-term devastating impact on health and mental health due to the chronicity of these physiological states.

5. Mental health features of the CSA survivor that impede their health outcomes

CSA survivors may experience shame and self-blame regarding the sexual abuse and approach both mental health practitioners and health professionals with distrust, fear, and anxiety. CSA survivors may also experience a range of PTSD symptomatology that includes avoidant behaviors, depression, and dissociation.

The survivor may not have had good health care models to emulate or his or her health care needs may have been neglected and minimized. Cycles of negative emotions, stress, pain and self-defeating beliefs may perpetuate physical problems. Years of avoidant behavior regarding health issues may have passed before the CSA survivor reaches the health care professional, thus warranting more intensive and costly treatment.

6. Health risk behaviors

In an effort to self-soothe, the CSA survivor may have tried to self-medicate using a variety of maladaptive behaviors and methods. No one would doubt that the prevalence of addiction difficulties with substances such as drugs and alcohol in the United States is of epidemic proportion. Eating disorders, closely correlated with sexual abuse, is a mental health difficulty with severe physical consequences. Unprotected sex, sexually risky behaviors, and prostitution have their etiology in sexual abuse trauma (Tarakeshwar, Fox, Ferro, Khawaja, Kochman, Sikkema, 2005). Self-injurious behavior such as skin carving has long been thought to alleviate some of the internal stress experienced by CSA survivors.

7. Medical issues

Before reviewing the medical issues of CSA survivors one must consider the often mistaken assumption that the somatic complaints of the survivor have no physical etiology, and therefore they are often overlooked and/or misdiagnosed. This phenomenon occurs both with the health and mental health care professional as well as the CSA survivor.

Psycho-physiological changes coupled with psychological changes create multi-systemic problems common to CSA survivors. The American Medical Association 1992 addresses these changes when they state,

> The event has such physiological and psychological intensity that it overrides and impairs the individual's neurophysiological mechanisms of adaptation. The resulting damage is not merely emotional. The person's biological capacity to tolerate and regulate internal and external stimulation can be altered. These changes, in turn, compromise the person's ability to organize perceptual stimuli and cognitive information, making them susceptible to a range of somatic illnesses and a spectrum of anxiety and depressive disorders (p 35).

Psychological distress also contributes to the CSA survivor having an impaired view of their health either through somatization and/or dissociation.

8. Types of health issues

Gastrointestinal symptomatology and disorders have been correlated with childhood sexual abuse. Gastrointestinal disorders include irritable bowel syndrome which is known to affect as many as 10%-20% of adults living in the United States (Hymowitz, 2011). Heim (2002), Drossman (1998), and Levy (2005) have discussed the relationship of genetic and environmental factors, joining with life stressors that influence physiological factors such as the Central Nervous System (CNS), and the Enteric Nervous System (ENS) (Hymowitz,

2011). All of these factors modulate functional aspects of the gastrointestinal system and later, symptoms. While IBS is influenced by several factors such as genetics, environment, and family environment, childhood sexual abuse is a contributing factor.

Gynecological problems such as difficult menses and pain when having sexual intercourse, sexual performance, as well as promiscuity, may also contribute to poor reproductive health outcomes.

CSA survivors may also suffer from Immune System Dysfunction, musculoskeletal difficulties, respiratory ailments such as Asthma, and rheumatic disorders. CSA survivors can also experience what is called Medically Unexplained Symptoms (MUS) such as fibromyalgia (Roelofs & Spinhoeven (2009). Other types of difficulties include urinary tract infections, migraine headaches, chronic pelvic pain and pain intolerance or sensitivity.

Addictive behaviors that lead to poor health outcomes are also associated with childhood sexual abuse such as eating disorders (anorexia, bulimia, and obesity), substance abuse (alcohol and/or drugs), and cigarette smoking. Table 1 lists the most common medical conditions for CSA survivors.

Autoimmune Diseases
Cardiovascular Disease
Pain Perception and Chronic Pain
Compromised Reproductive Health
Gynecological Issues
Diabetes
Eating Disorders (Anorexia, Obesity, Bulimia)
Gastrointestinal Disorders (Irritable Bowel Syndrome)
Immune System Dysfunction
Musculoskeletal difficulties
Respiratory Ailments (Asthma)
Medically Unexplained Symptoms (MUS) e.g., fibromyalgia
Rheumatic Disorders

Table 1. Common Medical Difficulties Reported By CSA Survivors

9. Dental health issues for CSA survivors

Dental health has gained increasing attention as a primary factor supporting overall health. Periodontal disease is now associated with upper respiratory illnesses such as pneumonia and cardiac conditions, even premature death (Eke, Thornton-Evans, Wei, Borgnakke, Dye, 2010). Given the importance of dental health in overall well-being, it is significant that by and large CSA Survivors have poor dental health, health seeking behaviors, and follow through with dental protocols (Hays & Stanley, 1996; Leeners, Stiller, Block, Gorres, Imthurn, Rath, 2009; Monahan & Forgash, 2000; Willumsen, 2004). As with physical health, dental health seeking behaviors can be defined as recognizing the necessity for dental care, making and keeping appointments with the dentist, follow-through with dental advice and hygiene, e.g., brushing teeth, flossing daily, annual visits, and finally, follow through with necessary procedures.

CSA Survivors are resistant to dental treatment for much of the same reasons that they have difficulty with health issues. Feelings of un-deservedness, low self-esteem and self-worth, poor parental modeling and instruction of good dental care, and denial of dental health care needs are the primary issues that underscore the CSA Survivors lack of dental care.

Several other issues factor into the CSA Survivors lack of dental care. While the general population may experience reluctance and even phobia when it comes to dental care, the survivor may have experienced oral rape and this compounds her reluctance to seek dental care. Additionally, because of her overall fear and trepidation about the dental experience she may have experienced trauma in the dental chair, with a dentist unfamiliar with trauma victims. Lack of knowledge, experience, and patience in dealing with this type of situation, can cause iatrogenic trauma. Table 2 lists some of these issues.

Poor Dental Health Seeking: • Lack of or inconsistency in dental hygiene • Few to no dental check-ups in childhood or adulthood
Untreated Dental Pain, Periodontal Problems, TMJ, Malocclusions
Difficulty Sitting and Reclining in the Dental Chair
Difficulty Communicating dental fear or abuse history

This table was compiled using data from AMA, *Diagnostic & Treatment Guidelines on Mental Health Effects of Family Violence*, Chicago, IL.: AMA, 1995; Hays, K.F. & Stanley, S.F. (1996). The Impact of Childhood Sexual Abuse on Women's Dental Experiences. *Journal of Child Sexual Abuse*, 5, 65-74; Monahan & Forgash, (2000). Enhancing the Health Care Experiences of Adult Female Survivors of Childhood Sexual Abuse, *Women & Health*, 30(4), 27-41; Randomsky, N., *Lost Voices, Women, Chronic Pain and Abuse*. New York, NY: Harrington Park Press, 1995; Sidran Institute, Dental Tips for Sexual Abuse Survivors

Table 2. Common Dental Difficulties Reported By CSA Survivors

Several studies indicate that respondents have experienced at least one painful dental encounter (Klepac et al, 1980; Vassend, 1993) and the general population still approaches dental experiences with some level of dental fear. Childhood sexual abuse survivors may experience a *pronounced* level of fear emanating from oral rape and therefore it is important to understand that sexual assault that involved the mouth may result in CSA survivors' reluctance to address their dental health needs and avoid visits to dental health practitioners. (Stalker, Russell, Teram, Schachter, 2005; Teram; Leeners, Stiller, Block, Görres, Imthurn, Rath, 2007) Other reasons may include: viewing the experience as intrusive, experiencing loss of control coupled with a sense of powerlessness, and, most importantly, procedures that may be symbolic and trigger painful memories of childhood abuse (Monahan & Forgash, 2000; 2011).

Much of the same history gathering, rapport building, stabilization and collaboration is the same in cases of dental health for CSA survivors as with health issues. Educating both the CSA survivor and the dental and health practitioner regarding expectable reactions post-trauma and how to begin a purposeful, goal directed program toward health should be the primary goal. The following is a case example, from the second author, of earlier iatrogenic trauma and collaboration between the dentist and the mental health practitioner.

Mrs. C , 35 years old, had avoided dental treatment since moving out of her family home when she married at age 25. As a small child she was sexually abused by her grandfather who lived with the family. He frequently orally raped her and threatened to beat her if she ever told anyone about it. This abuse went on until he was moved to a nursing home when she was 10 years old. The family dentist did not believe in any analgesia for pain when he had to fill cavities or pull any diseased teeth. She felt that the dentist was being "mean to her" like her grandfather. By her teens she had dissociative amnesia concerning the abuse by her grandfather. She disliked going to the dentist and was very consistent in her dental hygiene, hoping to avoid cavities. By the time she was 35, she had entered therapy with symptoms of PTSD . She reported that was having a toothache, and bleeding from her gums. She had begun to remember some fragments of the sexual abuse and the harsh dental treatment from childhood. Her therapist taught her relaxation techniques, to alleviate some anxiety. She spoke with the dentist her husband saw who assured her he would do everything he could to make the experience as painless as possible. Her therapist coached her to tell him some general information about her abuse and early dental trauma. The therapist and dentist telephone conferenced and discussed some strategies to help the patient during and after the session in the dental chair.

The dentist was also well versed in relaxation techniques and was able to talk the patient through some exercises. He provided her with headphones and soft music of her choice. In her next therapy session, the therapist and patient reviewed what had gone well and planned for any additional skills the patient felt she needed. They both felt that the patient felt stabilized and safe enough to begin trauma work on the sexual abuse by her grandfather. The therapist was trained in a phased model of trauma treatment to work through and resolve the trauma. The patient also, with the help of the current positive dental experience, resolved the earlier dental trauma to the point that she was able to plan for long term dental and periodontal treatment. However, there were severe problems, notably, damage from clenching, grinding and teeth broken off at the gum line and bone loss from periodontal disease. This was the legacy of years of avoidance of dental care and the dental / childhood trauma.

Techniques for being a good health care consumer

As part of psychotherapy with this population, reviewing how trauma has impacted their health seeking behaviors and, ultimately their health, is imperative. As mentioned, CSA survivors may not have viewed their trauma histories as having any bearing on their conduct with their health, and/or believing that they do not deserve good health outcomes. Additionally, they may believe that they should not be assertive with health care professionals, have the right to ask questions, or get a second opinion. CSA survivors may demonstrate a lack of cooperation, poor decision making, or even the inability to retain important health information, and it is important for the health care professional to understand that this lack of health assertive behavior emanates from fear, confusion, dissociation, poor health care modeling, and an over all sense that he/she does not deserve attention or good health care. Additionally, the psychotherapist can share and discuss information and how-to techniques on becoming a healthcare consumer with the patient. Many organizations produce informational brochures and flyers on health consumerism for sexual abuse survivors.

Psycho-education regarding health care needs and developing assertive behavior with health care professionals can improve the health outcomes for CSA survivors and is a necessary part of psychotherapy with the CSA survivor.

Teaching the CSA survivor how to modulate stress and improve health outcomes through psychotherapy

Psychotherapy with CSA survivors is generally constructed around a three-stage approach that begins with establishing safety, stabilization and emotional regulation (Ford, Courtois, Steele, van der Hart, Nijenhuis, 2005). While there are a variety of treatment models addressing the issues of trauma available today, most of these treatments are phase-oriented and focus initially on establishing safety for the patient and the therapeutic relationship as the foundation of the work in which processing trauma occurs. The therapeutic relationship becomes the "container" - the holder of painful memories, thoughts, and issues related to the traumatic event. More importantly, the mental health practitioner becomes the model for containment through support that is consistent, boundaries that are well established, and empathic interest in the patient (Ford et al, 2005). The patient will explore and reprocess the traumatic events and finally, achieve mastery and resolution of life issues.

The mental health practitioner should be a warm, genuine individual who can provide an empathic stance, thus formulating the foundation for a therapeutic alliance. It is important for the therapist to retain this empathic demeanor as well as a calm façade when hearing distressing histories from the CSA survivor, generally not a minor feat to accomplish. Sessions should be consistent and the mental health practitioner should provide the CSA survivor with what has been called, "a corrective emotional experience" (Alexander & French, 1946) throughout the course of therapy.

10. Phase I

There are many important components of the first phase. One is to take a history of the patient making sure to note previous abuse incidents and outcomes. Assessment should include patient symptomatology, previous treatment and/or hospitalizations, family history and current contact, health history, and vocational status. Psycho-education includes defining and normalizing triggers, flashbacks, dissociative symptoms and problems in controlling emotions as part of the normal reaction to traumatic events, and can reveal strengths. Ford et al (2005) state, "The client's response to education also reveals strengths that can become a basis for overcoming helplessness without invalidating unmet dependency needs" (p. 438) (See also Steele, Van der Hart, Nijemhuis, 2001). Safety is established in this phase and issues such as suicidality, and maladaptive behaviors such as unhealthy risk taking and self-harm are addressed (Pearlman & Courtois, 2005; Ford, et al, 2005). The patient will learn and practice skills to manage these symptoms as necessary preparation for phase two: trauma treatment. In this phase collaboration with existing support networks or developing them begins (Ford et al, 2005).

11. Phase II

Once safety and stability have been well established, identifying, exploring, and processing the traumatic experiences can take place. Additionally, emotions such as shame, guilt, and helplessness need to be understood and processed. As acceptance of past actions takes place, and responsibility for abuse is correctly assigned to the perpetrator, internal conflicts can be addressed and resolved. The patient can slowly begin to give up the victim role, practice new more assertive behaviors and beliefs, and begin to 'deserve' good health. Additionally, the patient begins to review and predict where in this process they may have difficulty, and apply some of the basic principles of "relapse" prevention, e.g, falling back to old behaviors that negated his/her rights to good health.

12. Phase III

In this phase, patients work to regain control of their lives and achieve healthy functioning and efficacy in life domains. They work on gaining positive self worth and identity and a sense of empowerment. The patient often reports seeing old events and relationships from more of an adult perspective. Additionally, they express feelings of competence and can attend to their healthcare needs as an adult.

It should be noted that in all phases of this work, but particularly in the beginning, the patient may test the mental health professional as part of reenactment of earlier rejection and betrayal by family members, or insecure attachment styles. The mental health practitioner may find that attunement through non-verbal, affective, and bodily communication takes on heightened importance (Ford et al, 2005; Fosha, 2000; Ogden, & Minton, 2000) during all the phases of therapy.

Collaboration between the healthcare professional and the mental health practitioner

Collaboration or a team approach provides a more comprehensive and successful outcome for the CSA survivor in accessing and following through with health care needs. Ethical practice always demands that consent be obtained to contact another treating professional. But more importantly, once a team approach is decided upon, obtaining consent from the CSA survivor to contact another health professional, often provides her with a sense of control.

The mental health professional can act as the patient's advocate and assist in explaining background, symptoms, and specific needs. The mental health practitioner may also explain some of the abuse issues and problems stemming from the trauma. In situations where flashbacks and dissociation are prominent, the mental health practitioner can explain these reactions and assist the health care professional in what to do. The mental health practitioner can let the health professional know the patient's stage of treatment and how that will impact medical treatment. The following case example describes collaboration between the mental health practitioner, the medical specialist, and the patient.

Mrs. N, 65 years old, woke up in the recovery room after a colonoscopy, screaming that a man was coming after her. The doctor was called in after the nurse could not calm her. She was able to tell the doctor that the man was a neighbor who had attacked her sexually and that she had not remembered anything about him in almost 60 years. She became very disoriented, weepy and had to be sedated. For several weeks she did not "feel like herself" and her family doctor referred her to a psychiatrist who medicated her and recommended that she see a trauma therapist. She grew to trust the therapist who was soft spoken and reminded her of her grandmother, even though the therapist was younger than Mrs. N. The therapist normalized the long-term dissociation and amnesia as survival techniques for a little girl who had alcoholic, unprotective parents. Mrs. N. stated that they were usually too drunk to listen or protect her and her siblings. The therapist was trained in Eye Movement Desensitization and Reprocessing (EMDR) a phase-oriented therapy validated for the treatment of PTSD. It included all of the three phases of trauma treatment as mentioned above plus a desensitization, reprocessing, and evaluation phases. As she learned relaxation exercises and practiced them in between sessions, she felt stronger and more in control of her life. She learned about triggers and made the connection between the colonoscopy and the childhood anal rape. Several months after, she felt strong enough to rehearse a planned visit to a gynecologist to discuss exploratory laparoscopic surgery for ovarian cysts. Both she and the therapist felt that she had completed the trauma work and would not be triggered by the procedure. She did tell the doctor about the earlier abuse and the incident triggered by the colonoscopy. They planned that the nurse would sit with her in the recovery room and say to her, "Hello Mrs. N. I'm here with you now. Would you like a drink of water?" That would be a cue that she was in the present, a common grounding technique. Her husband would also be brought right in and would hold her hand to provide comfort. There were several weeks of rehearsal and the medical protocol went well.

13. Conclusion

During the past ten years there has been a proliferation of research and clinical studies in the medical, dental, and mental health journals that unequivocally supports that childhood sexual abuse is epidemic and detrimental to the mental, physical and dental health of survivors. It has been defined as a public health issue, yet changes in bringing this knowledge and clinical expertise to core curricula (and not as an elective or special course) in Medical, Dental, Mental Health or Nursing Graduate programs has been slow. Collaboration with health professionals and mental health practitioners increases the probability that CSA survivors will begin to enjoy good health. One means toward that end is educating practitioners from all health fields on the issues of child sexual abuse and negative health outcomes.

The incidence and prevalence rates of child sexual abuse have held constant since we began collecting statistics in the late sixties. The human suffering and negative health outcomes of so many are only one part of this social problem. The financial expenses of medical and pharmaceutical needs, time lost at work, psychotherapy costs and substance abuse treatment, family support and help for survivors' children makes this a social problem whose immediacy cannot be ignored. Isn't it time to turn lead into gold?

14. References

American Medical Association, Council on Scientific Affairs (1992). Guidelines for Medical Settings Regarding Violence Against Women. Chicago, IL: AMA.

Alexander, F.G. & French, T.M. (1946). *Psychoanalytic Therapy, Principles and Application*, University of Nebraska Press, John Wiley.

American Medical Association (1995). *Diagnostic & Treatment Guidelines on Mental Health Effects of Family Violence*. Chicago, IL: AMA.

American Psychiatric Association. *Diagnostic and Statistical Manual of Mental Disorders, 4th ed, text revision*. Washington, D.C: American Psychiatric Association, 2000

Bergmann, U. (2011). *Foundations of Neurobiology for EMDR Practice*. New York: Springer Publishing.

Boscarino, J. A. (2004). Posttraumatic Stress Disorder and Physical Illness, Results from Clinical and Epidemiologic Studies, *Annals of the New York Academy of Science*, 1032, 141-153.

Bowlby, J. (1980). *Attachment and Loss, Vol 3*. New York, N.Y.: Basic Books

Briere, J. & Elliott, D.M. (2003). Prevalence and symptomatic sequelae of self-reported childhood physical and sexual abuse in a general population sample of men and women. *Child Abuse & Neglect*, 27, 1205-1222.

Briere J. & Scott, C. (2006). *Principles of Trauma Therapy*. Thousand Oaks, CA: Sage Publications.

Briere, J., Scott, C., & Weathers, F. (2005). Peritraumatic and persistent dissociation in the presumed etiology of PTSD. *American Journal of Psychiatry*, 162, 2295-2301.

Brown, D. (2009). Assessment of attachment and abuse history, and adult attachment style. In *Treating Complex Traumatic Stress Disorders, An Evidence-Based Guide*. Christine A. Courtois and Julian D. Ford (Eds.). New York: Guilford Press, pp. 124- 126.

Browne, A. & Finkelhor, D. (1986). The impact of child sexual abuse: A review of the literature. *Psychological Bulletin*, 99(1), 66-77.

Cicchetti, D. & Blender, J.A. (2004). A Multiple-Levels-of-Analysis Approach to the Study of Developmental Processes In Maltreated Children. *Proceedings of the National Academy of Sciences*, December.

Courtois, C. (2005). When One Parent Has been Sexually Abused As A Child. Family *Stressors, Interventions for Stress and Trauma*. Don R. Catherall (Ed). New York, N.Y: Taylor & Francis, pp. 95-111.

Chartier, M.J., Walker, J., & Naimark, B. (2008). Health Risk Behaviors and Mental Health Problems as Mediators of the Relationship Between Childhood Abuse and Adult Health. *American Journal of Public Health*, 10.2105/AJPH.2007.122408.

Cook, A., Spinazzola, J., Ford, J., Lanktree, C., Blaustein, M., Cloitre, M., DeRosa, R. et al (2005). Complex Trauma in Children and Adolescents. *Psychiatric Annals*, 35(5), 390-398.

Drossman, D. (1994). Physical and Sexual Abuse and Gastrointestinal illness: What is the Link? *American Journal of Medicine*, 97, 105-107.

Eke, P.I, Thornton-Evans, G.O., Wei, L, Borgnakke, W.S., Dye, B,A. (2010). Accuracy of NHANES Periodontal Examination Protocols, *Journal of Dental Research*,

Finkelhor, D. (1984). *Child Sexual Abuse: New Theory and Research*, New York: The Free Press.

Felitti, V.J., Anda, RF, Nordenberg, D., Williamson, DF, Spitz, AM, Edwards, V, Koss, M.P, Marks, J.S. (1998). The Relationship of Adult Health Status to Childhood Abuse and

Household Dysfunction. *American Journal of Preventative Medicine,* vol. 14, no 4, pp. 245-258.
Filetti, V.J. (2001). Reverse Alchemy in Childhood: Turning Gold Into Lead. The Family Violence Prevention Fund, 8(1), 1—4.
Ford, J., Courtois, C., Steele, K., van der Hart, Nijenhuis, E. (2005). Treatment of Complex Posttraumatic Self-Dysregulation, *Journal of Traumatic Stress,* 18(5) , 437- 447.
Forgash, C. & Copeley, M. (Eds.) *Healing The Heart of Trauma.* N.Y.: Springer, 2008.
Fosha, D. (2000). *The Transforming Power of Affect.* New York: Basic Books.
Hays, K.F. & Stanley, S.F. (1996). The Impact of Childhood Sexual Abuse on Women's Dental Experiences. *Journal of Child Sex Abuse,* 5, 65-74.
Heim, C., Newport, D.J., Heit, S., Graham, Y.P., Wilcox, M., Bonsall, R. (2000). Pituitary-adrenal and autonomic responses to stress in Adult Women with Sexual and Physical Abuse In Childhood. *Journal of the American Medical Association,* 284, 592-597.
Herman, J. L. (1992a).Complex PTSD: A Syndrome In Survivors of Prolonged and Repeated Trauma. *Journal of Traumatic Stress,* 5, 377-391.
Herman, J. L. (1992b). *Trauma and Recovery: The Aftermath of Violence From Domestic To Political Terror.* New York: Basic Books.
Howard, P.J. (2006). *The Owner's Manual for The Brain, 3rd Edition.* Austin, TX: Bard Press.
Hymowitz, G. (2011). Do Previous Life Experiences and Family History Moderate Gastrointestinal Symptoms, Somatic Symptoms, and Stress in Response to Transient Stressors? Unpublished Dissertation, Psychology Department, Stony Brook University, Stony Brook, N.Y. 11794
Irish, L., Kobayashi, M.S., Delhanty, D.L. (2010). Long-term Physical Health Consequences of Childhood Sexual Abuse: A Meta-Analysis. *Journal of Pediatric Psychology,* 35(5), pp. 450-461.
Jehu, D. (1989). Sexual Dysfunctions among women clients who were Sexually Abused in Childhood. *Behavioral Psychotherapy,* 17, 53-70.
Kazaks, A. & Stern, J.S. (2005). Diet, Physical Activity, And Behavior. In *Pharmacotherapy of Obesity, Options and Alternatives.* K. Hofbauer, U. Keller, and O. Boss (Eds.), Taylor & Francis, http://www.ebookstore.tandf.co.uk/
Klepac, R.K., McDonald, M., Hauge, G., Dowling, J. (1980). Reactions to Pain Among Subjects High and Low In Dental Fear. *Journal of Behavioral Medicine,* 3, 373-384.
Leeners, B., Stiller, R., Block, E., Gorres, G., Imthurn, B., Rath, W. (2009). Consequences of childhood sexual abuse experiences on dental care. *Journal of Psychosomatic Research,* 62(5), 581-588.
Levy, R., Olden, K., Naliboff, B.L.B., Francisconi, C., Drossman,D. et al (2005). Psychsocial Aspects of the Functional Gastrointestinal Disorders. *Gastroenterology,* 130(5), 1447-1458.
Liebschutz, J.M., Feinman, G., Sullivan, L., Stein, M., & Samet, J. (2000). Physical and Sexual Abuse in Women Infected with the Human Immunodeficiency Virus: Increased Illness and Health Care Organization. *Archives of Internal Medicine,* 160(11), 1659-1664.
London, K., Bruck, M., Ceci, S. & Shuman, D. (2005). Disclosure of child sexual abuse: What does the research tell us about the ways that children tell? *Psychology, Public Policy, and Law,* 11, 194-226.

McEwen, B.S. (2008). Central Effects of Stress Hormones in Health and Disease: Understanding the Protective and Damaging Effects of Stress and Stress Mediators. *European Journal of Pharmacology*, 583, 174-185.

Meade, C.S., Kershaw, T., Hansen, N.B., Sikkema, K. (2009). Long-Term Correlates of Childhood Abuse Among Adults With Severe Mental Illness: Adult Victimization, Substance Abuse, and HIV Sexual Risk Behavior.

Monahan, K. & Forgash, C. (2000). Enhancing the health care experiences of adult female sexual abuse survivors of childhood sexual abuse. *Women & Health*, 30(4), 27-41.

Monahan, K. & Forgash C. (2011). Enhancing the Dental Health Care Experiences of Adult Sexual Abuse Survivors. Unpublished paper.

Neigh, G.N., Gillespie, C., Nemeroff, C.B. (2009). The Neurobiological Toll of Child Abuse and Neglect. *Trauma, Violence, & Abuse*, 10(4), 389-410.

Ogden, P. & Minton, K. (2000). Sensorimotor Psychotherapy. *Traumatology*, 6, 149-173.

Owens, G.P. & Chard, K.M. (2001). Cognitive Distortions Among Women Reporting Childhood Sexual Abuse. *Journal of Interpersonal Violence*, 16(2), 178-191.

Paine, M.L. & Hansen, D.J. (2002). Factors influencing children to self-disclose sexual abuse. *Clinical Psychology Review*, 22, 271-295.

Pearlman, L.A. & Courtois, C. (2005). Clinical Applications of the Attachment Framework: Relational Treatment of Complex Trauma. *Journal of Traumatic Stress*, 18, 449-459.

Priebe, G & Svedin, C. (2008). Child sexual abuse is largely hidden from the adult society, An epidemiological study of adolescents' disclosures. *Child Abuse & Neglect*, 32, 1095-1108.

Roelofs, K. & Spinhoeven, P. (2009). EMDR in the Treatment of Medically Unexplained Symptoms. *JEMDRA*, 3(4), 248-263.

Schnurr, P. (1996). Trauma, PTSD, and Physical Health. *The PTSD Research Quarterly*. The National Center for Post-Traumatic Stress Disorder

Sprei, & Courtois, C. (1988). The Treatment of Women's Sexual Dysfunctions Arising from Sexual Assault. In R.A. Brown & J. R. Fields (Eds.) , *Treatment of Sexual Problems in Individuals and Couple Therapy* (pp. 267-299). New York: Aperture.

Stalker, C.A., Russell, B.D., Teram, E., Schachter, C.L. (2005). Providing Dental Care to Survivors of childhood Sexual Abuse: Treatment Considerations for the Practitioner. *Journal of American Dental Association*, 136, 1277-1281.

Steele, K., Van der Hart, O., Nijemhuis, E.R.S. (2001). Dependence in the Treatment of Complex Posttraumatic Stress Disorder and Dissociative Disorders. *Journal of Trauma and Dissociation*, 2(4), 79-116.

Tarakeshwar, N., Fox, A. Ferro, C., Khawaja, S., Kochman, A.,Sikkema, K. (2005). The Connections Between Childhood Sexual Abuse and Humman Immunodeficiency Virus Infection: Implications. *Journal of Community Psychology*, 33(6), 655-672.

Teicher, M.H., Andersen, S.L., Polcari, A., Anderson, C.M., Navalta, C.P. (2002). Developmental Neurobiology of Childhood Stress and Trauma. *Psychiatric Clin North America*, 25(2), 397-426.

Teram; Leeners, Stiller, Block, Görres, Imthurn, Rath, (2007) Providing Dental Care to Survivors of Childhood Sexual Abuse: Treatment Considerations for the Practitioner. *Journal of American Dental Association*, 136, 1277- 1281.

Van der Kolk, B. (2011). Developmental Trauma Disorder, *Psychiatric Annals*, 35(5), 401-408.

Vassend, O. (1993). Anxiety, Pain and Discomfort Associated with Dental Treatment. Behavioral Res Therapy, 31, 659-666.

Willumsen, T. (2004). The Impact of Childhood Sexual Abuse on Dental Fear. *Community Dentistry and Oral Epidemiology*, 32, 73-79.

10

Child Sexual Abuse and Its Implications for Children's Health

Lia Leão Ciuffo and Benedita Maria Rêgo Deusdará Rodrigues
University of the State of Rio de Janeiro
Brazil

1. Introduction

1.1 Contextualizing violence and child sexual abuse

The violence is present in the everyday life of citizens all over the world and in national and regional level too, affecting interpersonal relationships and influencing people's way of acting and thinking.

Violence is presented as a complex problem that affects, everybody without distinction, independent of social class, race, religion, sex or age. Today it is more studied, investigated and divulged and because of that it has acquired an important social meaning in the few years. (Moura & Lisboa, 2005)

The factors that contribute to violent responses - whether they are factors of attitude and behavior or related to larger social, economic, political and cultural conditions - can be changed. In this perspective, understanding the factors that increase the risk of young people being the victims or perpetrators of violence is essential for developing effective policies and programmes to prevent violence. (Krug et al, 2002)

However, we can note that the boundaries between different types of violence aren't well defined, so we must carefully examine all aspects of family violence, and particularly sexual abuse cases, seeking to get a better comprehension about the framework that professional faces. (Ciuffo, 2008)

In general, hearing about real cases of sexual abuse cause on people a feeling of malaise. Sexual violence affects many layers of society and people of different ages, including children and adolescents. Reports of such aggression against a child who probably had been induced or coerced and even forced to participate in such an act unfortunately are common.

In this sense, report and prevent child sexual abuse and other crimes against children is a worldwide concern. The cases reported on television and in newspapers of general circulation represent only the tip of the iceberg. If thoroughly investigated, it may be noted that a large number of boys and girls are subjected to violence of all kinds in their daily lives. (Ciuffo, 2008)

The interactions that individuals establish in society, economic issues, policies and legal requirements that govern society help us understand more clearly the various forms of violence and, among them, child sexual violence.

2. Methodology

This chapter was structured on the proposal of a systematic review of national and international publications on childhood sexual abuse. The focus of this systematic review is directed towards gathering, discuss critically and conduct a synthesis of results of primary studies on the subject. For this purpose we used systematic methods that enabled to identify, select and promote critical and reflective discussion as well as to collect and analyze data from these selected studies.

A systematic review consists on a rigorous synthesis of all researches related to a specific question. The question may be about cause, diagnosis, prognosis of a health problem, but often involves the effectiveness of an intervention to solve this. In this sense, the systematic review is an important resource in evidence-based practice, which consists in a form of synthesizing the research results related to a specific problem. (Galvão et al, 2004)

The review was carried out from March to June 2011, period that I am still developing my thesis in order to obtain the Doctor's degree on Nursing of the Nursing College in University of the State of Rio de Janeiro. To do so, I am counting on the support and guidance of my teacher who works at this University.

The literature search was conducted in the databases LILACS (which is the most important and comprehensive index of scientific and technical literature in Latin America and the Caribbean) and MEDLINE (Medical Literature Analysis and Retrieval System Online). We used descriptors such as: violence, abuse, sexual abuse, child care and nursing. The inclusion criteria were published articles that contemplate the issue of violence and sexual abuse against children, in English or Portuguese between the years 2000 to 2010, available entirety online. Publications were excluded when not meet these criteria.

For the selection of productions, we observed the inclusion criteria, at a first moment. Later, we carried out a selection based on title and / or abstract and, finally, evaluated the study in full.

The survey of this study has 154 publications, 31 (20.13%) were repeated, 108 (70.13%) publications were unrelated to the topic of study. Finally, we selected 15 publcations (9.74%) by adherence to the theme of the study.

Moreover, in order to solidify and consolidate knowledge in this field, we also used in the construction of this chapter books, thesis, dissertations, and national and international documents that addressed the issue of violence against children. The content analysis of studies enabled us to organize knowledge on the subject according to the different aspects that follow in section 3.

3. Discussing literature relevant aspects

3.1 Contextualizing child sexual abuse and its implications for children's health

In this section we are going to understand better the concept of sexual abuse and it's implications for children's health . In this perspective, sexual abuse is the sexual act that occurs in heterosexual or homosexual, whose abuser is in an earlier stage of psychosexual development than the child or adolescent. The abuser or perpetrator has the intention to stimulate a child sexually or use it for sexual satisfaction. These erotic and sexual practices are imposed on children by physical violence, threats or inducements to his will / desire. (Krug et al, 2002).

Child sexual abuse is one of the most perverse forms of abuse that victimizes children and adolescents. The healthy life expectancy is severely threatened by the consequences of this experience.

Sexual violence, among all expressions of violence, brings more consequences for the child's life, considering that besides involving the physical part, it also affects deeply the emotional part, leading to brand that will be taken to adulthood.(Woiski & Rocha, 2010)

Analyzing sexual violence, it is worth highlighting the inadequacy of isolating it from the psychological and physical violence. This can be explained because often other types of violence are associated, and the effects sometimes are worse than sexual violence only.

The threat was the most used (41.93%), followed by the use of physical force (29.03%) and seduction (16.12%) and there were no cases of use of a weapon of any kind. The threats often refer to the fact that the aggressor say to the children that they could not tell anything to the parents. In addition, many offenders make the victim feel guilty for the act committed by him (Inoue & Ristum, 2008).

Thinking about threats or physical abuse and their relation to sexual violence is essential and should not be forgotten. Therefore, it is necessary to contextualize the situations in which such act happened.

The data about this issue is worrying, as evidenced in this study, where the results indicate that children and adolescents victims of sexual abuse were, in most cases, female, 80.9%. The age of onset of abuse has focused on three age groups, with 10.6% of children ranging from 2 to 5 years old, 36.2% of these were between 5 and 10 years old and 19.1% were between 10 and 12 years old. Most children, 26.6% were attending primary school at the beginning of the aggression. (Habigzang et al, 2005)

Considering the links between actors of this delicate situation can best direct us to confirm the diagnosis. An important aspect about child sexual abuse is the fact that in most cases the abuser is someone known to the child, so he approaches quiet easily and has great persuasive power. Generally, the main objective is to convince the child to do what they want in secret. (Ciuffo, 2008)

Child sexual abuse sets up a phenomenon that affects the entire family, and often exacerbates family disintegration, especially when dealing with sexual abuse that occurs within families. (Carvalho et al, 2009)

The perception of victims are related to the abuser shows that the majority of children and adolescents expressed the desire to stay away from the aggressor (41.8%) and were afraid of them (38.2%). Regarding the perception of aggression (31.9%) of the submitted information and documents examined, the children said they would not be conducive to the situation, or haven't consented, trying to avoid it, or expressed their lack of understanding of the abuse experience. (Habigzang et al, 2005)

According to the records of the Guardianship Councils, between the years 2003 and 2004, were reported of 1,293 cases of violence, 1,011 (78.1%), originated in the home. The most frequent types of violence were: neglect (727), failure to provide basic care (304) and abandonment (259); physical violence (455), beatings (392) between 2 and 13 years old; psychological violence (374) through threats (219); sexual violence (68) through abuse (58), mainly among adolescents. (Costa et al, 2007)

The same authors above clarify that sexual violence reached 68 cases, 58 were cases of abuse and 10 of them were sexual exploitation. The abuse occurred in all age groups, with 20 cases in the range of 10 to 13 years, 12 cases from 14 to 16 years and 9 cases from 6 to 9 years.

In a study which has a sample of 124 cases of suspected sexual abuse was selected, both male and female, aged from 0 to 17 years, the authors reveal that the relationship between victim / perpetrator was the father / stepfather / guardian - a total of 20 cases (16.13%) where 16 cases were female. When the abuser is a relative / acquaintance - the authors found 35 cases (28.23%), where 28 cases were female. When the perpetrator is unknown - was found in 17 cases (13.71%), where 16 cases were female. And finally, also has returned when the offender is not informed - we obtained a total of 38 cases (30.65%), 30 cases were female. (Aded et al, 2007)

The prevalence of reported child sexual abuse in the sample studied was 3.9%, higher among girls (5.6%) than boys (1.6%). Over 80% of all reported first sexual abuse episodes took place before reaching 19 years of age; 63% happened before 15 years; 49% before 13 years; 27% before the children were 8 years old; and 6% before reaching 4 years of age. Among the respondents reporting being victims of sexual abuse before 19 years of age, 7.6% reported being less than 4 years old at the time; 37% were less than 8 years; 60% were less than 13 years; and 89% were less than 15 years. (Aded et al, 2007)

The prevalence of self-reported sexual abuse before 12 years of age is higher among girls (1.7%) than boys (0.5%) and similarly higher among girls 12 years of age and older (1.5% vs. 0.3%). Girls experienced the majority of the total burden of child sexual abuse reported by the study participants (80% of the child sexual abuse before age 12, and 84.1% of it after age 12). While 53% of all reports of child sexual abuse for boys happened from ages 0 to 7, for girls, 33% of the child sexual abuse happened before age 8 and peaked around ages 8 to 15, when 88% of all reported abuses had already taken place. (Bassani et al , 2009)

As a result of their study about the incidence of sexual abuse with children in Rio de Janeiro, found that the abusers had some link with their victims in 55 cases: 20 cases (16.13 %) were assigned to responsible parents or stepparents, and in 35 (28.23%), relatives (uncles, grandfathers, cousins) or acquaintances. (Aded et al 2007)

Subsidized by the assertive in the study cited above, we could conclude that although there is a representation of the abusers at all levels of schooling, there is a higher prevalence among those with low education. Therefore, we must give attention to the issue of health education and more specifically for this population group, stimulating abusers a change of attitude towards children by getting them to understand that every child needs to grow and develop healthily, free from violence and surrounded by people who want their welfare.

Drezett (2007) states that child sexual abuse is usually committed by people trusted by the child, prevailing parents, stepfathers, uncles and grandfathers as the main aggressors. A study on characterization and analysis of sexual violence cases performed at school revealed to the linkage between aggressor and victim, a higher frequency of domestic violence (56.0%) prevailed. The second most frequent category, this study was entitled "acquaintance" (40.0%) and refers to known offenders, but without any relationship with the victim. (Inoue &, Ristum, 2008) .

In a study it was verified that practically all offenders were known to the victim, with only one case of unidentified. The aggressors, all male, numbered a total of 25, since in two cases there was more of an aggressor. There was a predominance of ages "over 40" years (36.36%), followed by ages of 31 to 40 years "(22.72%) and" 20 years "(22.72%), with a variation 15 to 54 years. The forms of coercion or intimidation used by the aggressors were a threat, physical force, seduction and other unidentified. It was observed that in some situations, the aggressor used more than one form of coercion. The threat was the most used (41.93%), followed by the use of physical force (29.03%) and seduction (16.12%). (Inoue & Ristum, 2008)

Although people believe that sexual violence is practiced by unknown people, most crimes are actually practiced by someone close to the victim. In this study, regarding age, there was a predominance of attendance for children (42%) and teenagers (36%). Considering separately by sex, was found higher frequency for female adolescents (40%). For males, higher frequency of sexual abuse was among children (79%). About the identification of the aggressor, it was found that 700 (76%) were identified by the victims. Among these, a greater proportion of the category friend / acquaintance (19.2%) was followed by a stepfather (12.4%), father (11.7%), neighbor (11.4%) and uncle (8 3%). (Campos & Schor, 2008)

There are common feelings of fear, anger and shame of the victim regarding the abuser, especially in cases of sexual abuse because there is a disruption of the trust and bonding due to violence.(Habigzng et al, 2005)

One of the most critical issue of this alarming situation is that in our society, often, the child becomes a victim of this assault for a long time. The attack remains hidden because the prevailing feeling of fear of suffering rebukes by the abuser. (Ciuffo, 2008)

However, it is important not to make a pre-judgment of the abuser, but take into account that in some cases, victims didn't resist, others remain passive and others may encourage the abuser, in order to search for love and affection denied by them. But the fact is that most sexual exchanges between adult and child is initiated by the adult. (Ciuffo et al, 2009).

3.2 Most frequent forms of sexual abuse

Sexual abuse against children and adolescents can be subdivided, (Magalhães, 2005):

- Verbal sexual abuse can be characterized by the conversations about sexual activities with the aim of arousing the interest of the child and adolescent and shocking them;
- Sexual harassment is configured in the proposals of sexual contact, which in most cases the victim is blackmailed by the position of power occupied by the aggressor;
- Exhibitionism has the intention to shock the victim whereas the exhibitionist shows the parts of his body and makes obscene gestures;
- Voyeurism is characterized by the gratification through the observation of sexual acts or sex organs of other people;
- Physical-genital acts include sex vaginal penetration or attempted sexual relations, handling of genitals, oral sex and anal penetration;
- Rape cases are situations where vaginal penetration occurs with the use of violence or serious theats;
- Incest is the situation where there is a family tie or not and it involves a sexual relationship between adults and children, adolescents and children or between adolescents;
- Indecent assault means to embarrass someone to practice sexual acts without vaginal intercourse, using violence or serious threat, being practiced in children over 14 years old;
- Pornography refers to the use of children and adolescents as actors or models in obscene pictures and videos, usually for economic purposes, and
- Prostitution concerns the participation of children and adolescents in sexual acts with adults or other minors, where there is not necessarily physical strength, but in this kind of situation there might be coercion.

The biopsychosocial consequences in situations of abuse are often related to factors such as the conditions in which it occurs, the child's age, degree of intimacy between the child and the abuser and others. So, it is essential that there are measures that seek to protect children and minimize the possibilities of new occurrences.

3.3 The nurse's role face child sexual abuse suspicion

Children constitute a group with high vulnerability and exposure to situations of maltreatment, and especially child sexual abuse, which is often imposed to the children by physical violence, threat or inducements to their will. (Ciuffo et al 2009)

Obtaining of information and care directed to a sick child requires from the professional, much more than technical care, but subjective care too, since it considers the singularity and individuality of each child and also the expression of their feelings and emotions. It is important to consider the child victim of sexual violence story, in light to know how the child relates to the context in which violence occurred and all the symbols and meanings that this event means to her.(Woiski & Rocha, 2010)

It is worth to emphasize that among the professionals involved in this context are the nurses and the nursing staff. These professionals have an important role in the treatment of children with suspected sexual abuse because they can, through care, child support, spread the love and security the child needs to face this situation. .(Woiski & Rocha, 2010)

Moreover, nursing, considered as a social practice and committed to emancipation and human development, cannot be performed outside the perspective of the complexity of transformations in the contemporary social context, which includes the integral and multidisciplinary approach of domestic violence against children. (Silva & Ferriani, 2007)

It must be considered that nurses can and should have a decisive action when fighting the everyday reality of sexual abuse against children, considering that, besides recognizing and identifying signs of abuse of they should be aware of laws protecting the rights of children's health and attitudes to be taken in these cases. Thus, it enables monitoring the situation of children and their families during and after children care and legal ramifications involved when one considers the suspected sexual abuse. (Ciuffo et al, 2009)

It is necessary to understand that nurses must strive themselves working on a service geared to the real needs of the child and his family, seeking health education as a key point in all stages of care. Nurses' role as elements in the health team, imply in a more active attitude, appropriating new knowledge for nursing and practices. (Silva & Ferriani, 2007)

Knowing the perception that children who are victims of domestic violence have on family care is crucial to understand their development and relationship with other people. The authors add that this issue is also important to develop more specific and resolutive care strategies. These strategies should be guided the rebuilding of relationships and possibilities preservation of parental bonds and family reintegration. (Gababtz et al, 2010)

So, the planning, setting priorities, the survey of available resources are nursing actions that work as a lever to achieve the goals of health care for children and their families. For this, the family's involvement in all stages contributes to the success of care.

The singularity, habits, family dynamics, culture and social and financial situation of the family should be studied carefully so that the inclusion of nursing and health team for children and their caregivers are in line with the reality in which they live.

It is also important to emphasize that understanding an in-depth study of this phenomenon, taking into account its specificity, help nurses to think and act in a timely and proper posture in front of the child.(Ciuffo, 2008)

In this perspective, one aspect of great importance regarding the nurse's role when treating a child with suspected sexual abuse is the "care from the perspective of another." The authors noted that preserving patient avoiding them to be exposed in the ward, in order to minimize the trauma suffered with a sensitive and a special look that includes the family, is part of nursing care. (Ciuffo et al, 2009)

The nursing care has a broader significance for the human beings because it involves the relationship and interaction between people. When a nurse or any other professional is willing to help others to grow, to feel better, teaching them to become more independent they are taking care of them.

During the assistance of children with sexual abuse suspicion, the nurse has a valuable role and should seek to apply their scientific and technical knowledge to perform global care. So, it requires a deep study about this major public health problem in order to better direct nursing actions, making them more effective and focusing mainly on early detection and reducing the consequences.

Furhermore, research in the field of nursing focused on care for the child victim of sexual violence is of great importance, because it allows, not only to understand better experience of caring a child that lived such impacting phenomenon, but also to think about nurse's performance in this cases in order to improve it. (Voiski & Rocha, 2010)

We believe that listening carefully to the reports, explaining the consequences of sexual abuse in child health for the family are fundamental steps. In addition, using an appropriate vocabulary respecting the social and cultural context and beliefs is an interesting posture to be adopted by the nurse in their daily practice.

It is clear for us that if nurses act this way they will have more possibilities to increase the chances of making a follow-up with the child, ensuring continuity and systematization of nursing care.

Professional role is to guide families to other ways to educate and communicate with their children, and accompany them with respect and attention. However, there are aspects of social and economic context that transcend individual or family behavior. The community or social group where the children and adolescents live with their families affects directly their behavior. In this reasoning line it is essential to think about the role of social networks support as important fronts for work and interaction with family from the perspective of protection, defense and guarantee the rights of children and adolescents. (Brasil, 2010)

The professional intervention promotes physical and emotional health of children and adolescents in their process of growth and development, especially during times of major changes. So in the course of professional assistance, it is useful to highlight that the speech, the look, gestures, the information communicated in simple and accessible language can make a huge difference in building raport with the child. (Brasil, 2010)

Sexual violence must also be worked preventively, together with the family and their children. It is possible to make an approachment, using language that is appropriate to their ages and explaining the issue of sexuality and also the body touches socially appropriate and inappropriate between a child and someone older or adult. (Brasil, 2010)

3.4 The interdisciplinarity in the performance of health professionals in relation to suspected or confirmed cases of child sexual abuse

The detection sexual violence cases is a very important step, however, the institutions where children are assisted have to prepare and train professionals to offer an appropriate care for the child and his family. To help unravel the principle that the data are hidden in the cases treated, it is missing the vision of multiple causes of such violence. (Ciuffo, 2008)

Nursing actions can be thought as a driving force that propels nurses to develop researches in child health field. These researches may influence in a healthy growth and development in childhood. So, we agree that group actions with other professionals who work in the health care team are very important, because the chances of identifying health problems and needs related to them increases a lot.

Promoting interdisciplinary actions is vital to delivering an appropriate support, whose efforts should focus not only on physical examination and diagnosis, but also emotional and psychological support for the well-being of the individual, and in particular child who suffered domestic violence. The victimized child is very vulnerable because childhood is a stage of life where the greatest changes occur physically and psychologically. By these cahnges need to be followed in order to promote and maintain health, as well as the intervention on factors that could compromise it.(Grüdtner, 2005)

Nurses and others health professionals must understand that children may be brought to professional attention because of physical or behavioural concerns that, on further investigation, turn out to result from sexual abuse. (Krug et al, 2002)

In addiction, the authors above also affirm that to be able to detect child sexual abuse requires a high index of suspicion and familiarity with the verbal, behavioural and physical indicators of abuse. It is possible that many children will disclose abuse to caregivers or others spontaneously, though there may also be indirect physical or behavioural signs.

As a result of the study on nursing care of children with suspected sexual abuse, one of the categories that emerged from interviewees' speech was entitled "interact with other professionals in child care," where many subjects emphasized in their speeches that a step of great importance in the care of children who suffered sexual abuse lies in interdisciplinarity.(Ciuffo, 2008)

Joining forces with other professionals to provide a better service that is comprehensive, focused on the social, emotional and psychological aspects. In this perspective, it is possible to characterize the contribution of professionals of many different formations in attendance. (Ciuffo, 2008)

It is of great importance that the team of professionals from different fields comply with the trauma and pain produced by violence, considering that this phenomenon goes beyond the socio-cultural factors and also the legal, since violence interferes in the victim's psychological field and also in their family structure. (Carvalho et al 2009)

In the study on labor relations in interdisciplinary teams, the authors emphasize that the contribution of new forms of work organization in health. As a result of their study it was found that there are several factors that influence in improving the relationship between professionals and clients, some of them include: bonding, acceptance and quality care. (Matos et al 2009)

In this sense, it is possible to say that the routine of health professionals should include recognition of signs of various forms of violence against children. They also need to be aware that the approach of these situations involves the complexity . So, when suspecting or confirming the existence of ill treatment, try to keep in mind that not only skill is necessary, but also sensitivity and commitment to this cause. (Voiski & Rocha, 2010).

Undoubtedly, the above mentioned factors are of great importance in assisting interdisciplinary teams in health practice and also in attention to child and family. We would also add empathy, willingness to help, to hear and a comprehensive view at the problems of others. (Ciuffo, 2008)

The interdisciplinary team should seek to achieve weekly meetings in order to discuss the cases treated to facilitate and ensure the timing in attendance, allowing an integral and homogeneous comprehension by all professionals on every patient seen. Also according to these authors, "this work dynamic enables an actual vision of each work on violence, while ensuring higher quality of care to victims. (Mattar et al 2007)

Nurses should understand and prioritize the need of interaction with other professionals in attendance, seeking to find better solutions for their actions. Thus, it is also an opportunity to gain more support and acquire new knowledge from this interaction with other professionals. (Ciuffo, 2008)

There are many socio-cultural contradictions, family conflicts and professional dilemmas involved in violence situations. Exploring these interfaces represent that the professional has a commitment with the family, the aggressor and the child that experience violence in everyday life (Pierantoni, 2007). Thus, the task of monitoring the situations of violence requires the nurse and the interdisciplinary team to work in health education and skill development to each case of violence, the use of group discussions and a deep study to apply prevention and intervention of this issue towards a more effective approachment.

Every health professional has special moments of contact with children, adolescents and their families. For example: receipt, vaccines, bandages, health education and medical, dental, nursing or psychological care, home visits, among others.

The moments described above are appropriate and create favorable conditions to observe the existence of signs and symptoms that may be resultant of a violent situation. Also they promote the required care for the protection and welfare of the child and it is an opportunity to give orientation to families about prevention and how to overcome the violence. (Brasil, 2010)

It is necessary to develop reflections about the needs of studies that seek understand more clearly the complexity of different realities where violence occurs. However, there is a difficulty in understanding violence in different contexts, because each professional has a point of view of someone who has experienced it. But we also must expand our knowledge and also see the violence as a consequence of a complex relational dynamic. (Nunes et al 2008)

4. Conclusion

Through the present study, we could conclude that nursing staff and the multidicisciplinar team must be motivated by this problematic, directing the service for the necessities of the child who suffered violence. It is important to adopt a posture that enables the professional to give specialized attention, to listen and to agree on possible solutions for the problem, building an assistance with better quality.

Furthermore, we believe that extensive research in this area provides a broader perspective, which not only addresses to the symptoms and signs, but also searches tools to identify the clinical features and history of violence.

Nurses should contribute with the nursing staff guiding their care. It is primordial exercise an especially attentive listening and careful observation for the child who suffered sexual violence. It is also important to be available to understand the attitudes, postures, verbal and non verbal expressions of children and their families, which might have significant meanings.

Nursing is considered as a social practice which is committed to emancipation and human development. In this thought line, it cannot be performed outside the perspective of the complexity of transformations in the contemporary social context. So, it must include the integral and multidisciplinary approach of domestic violence against children. (Silva & Ferriani, 2007)

In this sense, studies are necessary for establishing national and international parameters and more precise drawings about the risk factors and prevention. We believe that still exist a gap in nursing actions. So, the studies in this area are very important, since every time the nurses can't detect a sexual abuse suspicion, they are colluding with the possible recurrences. It is important to remember that other types of violence may also be present in that child's life.

In addition, we believe it is essential to rethink public health policies in order to develop new actions that would not only prevent the phenomenon, but also protect the victims, avoiding the appearance of new recurrences and promoting the health of children and their families.

The situation of child sexual abuse is undoubtedly a great challenge today. If society isn't interest in understanding violence, its magnitude and its density, there will never be appropriate tools to fight it, or care for its victims. (Carvalho et al, 2009)

It can be reaffirmed that domestic violence against children and its nuances impose themselves as an exercise to understand the current dynamics of the family and society. The theme is complex and, given its complexity, knowledge about it is still under construction. (Silva & Ferriani, 2007)

The study above aimed at assessing information systems to accompany the magnitude of the problem, that attempt to improve a theoretical-analytic reference framework that is capable of permitting an understanding of the specific nature of this phenomenon today, the vulnerability and protection factors which different cultures and societies have in common.

The restitution of the child's self-esteem, reframing the moral values of children and family and a deep reflection on the training of individuals in society are points to be observed, studied and analyzed by all of us as human beings.

It is necessary trained professionals who can investigate and take appropriate tools to apply in resolving this type of violence, we must take the allegations seriously. We believe it is substantial special units in police departments, special public prosecutor to alert the school professionals to be vigilant to signs of identification of cases.

Cases of violence are increasingly closer to the daily lives of people. Every day appears stories of violence in media and this phenomenon has assumed a social problem. Thus, health professionals can not be indifferent to this situation and should position itself as a facilitator and organizer in the network of support and protection for victims. (Luna et al, 2010)

We understand that child sexual abuse and various types of family violence can be avoided if health professionals, with the support of education professionals, police, government officials know how to recognize suggestive signs in these situations.

The development of multisectoral and multidisciplinary actions in order to have a closer look into the risk factors of sexual violence in childhood allied to prevention of recurrence of the cases can be a feasible path to help solve this collective problem.

Governments have an important role to play in public education efforts, national and also international campaigns carrying the message that abused children have rights and that there are ways to prevent and avoid not only sexual abuse but all aspects expressed by violence.

From the statement above is interesting to reflect on possibilities to act in advance. We must think about prevention, the way is by investigating profiles and main characteristics of violence. Moreover, understanding the context and the circumstances in which the violence occurs facilitates the intervention's planning.

In this perspective, we must pay attention to the risk factors above when we are in nursing assistance. It is also of great importance hearing the victim's story and try to contextualize the problem, seeking the most appropriate solutions.

Challenging violence requires an effective integration of different sectors such as health, security, justice and education, as well as the involvement of civil society organizations. (Inoue & Ristum, 2008)

As conclusion it was point out the relevance of this theme. Everyone can exercise their co-participation in the protection of children, who are in the phase of growth and development. This study also suggests new researches to supplement gaps in knowledge and improve children's quality of life. (Martins, 2010)

Professionals who deal with children need to be engaged in various everyday issues that affect the lives and health of human beings. For that to happen, there must be an "awakening of consciousness" through studies, training and practice that every day throws us new challenges to overcome. We think that life itself invites us to learn new lessons every obstacle, thus enabling the reflection, a rethinking of old concepts no longer apply to the practice, and the need to be guided by the construction of new knowledges considering the inexorable changes in society and science advances.

5. References

Aded, N.; Dalcin, B.; Cavalcante, M. (2007) Sexual abuse of children and adolescents in Rio de Janeiro, Brazil: an incidence study. *Cad. Saúde Pública*, vol.23, no.8, (August. 2007). pp.1971-1975. ISSN 0102-311X

Bassani, D et al. (2009).Child sexual abuse in southern Brazil and associated factors: a population-based study. *BMC Public Health,* vol.9 , no. 133 (May 2009) Available at : http://www.biomedcentral.com/1471-2458/9/133/prepub

Brasil. (2002). *Notification of maltreatment against children and adolescents by health professionals: a further step toward citizenship in health.* Brasília: Ministério da Saúde, ISBN 85-334-0499-9. Brasília.

Brasil. (2010). *Line of care for integral health care of children, adolescents and their families in situations of violence: guidance for managers and health professionals.* Brasília: Ministério da Saúde, ISBN 978-85-334-1688-8. Brasília.

Carvalho, Q; Galvão, M; Cardoso, M. Child sexual abuse: The perceptions of mothers concerning their daughters' sexual abuse. *Rev. Latino-Am. Enfermagem*, vol. 17, no.4, (July/August 2009) pp.501-506. ISSN 0104-1169

Ciuffo, L.(2008). *Nursing care of children with suspected sexual abuse.* . Dissertation Rio de Janeiro, Brazil.

Ciuffo, L., Rodrigues, B., Cunha, J. (2009). The nurse in sexual abuse child suspicion attention: a phenomenology approach. *Online Brazilian Journal of Nursing,* vol. 8, no.3 (November 2009) ISSN 1676-4285 Available at: <http://www.objnursing.uff.br/index.php/nursing/article/view/j.1676-4285.2009.2665/572>.

Drezett, J. (2007). Sexual violence as a public health problem.. In: TAQUETTE, S. (Org.). *Violence against women, adolescent/young.* UERJ, ISBN 978-85-7511-107-9.

Gabatz, R.; Neves, E; Beuter, M; Padoin, S. (2010). The meaning of care for children victims of domestic violence. *Esc Anna Nery Rev Enferm,* vol. 14, no.1, (January/ Febuary 2010) pp 135-42, ISSN 1414-8145

Galvão, C.; Sawada, N.; Trevisan, M (2004). Systematic review: a resource that allows for the incorporation of evidence into nursing practice. *Rev. Latino-Am. Enfermagem,* vol.12, no.3, (May/ June 2004) pp.549-556. ISSN 0104-1169

Grüdtner, D.I. (2005) *Domestic Violence against children and adolescents: reflections on nurses' care.* Thesis. Florianópolis, Brazil.

Habigzang, L. et al. (2005) . Sexual Abuse Against Children and Family Dynamics: Juridical Processes of a Public Prosecution Service. *Psic.: Teor e Pesq.,* vol. 21, no. .3, (December 2005) pp.341- 348. ISSN 0102-3772

Inoue, S.; Ristum, M.(2008) Sexual violence: description and analysis of cases detected in the school environment. *Estud. psicol.,* vol.25, no.1 (January./March 2008) pp.11-21. ISSN 0103-166X

Krug, E. et al. (2002). *World report on violence and health.* World Health Organization, ISBN 92 4 154561 5, Geneva.

Luna, G; Parente, E; Moreira, D; Vieira, L. (2010). Reporting child and adolescent maltreatment: official discourse and professional practice. *Rev. enferm. UERJ,* vol. 18, no. 1 (January / March 2010) pp 148-152. ISSN 0104-3552

Magalhães, A. (2005). *Incestuous sexual abuse: a theme centered on the child and family.* Letra Capital, ISBN 9788586568671, Rio de Janeiro.

Martins, C.(2010). Maltreatmens against children and teenagers. *Rev. bras. enferm.* vol. 63, no.4 ,(July / August 2010) pp. 660-665. ISSN 0034-7167

Matos, E; Pires, D; Campos, G. (2009). Work relationships among interdisciplinary teams: contributions for new methods of organization in health work. *Rev Brás Enferm,* vol. 62, no. 6, (November/ December 2009) pp. 863-869. ISSN 0034-7167

Mattar, R et al. (2007). Multidisciplinary care for victims of sexual assault: the experience at the Federal University in São Paulo, Brazil. *Cad. Saúde Pública,* vol.23, no.2,(February. 2007) pp. 459-464. ISSN 0102-311X

Moura, F ; Lisboa, M. (2005). Violence, the workplace and public health nurse. *Esc. Anna Nery. R. Enferm.,* vol. 9, no.1, (April 2005) pp. 108 -115. ISSN 1414-8145 .

Nunes, C; Sarti, C; Ohara C. (2008) Conceptions held by health professionals on violence against children and adolescents within the family. *Rev Latino-am Enfermagem,* vol. 16, no. 1 (January / March 2008) pp 136-141. ISSN 0104-1169

Pierantoni, L.(2007). *(Des) paths guard of children in violent situations: subsidies for nursing action in the health team*. Dissertation. Rio de Janeiro, Brazil.

Silva, M; Ferriani, M.(2007) Domestic violence: from the visible to the invisible. *Rev. Latino-Am. Enfermagem* vol.15, no.2 (March./April 2007) pp.275-281. ISSN 0104-1169

Woiski, R; Rocha, D. (2010). Nursing care for sexually abused children in hospital emergency units. *Esc. Anna Nery*, vol.14, no.1, (January/March 2010) pp. 143-150..ISSN 1414-8145

Part 3

Culturally Diverse Attitudes in Coping with Assault

11

Coping with an Experience of Child Sexual Abuse: Perspectives of Young Female Survivors in South Africa

Nareadi Phasha
University of South Africa
South Africa

1. Introduction

An experience of sexual abuse in childhood is known to be associated with negative emotional, psychological, health/physical, and educational repercussions. Internationally, research suggests that the repercussions may be immediate and/or long term (Finkelhor, 1979; 1984; 1988, 1984; Sgroi, 1982). Similar findings were evident in South African studies (Russell, 1995; Collings, 1995, Madu & Peltzer, 2001, Human Rights Watch, 2001). Studies have gone further to reveal that some survivors turn out to be resilient (Barbarin, Ritcher & de Wet, 2003; van Rensburg & Barnard, 2005). The suggestion thereof is that survivors cope with the problem in different ways which may or may not be detrimental to their development.

This chapter will focus on strategies which some of the young survivors of child sexual abuse utilised to cope with their experiences and emotions associated with it. Coping strategies warrant a deeper understanding for the sake of helping survivors heal the wounds created by an experience of child sexual abuse, to prevent chances of re-victimization, and to facilitate wellness. For the purpose of this chapter, coping refers to a conscious process for managing a problem and regulating the attendant emotion (Gipple, Lee & Puig, 2006).

2. Coping strategies

Different coping strategies which could be classified under two broad categories were noted in the literature consulted, namely: emotion-focused and problem-focused. According to Gipple *et al.* (2006), emotion-focused coping strategies include purposeful attempts to retreat from unpleasant stimuli, or individuals' attempt to regulate their emotions in dealing with the stressor; while problem-focused strategies entail manipulation, reflection and application of instrumental responses of the stressor.

Studies suggest frequent tendencies to use emotion-focused. This was so in the study that involved female incest survivors as participants (Brands & Alexander, 2003). In particular, avoidance was the most preferred coping strategy, which participants indicated to have used in childhood when the abuse was occurring and later in adult life when the feelings resurfaced. Also, Sigmond, Greene, Rohan, and Nichols (1996) revealed that whether the abuse was recent or had occurred a long time ago, participants' preference for emotion-focused coping strategies remained evident, and even at the time of the study participants were still using those strategies.

Csoboth, Birtas and Purebl's (2003) findings obtained from women with histories of physical and sexual abuse, revealed tendencies to indulge in heavy eating, drinking and smoking habits in comparison to their non-abused counterparts. Interestingly, women with experiences of sexual abuse consumed larger amounts of alcohol than those with physical abuse histories and their non-abused counterparts. In addition, sexual abuse by an important person, such as one's close relative, and a fear of someone in the environment contributed to increased alcohol consumption. Tendencies to resort to high consumptions of alcohol and substances in order to dull and numb painful emotions were also identified amongst male survivors of sexual abuse (Valente, 2005). Alongside such tendencies were also suicide and self-mutilation which surfaced when feelings of anxiety and self-loathing were overwhelming. Resorting to self-injurious behaviours and suicidal ideation and attempts were common coping strategies amongst younger males (16 years) and female survivors who were highly depressed as a result of feeling despair and lacking a sense of hopefulness (Swanston, Nunn, Oates, Tebbut & O'Toole, 1999). Dissociation was adopted amongst participants with intense feeling of shame (Talbot, Talbot & Tu Xi, 2004). Instances of resorting to dispositional optimism were noted in a sample, whose experiences of traumatic events, including sexual abuse, yielded intense feelings of depression (Brodhagen & Wise, 2008).

Some male survivors coped with the experience of sexual abuse by assuming the role of a passive victim syndrome, becoming angry avenger especially if they believed someone has to pay for what had happened to them, seeking emotional ties with people of the same age as their abuser with the hope of rebuilding the disrupted emotional ties, and/or becoming conformists to cover up their insecurities by blocking out the memories of the abuse and so creating a persona of the 'normal guy next door' (Valente, 2005). Frazier and Burnett's (1994) study revealed four types of coping strategies, namely: (a) seeking social support, (b) talking about the rape, (c) getting counselling and (d) keeping busy. The most commonly used strategies included taking precautions and thinking positively. According to Fallot and Heckman (2005), there are some tendencies to resort to religious/spiritual coping among women survivors with mental health substance disorder. Unfortunately to most survivors of sexual abuse such religious strategies were more negative than positive. Also, there were reports of various positive resolutions such as: a learned experience, personal growth and development, spiritual, moral/religious growth, increased knowledge of sexual abuse, improved relationships with others, interpersonal sensitivity, such as being more accepting and less judgemental of others (Wright, Crawford & Sebastian, 2007).

3. Method

The coping strategies reported in this chapter were obtained from a qualitative study conducted in South Africa. Being qualitative in nature, the study endorsed an interpretative epistemological assumption which holds the view that research should attempt to grasp or understand the meaning of social phenomena (Schwandt, 1994), referring to interpretation in terms of participants' own beliefs, history and context (Babbie & Mouton, 2009). For that matter, data was collected in the form of words and the presentation of findings took the form of description (Neuman, 1994). The study followed an iterative process, which resembles the features of grounded theory in generative questions were posed, core theoretical concepts were developed and tentative relationships were developed by constantly comparing data throughout data collection (Glaser & Strauss, 1967).

3.1 Participants

This chapter presents the views of a fraction of the 22 students who took part in a study conducted in South Africa for the purpose of understanding the implications of childhood sexual abuse on school functioning. Their selection for this study was on the basis that interviews with them revealed information covering coping strategies. In addition, they participated in interviews on more than one occasions, and this afforded me an opportunity to probe and tease out emerging issues. Participants were 12 young female participants belonging to three racial groups in South Africa: White (4), Coloured/mixed racial parentage (4) and Blacks (4).

Participation was voluntary following a thorough explanation of the study and research ethics, namely: benefits of the study, the rights to withdraw from the study at anytime without negative consequences. Participants were assured confidentiality by explaining that raw data will not be shared with anyone, including institution-based social workers. However, I indicated my intention to share the research findings during conferences and in peer-reviewed journals. I assured them that their names will be protected by replacing them with fictitious names. Before data collection, I cautioned participants about uncomfortable emotions that could be evoked by the interviews, and also, mentioned that there would be therapeutic support. I also provided them with a list of psychological services in their areas, should they prefer to use them.

Participants' ages range between 16 and 23 years. Recruitment was by means of referrals, which began with social workers based at the institutions. The sample increased as participants invited others to the study by means of invitation letter prepared by the researcher. In the letter, I made it clear to them that I did not know them but the person who is handing them the letter was of the opinion that they might share views which are relevant to the study. Included in the invitation letter was a self-addressed stamped envelop to use when responding to the researcher. The referral strategy generated a quick sample in a relatively small time because it came out that they knew about each other's experiences as they often talk to one another about reasons for being placed at those institutions. They also meet during group session therapies an attend school together. Participant-perpetrator age gap was more than 5 years, and the abuse involved penetration of the private parts. Participants' detailed descriptions are provided on Table 1. To protect their identity the names used in this study are fictitious and different from those appearing in the main study.

Student	Race	Perpetrator	Age of abuse	Duration
Cathrine (15)	White	Neighbour	13 years	2 years
Izora (18)	White	Biological father	6 years	6 years
Reetha (16)	White	School principal	14 years	1 year
Violin (16)	White	Biological father	10 years	4 years
Patricia (15)	Coloured	Stepfather	10 years	4 years
Shawa (16)	Coloured	Stepfather	12 years	4 years
Galata (16)	Coloured	Biological father	13 years	4 years
Mighty (16)	Coloured	Biological father	14 years	2 years
Hippy (23)	Black	Uncle and Mother's boyfriend	6 years 16 years	6 years 2 years
Nachos (18)	Black	Abducted and gang-raped by four men	16 years	7 days
Pheladi (15)	Black	Abducted and raped	14 years	Two weeks
Moira (16)	Black	Biological father, and Foster father	7 years 12 years	3 years 1 year

Table 1. Description of participants

3.2 Instruments

The in-depth interview was a sole method used to collect data. The interviews took place with each participant at a private office specifically allocated for this purpose by each social welfare institution. The only student who was not living at any of the institutions was interviewed at her home when her mother was at work and her sister was at school. In-depth interviews facilitated openness on the part of participants because they did not have to worry about what the next person would say about their views. Data were collected in bits, guided by categories identified in the previous interview with the same or different participant. Interviews were tape-recorded with the permission of participants and the social workers who acted as a legal guardian (in case of participants younger than 18 years), following a detailed explanation about the study and adherence to research ethics. To enhance the credibility of the study, all participants were interviewed on more than two occasions. In this way, I was able to verify data collected in the previous interview with participants.

To facilitate prompt follow-up of interesting issues, I carried data collection and analysis simultaneously. I listen to each tape on number of occasions to identify what was emerging. This was followed by full transcription of the recorded tape. Transcribed data were sent back to them for verification. Data were then coded and categorised according to themes. Comparisons of categories and sub-categories occurred throughout data analysis, relationships and sequences of events were also established (Dey, 1993; Charmaz, 2006). To minimised researcher bias, a critical friend was asked to check the analysed data.

4. Results

In dealing with emotions created by an experience of child sexual abuse, participants adopted three forms of strategies, namely: (a) detachment from the sexual abuse or its impact, (b) distorted beliefs about the experience and (c) acknowledgement of sexual abuse. In presenting the results, participants' quotes were used. Readers should be aware that as English was not the home language of most participants, marked deviations from the standard forms of expression should be expected.

4.1 Detachment from sexual abuse or its impact

Detachment describes tendencies to dissociate from thinking about the experience of sexual abuse. A total of eight participants reported that they had achieved such a state by engaging in either one or two of the following strategies: (a) keeping busy at all times, (b) using drugs, (c) engaging in unhealthy eating habits and/or (d) self mutilation, so as to obliterate the memories of their experience.

Three participants, namely Pheladi, Mighty and Galata indicated keeping themselves busy in different ways. Pheladi (15), a Black girl, was raped on two occasions by different males. Her first experience of abuse involved abduction and rape for a week by a local young man when she was 13 years old. She mentioned that none of her relatives was supportive, but rather that they laughed at her and told her that she deserved it. Her second experience occurred when she was 14 years, and it involved being used for prostitution by a friend for a period of two weeks. She indicated that when the memories of sexual abuse surfaced, she kept herself busy by *"avoiding sitting alone because I know exactly that* (the memory of sexual abuse *it is going to come back to me. So, I'll rather be with other people and play, laugh and make jokes with them.* Similarly, *a* 16 year-old Coloured girl, Mighty, whose sexual abuse by her biological father began when she was 14 and lasted for 2 years, indicated that:

> *Playing with other children stops the thought about that man (her father). I just feel like a child again, and in that way, I forget for a while because we are talking about parties and other interesting things.*

Also, Galata (16), a Coloured girl who had been abused by her biological father for 4 years since the age of 13, highlighted that *"I just get up and walk around the class. Sometimes, I initiate a conversation with whoever is around me and this stops my mind from thinking about the abuse"*.

Evidently, actions to keep themselves busy were initiated when it was neither appropriate nor necessary, and the idea was to escape being quiet as such an opportunity could trigger memories of the abuse. It was common for their minds to wonder about the abuse during lessons, as that was the time they were required to be silent and attentive. However, any action taken to keep busy subjected them to punishment, as they were seen to be disturbing the lessons or their classmates.

Another strategy for detaching themselves from abuse involved indulging in unhealthy eating habits, whereby participants starved themselves or overate. Two survivors, Patricia and Hippy, adopted such a tendency when their thoughts about sexual abuse became intense. Patricia, a 15-year old Coloured girl who had been abused by her stepfather for 4 years since the age of 10, and later raped by a stranger in her own neighborhood, indicated that she had starved herself. She particularly highlighted coping by

> *"Vomiting and making sure that everything I eat does not go down my throat. Food just came out when I was trying to eat".*

In contrast, Hippy, (23) a black survivor, resorted to over-eating. She was abused by her uncle from age 6 - 12 when she moved to live with her aunt in another village. She indicated that the abuse by her uncle was frequent (almost every day). Following her parents' divorce at age 14, she moved from her aunt's place to stay with her mother, whose living-in boyfriend also abused Hippy frequently. She explained that:

> *I overate and I still do. If I do not have anyone to speak to, I eat a lot, and that is why I became this big. I consoled myself with food and I still do. I just eat and eat.*

A feature common to both these participants was that their perpetrators were close relatives other than their biological parents. Again, their abuse involved frequent episodes which occurred over a lengthy period. They were abused by more than one perpetrator. In addition, they both reported having received no support from their mothers. For example, Patricia's mother asked her to remain silent because the family depended on her stepfather for financial assistance. Also, Hippy's mother dismissed her disclosure of abuse by her uncle, and warned her that it would cause "trouble in the family". She was also accused by her mother and her other aunt of being a liar when she disclosed the abuse by her mother's boyfriend. These factors could have caused intense feelings of anger from being betrayed by a trusted parent who could not protect them from further abuse, and led the body to respond to the sexual demands of the perpetrator. As a way to escape the feelings that had been bottled up for long, they resorted to unhealthy eating habits.

To some participants, detachment from abuse was achieved by being involved in self-injurious behaviours. This was reported by two White students, namely, Cathrine (15) and Izora (18), who reported that they hurt themselves to suppress the overwhelming memories of sexual abuse. Cathrine had been sexually abused by a neighbour who babysitted her. The abuse went on for 2 year without being disclosed, and it occurred alongside threats to kill her mother if she ever attempted to disclose. Izora was abused by her biological father for a period of 6 years, when she and her three sisters were finally placed at a Safety Home for neglect. None of her relatives, including her mother, knew about the abuse. She only disclosed it to the social worker following her placement at a Safety Home. Unfortunately for her, she rarely discussed it, and the opportunities for therapy were not afforded to her. Cathrine indicated that "*I bite myself, and sometimes I cut my wrist to make myself feel better*". Similarly, Izora highlighted that:

> *A lot of times I bite myself on my hand because of this thing keeps on coming back and because I am feeling so stressed out. It is terrible. I think I hit my head once against the wall. But, otherwise I bite myself when I am tips up.*

A lack of space to share one's frustrations could trigger self-blaming attitudes, which could in turn manifest themselves in a sense of guilt. This is because speaking up enables one to release emotions which could have been bottled up for a long time. In addition, a person could get positive feedback to help him/her realize that the abuse was not her/his fault.

To Patricia and Reetha, drugs helped them repress the memories of sexual abuse. Reetha, a 16 year old White girl was molested by the school principal who acted as an adoptive parent during the time she and her sister were living in a Safety Home. The school principal often invited her (and her sister) to his farm during weekends and holidays, with the permission of the Safety Home (The Safety Home did not know about the abuse). Both Patricia and Reetha mentioned using one or more of the following: drug, cigarettes, dagga, benzene, glue, nail polish remover and alcohol. Patricia started using drugs and drinking liquor when she was 11 years old, whereas Reetha began at age 12. Patricia smoked dagga and cigarettes at home and at school. While she confessed that she smoked dagga every day, she also mentioned that:

> *I smoked glue and I was also smoking benzene, nail polish remover and drinking beers with my friends just to make myself feel happy, but I won't feel happy.*

Similarly, Reetha mentioned that:

> *I started smoking dagga and all sorts of things because I thought it will take my problems away. But if you are out of that thing, you will still remember what happened to you again.*

It is evident that both Patricia and Reetha started using drugs when abuse was occurring, which could imply that the strategy was motivated by the need to numb their feeling of powerlessness to stop it. As indicated in the previous section, Patricia's mother dismissed the disclosure on the basis that if it could be reported to authorities, her husband would be jailed and the family would loose their only source of income. Also, with Reetha, she feared losing the love and care of the principal who her and her sister had come to trust and regard as a parent figure. Moreover, her sister did not know about the abuse. The Safety Home saw the school principal as giving the girls an opportunity to be in a real home environment. Such a situation could have instilled feelings of anxiety stemming from frequent anticipation that the abuse could happen again. Also, an awareness that there was nothing they could do to stop the occurrence of abuse could render the victimized person powerless, and leave them with no choice but to respond to the sexual demands of the perpetrator. Feelings of powerlessness and anxiety could even heighten depressive feelings. Desperation to numb overwhelming depressive feelings and to avoid facing up to problems causing those feelings could easily push a person to use drugs as the quickest remedy (Leigh, 1998). It is therefore not unusual for sexually abused participants to use drugs when dealing with the emotions caused by such an experience.

4.2 Distorted beliefs about the experience of sexual abuse

There was evidence to suggest that some survivors coped with their experience and memories of sexual abuse by creating distorted "positive" beliefs about their experiences. This was evidenced by their positive talks about the abuser, seeking positive reasons for the occurrence of the abuse and a perception of the abuse as a learning experience. Four students reported such beliefs, namely, Galata, Hippy, Patricia and Violin. Distorted beliefs diminished feelings such as anger, self-blame, guilt, and ultimately led to forgiveness, and the proper functioning of an individual. Galata indicated that when the abuse stopped and she was placed at the Safety Home for over a year, she could no longer cry when the memory of her sexual abuse by her biological father surfaced. Rather, she found herself talking positively about her father and the good thing that he did for them before the abuse occurred. In her own words, she highlighted that *"I just talk about my father as if we had a good relationship. In particular, I would focus only on the good things and never talk about the bad things.*

Speaking positively about the abuser facilitated survivors' forgiveness. Distorted "positive" thinking was common amongst participants who had been living in the Safety Home for more than a year. Interestingly, such a thought occurred when participants found themselves in the midst of peers who had good relationships with their families. These included situations where their non-abused peers at school shared stories of activities they did with their parents during holidays, weekends and other times at their homes, and when parents had come to watch their children playing games at schools. In this way, it can be assumed that a longing to live in a real family situation facilitated distorted "positive" thinking about their abusive fathers.

Therapy and regular visits to home when the abusive parent was jailed for sexual abuse appeared to have facilitated a different perception about the abuser and the abuse itself. Two participants, namely Patricia and Violin provided good examples. Patricia, who was angry towards her mother who could not recue her from the abuse by her father, indicated that when she started visiting home regularly, she realized that "*It is not right for a child to not talk to her mother or father because there are no parents who do not like their own child*". On the same note, Violin (16), White and abused by her biological father for four years from the age of 10, she expressed being angry towards her mother for allowing her abusive father to come into their lives after abusing her for the second time. She particularly, mentioned that therapy had changed her negative thoughts about her father and made her believe and accept when her mother told her that she needed her father. She said:

> *After a while when my mum told me that she, my brother and I need my dad, I started thinking about that very seriously. I realized that a daughter cannot live without her dad and when I got to know my father better and went for therapy sessions, I learned a lot of things like, the daughter need a father for protection.*

Although the impact of therapy cannot be dismissed in having facilitated positive thoughts about their abusive parents, nor can the impact of their non-abusive mothers and home conditions be underestimated, particularly as they started visiting home during the holidays and at weekends. The time spent at home permitted the bond between their mothers to strengthen and their trust in them grew, so they accepted their mothers' plea to forgive their abusive fathers. In addition, as their non-abusive parents were not working, it might have been that when Patricia and Violin visited their homes, they realized that their families needed their fathers in order to survive. Clearly, the contribution all these factors might have contributed to Patricia and Violin's distorted beliefs about their abusive fathers.

A distorted belief about the experience of sexual abuse took a form of finding a reason for it to occur. This was demonstrated by Hippy, who suffered multiple experiences of sexual abuse at different times in her life. She mentioned that when the memories of sexual abuse were too intense, she told herself that "*God does not let things happen for no apparent reason*". She further indicated that she believed that God has allowed the abuse to happen to her so that one day "*when I know a little girl that is in the same situation as I was, then I would be able to help them*".

Hippy's perception of her experience made her stronger and even more hopeful of the future. She also realized that her uncle, who had abused her since she was 6, needed help, and indicated that she had forgiven her mother for failing to protect her from abuse.

4.3 Acknowledgments of the occurrence of abuse

In contrast to participants who created distorted "positive beliefs" about their experiences, some coped with the experience by coming to terms with its occurrence. Seven participants demonstrated this coping strategy in ways that reflected the following: (a) the perception of the abuse as a learning experience, and (b) talking about it, and adopting an optimistic view about life. An 18-year old Black survivor, Nacho, overcame the negative impact of her two weeks abduction and gang rape ordeal by four men, by viewing her experience as a learning curve, which opened her eyes to reality. During the interview session, she highlighted that she no longer took life for granted.

It changed me. I was naïve, not thinking that such a thing exists or it can ever happen to me. The rape taught me to be careful all the time, and that the world is not safe.

Nachos' perceptions of her sexual abuse could explain the reason she mentioned that she was eager to talk about her experiences in public, so as to enlighten other people about the existence of abuse. She mentioned that she wished to talk about her experiences on a television show, as well a having a book written about her experiences. Perceiving the experience of sexual abuse as a learning experience could be associated with the support that Nacho received from her mother and teachers at her school, including her former primary school. Support mitigated feelings of self-blame and guilt because a person comes to realizes that she is not held responsible for what happened. In that way, feelings of acceptance are facilitated.

Talking about the sexual abuse also signifies that a person has acknowledged what has happened and s/he is ready to move on. Patricia and Violin coped by talking to someone about their sexual abuse whenever they experienced flashbacks. People who were there to listen included peers, professionals, and parents. The effectiveness of such a strategy was clear when Patricia asserted that *"I just talk to my friends about it and I will forget for a while"*. On the same note, Violin indicated that *"I talk about my problems and when I do so, it makes me stronger and I want to go on with life again"*. Interestingly, Moira (16), who had been sexually abused by her biological father for three years from the age of 7 years, and later at 12 by a foster parent for a year, alluded to talking indirectly about her experiences.

I would tell someone that this friend of mine is going through this and that, what can I do to help her? But actually I was referring to myself. Then they would give me an advice. This method helped me bear the pain of the abuse.

Talking about the abuse is possible and could be effective when the listener is non-judgmental and s/he is capable of comforting the person who has experience of sexual abuse. As demonstrated in the previous section (distorted beliefs about the experience of sexual abuse), therapy played a major role in alleviating their feelings of anger and in helping the victims come to terms with their experience of sexual abuse. Such a situation could boost confidence to talk openly about their experiences of abuse.

On the other hand, three participants reported that they had adopted an optimistic attitude when they felt hopeless to stop the abuse and/or when the memories of their abuse were triggered. They hung on to the hope that their situation was temporary and that they would survive. Such an attitude was reported by Galata, Hippy and Shawa. Galata was unable to stop the sexual abuse because her father was hitting her and threatening to kill her mother if she attempted to disclose the abuse. Teachers did not belief her story but rather they protected her father who was their colleague. Her mother did not get to know about her abuse because she was not living with Galata and her abusive father. She was on her own. Galata mentioned that she was suicidal; however optimism had helped her to dismiss the thought of committing suicide. She declared that:

I told myself to be strong and that one day I will come out of it and I will open my heart and talk what is really going on with me. About the killing stuff [suicide], I just thought to myself that it is not a good idea. It won't solve my problem and where would my soul go? Well my body will go under the ground. Where will my soul go to because it will not rest?

Similarly, when Hippy's aunt and uncle ill-treated, insulted and threw her out of their house, she did not give up school. She mentioned that, as she was thrown out, the thought of becoming a prostitute came to her mind, but she dismissed it as she thought the practice would confirm her relatives' perceptions about her. She adopted the belief that things would change when she said:

Every time when things were tough, I used to say one day it will happen to me and I will be a better someone.

For example, when the social worker in Shawa's village did nothing about her disclosure and failed to honour the appointments she had made. Shawa demonstrated optimism when she persisted in finding protection rather than feeling discouraged. She sought help from a local clinic:

This year, I have decided that my whole life has been messed up. I do not want to see my social worker again because every time when I make appointments she says come on Monday or on Tuesday or Wednesday, and I would not find her. I promised myself that I will not give up on it. I am not going to give up on finding help for myself, but I am gonna leave this social worker and find someone else.

It is apparent that optimism was common among participants who lacked support and had received negative reactions when seeking help for their situation. In such circumstances, participants did not allow themselves to be discouraged.

5. Discussion

This study revealed strategies which fall into three categories, namely: (a) detachment from abuse, (b) distorted beliefs about the abuse/abuser, and (c) acknowledgement of the occurrence of abuse. Differences were noted in terms of strategies used when support was available and when there was no support. Detachment, the strategy that temporarily distances a person from the abuse, was often practiced by participants who had no form of support. These included participants who were abused by their parents and/or when their disclosure of sexual abuse was not believed or taken seriously by a trusted non-abusive parent/adult. This provides evidence for Kelly's (1988) assertion that forgetting is a consequence of a lack of understanding and social support. The suggestion is that they had no safe and comfortable platform to vent their frustrations, probably because of fear of family disruptions or defiling the family name. The fact that incestuous families tend to restrict the children's social interaction with non-family members (Finkelhor, 1979) could also be the reason some participants resorted to silence when there was no one to listen to their disclosure. Hence, they resorted to risky behaviours such as running away, drug use, self-injury and unhealthy eating habits.

Detachment from abuse and distorted beliefs are temporary strategies to suppress the emotional pain. Kelly (1988) warned that when someone tried to forget, he or she would repeatedly be reminded about their abuse through dreams and flashbacks. Physical pain inflicted on themselves in the form of self-injury and unhealthy eating habits signified participants' difficulty in coping with their memories and experiences of sexual abuse and are created by such an experience. Resorting to self-destructive behaviour helped them gain some relief from unbearable emotions related to the experience or memories of sexual abuse. For some victims it may be a way of attacking a despised object, namely their body, which they feel is defiled and no longer their own, whilst other victims are punishing themselves for their perceived guilt (Doyle, 1995).

Keeping busy and running away are strategies used to flee from realities of constant memories or persistent abuse. A child who has exhausted all sources of help believes that the only solution is to run away from home (Sgroi, 1982). Mrazek and Mrazek (1987) warned that although dissociation temporarily allows a child to function, if it persists it may have negative consequences for the development of future relationships. Remembering, acknowledging and working through experiences of sexual abuse are crucial processes if victims are to be able to deal positively with their past (Kelly, 1988: p.193). Indeed, participants in Hemelein and McElrath's (1996) study found that women who had adjusted well had talked about their sexual abuse to their friends or family members.

The perception of sexual abuse as a learning experience, talking about it, and expressing optimism reflect participants' acknowledgement of the sexual abuse. Participants who construe sexual abuse as a learning experience can review their own behaviour at the time of crisis and focus on more adaptive responses (Mrazek & Mrazek, 1987). However, they warned that if the strategy of treating the abuse as a learned experience is not checked, it could lead to a serious loss of reality. In the same vein, if talking about abuse is met with negativity, the survivor can further be damaged psychologically.

It was interesting to note racial differences in terms of the types of strategies adopted by participants. Black students avoided pain-inflicting tendencies, such as self-injury, drug use and starving. Instead, they justified the occurrence of the abuse, acknowledged its occurrence, and remained optimistic about the future. This could be rooted in African beliefs about misfortunes, tragedies and unpleasant events. Mbiti (1969:201) noted that in an African worldview, nothing harmful happens by chance; unpleasant events are caused by someone (a witch) and/or mystical power of religious nature. He further clarified that 'a divine authority' is perceived as the only solution to such misfortunes. Such beliefs could exert a greater impact in alleviating feelings of self-blame and guilt, in the sense that the responsibility for the occurrence of the abuse does not lie with the survivor. For that reason a person becomes motivated to fight the evil using religious-related strategies.

On the contrary, White and Coloured students reported self-injury and using drugs, talking about the abuse and distorted "positive" ideas about the abusers. These strategies could be linked to an individualistic worldview, commonly embraced by most White people, including Coloured people whom, Hickson and Kriegler (1999) indicated as having a culture more similar to Afrikaans speaking group than Africans or Indians in South Africa. In an individualistic worldview, self-reliance is greatly espoused. It centralizes the personal namely, personal goals, personal uniqueness, and personal control while peripheralizing the social (Williams, 2003: p.370). A human being is treated as capable of existing and flourishing on his/her own (Letseka, 2000). Evidently, an individualistic lifestyle could minimize the person's chances of benefiting from social support by people other than close relatives. For that matter, abused persons may struggle on their own to rescue themselves from the abusive situation. For young children with no resources or capability to deal with the situation it becomes easier for them to resort to "quick fix" strategies, especially if attempts to stop the abuse are frustrated.

6. Conclusion

Although based on the views of only a relatively small number of participants, this study provides clarity with regard to the ways survivors of child sexual abuse cope with their experiences and associated emotions, especially when support was and/or was not available. The study further revealed influence that could be exerted by idiosyncratic factors, such as one's racial/cultural background, in deciding on the type of strategies to adopt in dealing with a difficult situation. Cultural factors in particular, influence individuals' worldviews, and shape the way they see the world and their place in it. Most importantly, it shapes the way meanings are given to experiences and are passed between individuals, groups and generations (Eckersley, 2007). The implication for counselling is that one solution may not necessary be suitable for all cases. Interventions should consider the client's culture, and if not, they may not succeed or could lead to interventions that may cause damage to the clients (Cross-Tower, 2005). A suggestion to counselors, professionals and paraprofessionals is to obtain a broad knowledge of the beliefs and cultures of their clients before offering intervention services.

Several limitations to this study are evident. The sample size was too small to permit generalizations to a wider group of sexually abused survivors. Additionally, the views of male survivors were not captured, nor the views participants of all population groups in South Africa. Biases in the recruitment strategy are possible, as participants were only those who were based at the social welfare units. Survivors referred to such agencies are likely to have experienced serious forms of abuse and are receiving emotional support from the counseling services at the institutions where they are based. It would be interesting to capture views of survivors who have not yet received any form of emotional support.

7. References

Barbarin, O.A., Ritcher, L. & de Wet, T. (2001) Exposure to violence, coping resources, and psychological adjustment of South African children. American Journal of Orthopsychiatry 71 (1), 16-25.

Brand, B.L. & Alexandra, P.C. (2003). Coping with incest: the relationship between recollections of childhood coping and adult functioning in females survivors of Incest. Journal of Traumatic Stress, 16 (3), 285-293.

Brodhagen, A. & Wise, D. (2008). Optimism as a mediator between the experiences of child abuse, other traumatic events, and distress. Journal of Family Violence, 23 (6), 403-411.

Charmaz, K. (2006). Constructing grounded theory: A practical guide through qualitative analysis. London, England: Sage Publications.

Collings, S. J. (1995). The long-term effects of contact and non-contact forms of child sexual abuse in a sample of University men. Child Abuse and Neglect, 19 (1), 1-6.

Crossan-Tower, C. (2005). Understanding Child Abuse and Neglect (6th ed.). Pearson Education, Inc.

Csoboth C.T., Birkas, E. & Purebl, C. (2003). Physical and sexual abuse: risk factors for substance use among young Hungarian women. Behavioural Medicine, 28, 165-171.

Dey, I. (1993). Qualitative data analysis: A user friendly guide. London, England: Routledge

Doyle, C. (1995). Helping strategies for child sexual abuse. London. Whiting and Birch on behalf of the National children's Bureau.

Eckersley, R.M. (2007) Culture, Spirituality, religion and health: looking at the big picture. Medical Journal of Australia, 186 (10), 554- 556.

Fallot, R.D. & Heckman, J.P. (2005) Religious/Spiritual coping among women trauma survivors with mental health and substance use disorders. The Journal of Behavioral and Health Service and Research, 32 (2), 215-226.

Finkelhor, D. & Browne, A. (1985). The traumatic impact of child sexual abuse: A conceptualization. American Journal of Orthopsychiatry, 55 (4), pp. 530-541.

Finkelhor, D. (1979). Sexually victimized children. New York, NY: The Free Press, Inc

Finkelhor, D. (1984). Child sexual abuse: New Theory and Research. New York, NY: The Free Press, Inc.

Finkelhor, D. (1988). The trauma of child sexual abuse: Two models. In Wyatt, G.E. and Powell, G.J. (Eds). Lasting effects of child sexual abuse. Newbury Park, CA: Sage Publications.

Frazier, P.A. & Burnett, J.W. (1994). Immediate coping strategies among rape victims. Journal of Counseling and Development, 72, 633-639.

Gipple, D.E., Lee M.S. & Puig, A. (2006). Coping and dissociation among female college student: reporting childhood abuse experiences. Journal of College Counseling, 9, 33-45.

Grayson, C.E. & Nolen-Hoeksema, S. (2005). Motives to drink as mediators between childhood sexual assault and alcohol problems in adult women. Journal of Traumatic Stress, 18 (2), 137-145.

Herrenkohl, E.C., Herrenkohl, R.C, & Egolf, B. (1994). Resilient early school-age children from maltreating homes: outcomes in late adolescence. American Journal of Orthopsychiatry, (2), 301-309.

Hickson, J.& Kriegler, S. (1996). Multicultural Counseling in a divided and traumatized society. London, England: Routledge

Himelein, J.M. & McElrath, J.V. (1996). Resilient child sexual abuse survivors: Cognitive coping and illusion. Child Abuse and Neglect, 20 (8), pp, 747-758.

Human Rights Watch. (2001). Scared at School: Sexual Violence against girls in South African school. HRW: United States of America.

Kelly, L. (1988). Surviving Sexual Abuse. New York, NY: John Wiley and Sons.

Letseka, M. (2000). African philosophy and educational discourse. In P. Higgs, N.C. Vakalisa, T.V. Mda, and N.T. Assie-Lumumba. Cape Town, South Africa: Juta Publishers.

Madu, S.N. & Peltzer, K. (2001). Risk factors and child sexual abuse among secondary school students in Northern Province. Child Abuse and Neglect, 24 (2), 259-268.

Mzarek, P.J. & Mzarek, D.A. (1987). Resilience in child maltreatment victims: A conceptual exploration. Child Abuse and Neglect, 11, 357-366.

Russell, D. (1995). Incestuous Abuse: Its long-term effects. Human Sciences Research Council: Pretoria, South Africa. (ERIC Document Reproduction Service no.ED 354141).

Rutter, M. (1987). Psycho-social resilience and protective mechanisms. American Journal of Orthopsychiatry, 57 (3), 316-331.

Sgroi, S.M. (1982) Handbook of clinical intervention in child sexual abuse. (2nd ed). Massachusetts, MA: Lexington Books.

Sigmond, S.T.,, Greene, M.P., Rohan, K.J., & Nichols, J.E. (1996). Coping and Adjustment in male and female survivors of child sexual abuse. Journal of Child Sexual Abuse, 5 (3), 57-75.

Swanston, H.Y., Nunn, K.P., Oates R.K., Tebbut, J.S. & O'Toole, B.L. (1999). Hoping and coping in young people who have been sexually abused. European Child and Adolescent Psychiatry, 8, 134-142.

Talbot, J.A., Talbot, N.L. & Tu Xin. (2004). Shame-proneness as a diathesis for dissociation in women with histories of childhood sexual abuse. Journal of Traumatic Stress, 17 (5), 445-448.

Valente, S.M. (2005). Sexual abuse of boys. Journal of Child and Adolescent Psychiatric Nursing, 18 (1), 10 -16.

Van Rensburg, E. & Barnard, C. (2005). Psychological resilience among sexually-molested girls in the late middle-childhood: A case study approach. Child Abuse research in South Africa, 6 (1), 1-12.

Williams, B. (2003). The worldview dimensions of individualism and collectivism: Implications for counseling. Journal of Counseling and development 81, 370-374.

Wright, O,M., Crawford, E. & Sebastian, K. (2007). Positive Resolution of childhood sexual abuse experiences: the role of coping, benefit-finding and meaning-making. Journal of Family Violence, 22, 259-608.

12

What Went Wrong at Ohel Children's Home – and What Can Be Done About Its Failure to Protect Jewish Children from Abuse?

Amy Neustein and Michael Lesher
Help Us Regain The Children Legal Research Center
USA

1. Introduction

The cover-up of sex crimes at the expense of child victims has become an all-too-familiar story in many religious communities. The protection of priests accused of child molestation by the Catholic Church hierarchy is now a matter of record; more recent publicity has identified Orthodox Jewish communities as another locus of such misconduct (Dorff, 2009).

Central to such cover-ups is an institution powerful enough to suppress the evidence of abuse and motivated to do it. This chapter presents an analysis - for the first time - of the role in the suppression of child abuse scandals played by the American Orthodox Jewish community's most prominent child welfare agency. The agency, Ohel Children's Home and Family Services (hereafter, "Ohel"), is a large state-licensed agency located in a heavily Orthodox wedge of Brooklyn, New York, and performs foster care, adoption and counseling services. The Ohel agency first opened its doors in 1969. Rapidly, it grew into what the *Village Voice* in 1994 dubbed a "bulwark" of the Orthodox community (Barrett & Bowles, 1994), with a budget of over $4 million, and political ties that have brought U.S. Senators, Congressmen, state legislators and New York City mayors to its annual fundraising dinners.

Given the nature of its services - foster care was always one of its priorities - the agency dealt early with problems of child abuse. In early 1997, the agency doubled its investment in the issue by opening a program for child sex offenders. That program was shuttered after about five years (Winston, 2009b), but the agency continues to highlight its role in working with child victims of abuse. In April 2009, Ohel and the Brooklyn District Attorney, Charles J. Hynes, jointly announced the formation of a special program called "Kol Tzedek," the ostensible purpose of which was to encourage the highly insular Orthodox Jewish community in Brooklyn to recognize the seriousness of child sex abuse, and to confront the problem honestly - with steps including reporting all such abuse to appropriate city or state authorities (Winston, 2009a).

Lamentably, the agency's actual record belies these stated intentions. In February 2011, Ohel was skewered in an exposé reported by Hella Winston of the *Jewish Week*. Winston's article contained damning evidence that Ohel had blatantly ignored New York statutes requiring the reporting of suspected child abuse to state authorities. (Winston, 2011a).

The forum of the exposé was itself significant: the *Jewish Week* is anything but a fringe publication. On the contrary, it is a nationally distributed weekly magazine claiming over 100,000 subscribers to its hard copy weekly edition and a quarter of a million readers of its electronic version (updated daily). What is more, it is affiliated with the centrist Jewish Federation, a fact that tends to moderate its news reporting and makes it highly sensitive to criticism that it is singling out one religious group, such as Orthodox Jews, in its coverage.

Nevertheless, Winston's initial foray was soon followed by even more alarming allegations. In an article dated May 31, 2011, she revealed that Ohel, apparently in a frantic effort to clear its name from the charges contained in the earlier article, had shared confidential files about abuse cases with outsiders. Such conduct raised the hackles of a number of child welfare experts, as Winston reported:

> "Even if it were technically legal for Ohel to show the files to handpicked outside individuals, sharing patient information with consultants for the purpose of clearing the agency's name may be an inappropriate use of the Health Insurance Portability and Accountability Act, which governs privacy regulations, according to Abner Weintraub, a national authority on HIPAA. Mary Vandenack, another authority on HIPAA, told The Jewish Week that bringing in a consultant who is not an expert in the specific area or who has an interest in the outcome is unethical and may even constitute fraud if the agency and/or consultant make representations that the consultant is an expert" (Winston, 2011b).

In addition to what may have been a serious breach of confidentiality, Winston revealed that David Mandel, the agency's CEO, apparently implied to a group that reviewed those files "the prospect for future collaboration with and funding from Ohel." In other words, Ohel appears, in essence, to have bribed those who reviewed confidential files in order to elicit from them an assessment more favorable to the agency's public image. Sharing the files with outsiders in the first place was bad practice; the act threatened critical standards of confidentiality. Indeed, as Winston reported, it may have violated federal HIPAA laws. Coupled with an offer of financial benefit to the outside organization asked by Ohel to clear its name, the act took on a possibly criminal character. (Winston has told the authors that child advocates are asking law enforcement officials to investigate possible criminal violations perpetrated by Ohel.)

These startling details tell only part of the story. The authors – both as researchers and as members of the Orthodox Jewish community[1] – consider it imperative to examine the larger, systemic implications as well. How does Ohel's approach to reporting child sex abuse cases to authorities relate to its role vis-à-vis Orthodox Jewish communities in the United States, Canada and Israel, all of which financially (and politically) support the agency? How does the interlocking of Ohel and the Orthodox communities it serves contribute to the reification by which Ohel has become, as noted above, a "bulwark of the Orthodox Jewish community" (Barrett & Bowles, 1994)? Clearly, Ohel is a part of the Orthodox Jewish community rather than external to it. For this reason, our analysis of Ohel's conduct begins with a recognition of the agency as something integral to and generative of the community that has built, sustained and promoted it.

In this chapter, consequently, we will use the prominent and readily available example of Ohel to investigate the underlying reasons for the Orthodox community's all-too-frequent

[1] One of the authors is the daughter of the late Rabbi Dr. Abraham Neustein, a highly distinguished clergyman, educator and Talmudic scholar.

subordination of the rights of sexual abuse victims to the preservation of the community's good name. Similarly, we will examine the sociological background to the mounting evidence that Ohel, as part and parcel of the community it serves, has flouted state laws that require reporting of suspected sex abuse to authorities. It is worth stressing, in this connection, that when Ohel addresses its own community it goes out of its way to avoid any mention of such mandatory reporting, even in places where such mention should have been *de rigueur*. For example, in a promotional newsletter Ohel distributed in the summer of 2009, in which it quoted from a press release issued by Brooklyn's District Attorney announcing the new joint sex-abuse initiative with Ohel ("Kol Tzedek") mentioned above, the agency carefully removed from the press release every reference the D.A. had made to police, prosecutors and the reporting of sex crimes to secular authorities (Lesher, 2011).

We hope our example will inspire researchers to inquire along similar lines into other institutions, connected with religious communities, which may have failed to protect children from child sexual abuse. The effect of religion-based organizations taking on public functions is already receiving public attention: in the wake of the grisly murder in July 2011 of eight-year-old Leiby Kletzky in one Brooklyn's Orthodox neighborhoods, one of the authors was asked to write an editorial for New York City's most widely-read daily newspaper about the misuse of public money for Orthodox Jewish "citizen patrols" which, like Ohel, often refuse to report suspected Jewish offenders to police (Lesher, 2011).

The remainder of this chapter is divided into three main sections. First, we offer a sociological analysis of the Orthodox Jewish community's attitudes towards the reporting of offenders, as these related to a Jewish welfare agency like Ohel. Second, we examine the documented history of abuse or neglect cases apparently covered up either by Ohel officials or by professionals working with Ohel, such as pediatricians, counselors and their rabbinic advisors. Finally, we offer some suggestions for addressing the problems examined.

2. A case for denial

Ohel does not operate in a vacuum. Its actions reflect deeply held beliefs, attitudes and prejudices of the community it represents.

Although, strictly speaking, Jewish law requires adherence to governing secular law, in practice the observance of traditional Jewish piety is often at variance with secular laws requiring the reporting of suspected Jewish offenders to police. Let us examine how the Orthodox Jewish culture affects this sensitive issue.

2.1 Community homeostasis

Much as the physiological system of an organism maintains internal stability, owing to the coordinated response of its parts to any situation or stimulus tending to disturb its normal condition, Orthodox Jewish communities as a whole strive to maintain internal stability by rejecting or attacking any forces that threaten to disturb the community's perceived harmony. An important component of that harmony is the perception that the community continues to project a public image as a locale of behavior that is devout, sober, ethical, and so forth.

Sex abuse charges asserted against community figures such as teachers, rabbis, etc. can represent a serious threat to community homeostasis. To begin with, the accusation challenges ingrained hierarchies - rabbis above laymen, teachers above students, men above women, adults above children.

In addition, the accusation often threatens the livelihood of the accused in a community marked by the interdependence of community members. For instance, the teacher whose student credibly accuses him of sexual abuse will likely have to leave his teaching position. But where is the teacher to go? In truth, he (or she) is not likely to find a job in a secular environment, nor even to seek one, since religious Jews are socialized from an early age to stay within the Orthodox community; such insular Jewish communities look askance at socializing with non-Jews, or even non-religious Jews, for fear that the cultural norms that guide and regulate the everyday activities of Orthodox Jews might be questioned when members of such insular communities are exposed to outsiders. Consequently, exposure to the outside world is kept to a minimum. So, the community is faced with a stark choice between ignoring the alleged victim and jeopardizing the career of the teacher being accused. This weights the community's response heavily against the accuser.

Besides the loss to the accused, sex abuse charges threaten a loss to the community itself. The tight-knit social organization that has come to depend on each of its members for fulfilling religious obligations - participating in a quorum for communal prayer, assisting in ritual washing and burial of the dead, visiting the sick, consoling mourners, etc. - suddenly faces the possibility of losing a member's participation in the tasks that punctuate, define and regulate religious life. By the same token, a charge of sexual abuse endangers the participation of the accused's children in community life; if the charge is publicized, and still more if it is accepted as true, the children are no longer seen as desirable marriage prospects because of the taint of scandal looming over their family. And, on the other hand, unmarried life is very much frowned upon.

It may seem ironic that the same community that struggles to hold on to its members, even those accused of abuse, because of the vital role each Orthodox Jew plays in the social and religious communal structure, is ready, if need be, to ostracize (in some cases, even to expel) a victim of abuse who presses an accusation. But this too can be explained. The community's choices seem peculiar only in light of an assumed egalitarianism, which in fact the community rejects. As mentioned above, the Orthodox Jewish community constantly reinforces the inequality of the status and power of its members as a vital part of its homeostasis. When we consider that abusive dynamics traditionally involve an imbalance of power, it is not hard to see why homeostasis favors the more powerful. In fact, one highly-placed rabbi declared to one of the authors, "How would a school function if its principal or its teachers were expelled because of a sex abuse report made by a ten-year-old student?" That puts the whole case very neatly indeed. And when other officials offer patently inadequate excuses for disregarding child sex abuse reports (*e.g.*, "It takes time and money to find a replacement for a teacher"), they are implicitly affirming the same thing.

Erica Brown, a contributor to *Tempest in the Temple: Jewish Communities & Child Sex Scandals* – a collection of essays by rabbis, educators, mental health professionals and lawyers, published in 2009 - wrote passionately about the plight of clergy abuse victims when their complaints are disregarded or ignored:

> "That there are people who abuse authority for personal, immoral gain should not come as a shock. That some of these individuals have embraced a life of sacred service is extremely upsetting, but sadly, still not a surprise. . . . What we cannot excuse are those who stand on the outside and permit abuse because they do not call it by name. . . . The cry of clergy abuse victims is shattering. It breaks our hearts, and it can break our faith. . . . We must blame ourselves when we allow a religious leader to remain in place who has the power to break hearts and shatter souls" (Brown, 2009, p. 72).

A decade earlier, Sandra Butler, an expert on sexual abuse, addressed the same conspiracy of silence. Writing in 1999 in the *Journal of Religion and Abuse*, Butler wrote: "One urgent concern I have is that there are many in the rabbinic leadership who still hold tightly to the illusion 'not here,' 'not them,' 'not us,'" when faced with alleged sexual abuse in families, in yeshivas and in the synagogue (Butler, 1999, p. 107).

Even before this, Rabbi Irving ("Yitz") Greenberg challenged rabbinic leaders to take responsibility for crimes of sexual abuse in a 1990 article appearing in *Moment*. Rabbi Greenberg was unsparing in his address to his fellow Orthodox rabbis:

> "To be silent then is to incur the grave guilt of accessory after the fact. Spiritual leaders who ignore or even cover up the presence of sexual abuse, Jewish media that continue the conspiracy of silence by acting as if this does not happen in the Jewish community, those that cut off or isolate victims who dare speak out, bring upon themselves the judgment that the Torah places on the accessory and the bystander: 'Do not stand idly by the blood of your neighbor'" (Greenberg, 1990, p. 49.)[2]

Notwithstanding these warnings, it is clear that communal denial of sexual abuse is one way of maintaining homeostasis within the insular world of Orthodoxy. Denial may also be employed among Orthodox Jewish families - which exist as microcosms of the Orthodox community writ large - to deal with the disruption to homeostasis brought about when one family member charges sex abuse committed by another.

Massachusetts psychologist Joan M. Featherman demonstrates how the institution of the Jewish family is quick to eschew members who are alleged to disturb its harmony. In *Sexual Abuse in Nine North American Cultures: Treatment and Prevention*, Dr. Featherman wrote:

> "Jewish families tend to break off contact with family members who are perceived to have breached their commitment to the family harmony. These perceived breaches of commitment range from not attending a family event…to divorce, intermarriage…or *disclosing sexual abuse*" (Featherman, 1995, p. 130).

Baltimore psychologist Joyanna Silberg, who specializes in treating child sexual abuse trauma, reflected in "Out of the Jewish Closet," a co-written chapter appearing in Neustein's *Tempest in the Temple*, on the psychodynamics of Jewish families and their response of sexual abuse. After examining the accounts of various incest survivors, Silberg and her co-author, nurse practitioner Stephanie Dallam, showed how incest survivor Sue William Silverman described the ironic trap posed by the Jewish family structure:

---

[2] It should perhaps be noted that, although Rabbi Greenberg is Orthodox, he does not belong to the more religiously "right-wing" Orthodox body of opinion that governs the more traditional Orthodox communities.

"[T]he sacredness of the family unit in Jewish communities may make it impossible for even the adults to get help outside the family" (Silberg & Dallam, 2009, p. 93).

Silberg's own clinical experience bears out that claim. Writing in *Tempest*, Silberg and her co-author described how many clients originally sought family support when they discovered that their husbands were abusing their children. "They reported that, instead of giving support, their parents and friends encouraged them to look the other way, to 'stay with him,' or to work it out" (Silberg & Dallam, 2009, p. 93).

There is at least one more way in which a sex abuse accusation threatens community homeostasis. It challenges a principle of religious culture. The community considers it a touchstone of traditional Judaism that this ancient creed is perfect, answering to all needs and addressing all possible situations. Accordingly, Orthodox rabbinic leadership teaches (and enforces) the belief that whatever evil is encountered in Jewish life comes from "outside"; those raised entirely within Orthodoxy could not possibly be guilty of something as far from Jewish norms as sexual depravity. An accusation of child sexual abuse by an Orthodox Jew, particularly a rabbi or teacher, violates this basic principle and is therefore anathema. Judy Brown, who in 2009 (under the pseudonym "Eishes Chayil") authored a book about child sexual abuse specifically aimed at the Orthodox community, recently published a column (under the same pseudonym) in which she revealed that she and her publisher received threats from members of the community. "The message was clear," Brown wrote. "I had violated the rule that said victims must protect the community from their own crimes. Now, I would pay." And in Brown's candid assessment, it was just as clear what "message" the community preferred to send to Orthodox Jews in general:

"After I started meeting with victims and speaking with therapists, I began to encounter the community's wall of denial. These are things Jews don't do, I was told. . . .

"Some subjects are better left in silence, the rabbis said. Orthodox Jews did not need such words. Those were words for gentiles."

Brown wrote her book because, she says, "we [in the Orthodox community] forgot [to] look inside, to see that the most dangerous enemy always grows from within." Unfortunately, that is exactly the message that threatens the community's stability. (Chayil, 2011.)[3]

2.2 Sacrificing victims

In 2002, the Catholic Church child sex scandal made headlines around the world. At that time, presumably because of our high profile in speaking out about child sexual abuse in the Orthodox community (long before it became popular to do so), the authors suddenly found themselves invited by academic publishers, psychology journal editors and Jewish newspapers to comment in print, and now for a wider audience, on the perils of sex abuse within the Jewish clergy and the Jewish community writ large. We were asked, in particular, to address how such offenses were systematically covered up by the rabbinate, Jewish child care agencies, and powerful community organizations.

That year, the *Jewish Exponent*, a century-old paper serving metropolitan Philadelphia, invited us to write a guest editorial on the subject. We argued that child sex abuse was drastically

---

[3] Significantly, Brown explained in the column that she had published her book, *Hush*, under a pseudonym "to protect my family and friends from community retribution."

under-recognized in religious Jewish communities simply because, thanks to the communal fear of public exposure, too many victims met with cover-ups instead of compassion:

> "The denial by Jewish communities, and their leaders, that sexual abuse of all kinds does occur among Jews - with the ugly result that victims can pay a higher price than their tormentors when their accusations come to light. . . . In our examination of cases of alleged sex crimes by Jewish offenders in recent decades, we have found that both Jewish community figures and Jewish media lag behind in giving victims the support they deserve. This means that all too often the victims, not their alleged attackers, are sacrificed to the community's sense of shame. For instance, two years ago, a young boy in the ultra-Orthodox neighborhood of Borough Park, Brooklyn, accused a rabbi of having sexually abused him over a period of 18 months during private lessons. A child-abuse expert backed his story, but the Chasidic [piously religious] community was so eager to protect the accused rabbi -- whatever the facts -- that when a group of rabbis managed to persuade the District Attorney to drop the charges, the community celebrated publicly."

We concluded our editorial by asking the question:

> "How many victims must be sacrificed on the altar of the community's shame before this conspiracy [of silence] ends?" (Neustein & Lesher, 2002a, p. 37).

Around the same time, Dane Claussen published our chapter in his book *Sex, Religion, Media*, in which we demonstrated that Jewish media were still reluctant to run stories about child sexual abuse.

Unfortunately, it was clear to us - and still is - that the Orthodox Jewish community has a much larger problem in this respect than it has hitherto admitted. Nor have the emerging revelations of the disastrous consequences of cover-ups in the Catholic clergy done much to change the patterns of behavior in Jewish circles. Jewish media, which might conceivably act as an antidote to the community's taste for secrecy, have instead absorbed its distorted priorities. The religious leadership's need to block out the outside world, to protect itself from scrutiny by a society it regards as alien and dangerous, finds a parallel in the Jewish media's reluctance to publicize scandals among Jews (Neustein & Lesher, 2002b, p. 82).

Little had changed when, years later, we were invited to write an article for a special issue of the *Journal of Child Sexual Abuse* devoted to sex abuse committed by members of the clergy. The guest editors of this special issue - Drs. Robert A. McMackin, Terence M. Keane and Paul M. Kline - placed our paper prominently in this issue as the only contribution addressing abuse and cover-ups within the Jewish clergy: a compliment, perhaps, but also an ominous reminder that such analysis aimed at Jewish communities was still the exception. In our paper, titled "A Single Case Study of Rabbinic Sexual Abuse in the Orthodox Jewish Community," we analyzed abuse cover-ups within the Orthodox Jewish community by way of a detailed case history: a young, hearing-impaired Hasidic boy allegedly abused by his Hasidic tutor. The teacher, charged with 96 counts of serious child abuse, ultimately escaped even an indictment when, under pressure by a panel of rabbis, Brooklyn prosecutors dropped all charges against him. Afterward, the alleged victim's family faced so much ostracism from their Hasidic community that they were eventually forced to move away. Thus, the victim and his family - as so many prior cases - were sacrificed on the altar of the community's shame, paying the price for the community's misdeeds as its leaders suppressed an investigation in serious child abuse charges (Neustein & Lesher, 2008).

Our research has found that Orthodox Jewish community hostility to the publicizing of sex abuse charges can turn violent. In 1991, the day after a Stamford Hill (north London) rabbinic student was sentenced for sexually assaulting a five-year-old girl, a mob of between one and two hundred ultra-Orthodox Jews menaced the victim's family, hurling objects through their windows, causing the family to run for their lives. This was the fifth time they had been chased from their home during the criminal trial, which had lasted two years (Guardian staff reporter, 1991, p. 2).

Alas, this pattern has not abated with the passage of time. This year (2011), the authors were profiled once again in a Canadian television documentary called "Wall of Silence," which offered a close look at sex abuse cover-ups in Orthodox Jewish communities in the United States and Canada. Also featured in that documentary was a Brooklyn rabbi who alleges he was shot at with a pistol - and very nearly killed - by members of his community for speaking out about the plight of the abuse victim and the need to protect children from sexual predators within the community. He was also widely denounced in Williamsburg, New York (where he lives) on fliers distributed throughout his community depicting him as a poisonous snake (Mendelsohn, 2011). To date, no one in the community has apologized to the rabbi for any of these vicious attacks.

2.3 Conflicts of interest

As the facts above serve to illustrate, there is often a direct clash between the needs of abuse victims and the values brought to bear on their cases within Orthodox Jewish communities. Rabbi Dr. Mordechai Glick, vice president of an international organization of Orthodox Jewish health professionals, expressed this plainly when he complained eleven years ago, in a letter to *The Jewish Press*, that "if the police do get involved [in a case of alleged sex abuse], a massive cover-up and pressure campaign usually ensures that the case will either not get to trial or if it does, will be dropped because potential witnesses are pressured (code for threatened) to refuse to testify or outright lie" (Glick, 2000:87).

Recent developments confirm this pattern. This year, the entire Brooklyn Orthodox community mobilized in a search for a missing eight-year-old Hasidic boy named Leiby Kletzky. (In the end, lamentably, the boy was found dead: he had been abducted, smothered and then dismembered by an adult Orthodox Jew.) Even as masses of Orthodox community members scoured the streets for the abducted boy, one of the leading rabbis of Agudath Israel of America - America's single most influential ultra-Orthodox rabbinic body - insisted at a conference that any Orthodox Jew who suspects an act of child abuse must first turn to a rabbi, who will decide whether or not secular authorities should be contacted. What was especially remarkable about those comments is that the rabbi based them on the ruling of a highly-respected ultra-Orthodox authority that has been widely claimed as evidence of the Orthodox community's greater openness to the reporting of child sex abuse. Yet the requirement to take any question to an Orthodox rabbi *before* reporting to police effectively reaffirms that the community's leaders, not police, will decide the fate of a child abuse victim.

What is behind this apparent contradiction? Leading Orthodox rabbis have, indeed, begun to discuss publicly the problem of child sexual abuse in their communities - a sign of progress in itself, for as recently as the 1990s the head of a prominent Orthodox rabbinic organization in Brooklyn could still insist to one of the authors that child sexual abuse simply did not exist among Orthodox Jews. And it is true that Rabbi Y. S. Elyashiv, one of the world's most respected Orthodox authorities, issued a much-publicized ruling that clearly authorizes reporting cases of child sexual abuse to the police. No wonder that a spokesman for Agudath Israel of America has argued that his community has fully addressed the issue of child sex abuse (Shafran, 2006).

Yet it has not, for the Orthodox rabbinate's assumption of its own ultimate power is so strong, and so unacknowledged, that even the more "liberal" rulings with respect to reporting abuse are read within the community merely as permitting a *rabbi* to authorize the reporting of abuse in a specific case. The Orthodox rabbinate has not grasped that so long as it operates as gatekeeper between victims and secular authorities, rabbis still can - and will - choose to suppress evidence of sex abuse whenever they think it appropriate. That this problem has not even been recognized by the Orthodox community's leading authorities is an indication of the enduring strength of the very hierarchies and prejudices that, as we argued above, have always worked against victims of abuse.

That these hierarchies are alive and well at Ohel is evident from the fact that the agency continues to name Rabbi Dovid Cohen as its chief advisor on matters of Jewish law - including the reporting of suspected crimes to secular authorities - and, in fact, singled him out for honor at its annual dinner in February 2011. Reportedly, Rabbi Cohen has taught publicly that Jews may steal from non-Jews or defraud non-Jewish governments, "as long as one doesn't get caught, according to people in attendance" (*Jewish Week* staff reporter, 2009).

2.4 Religious rationalizations for non-reporting

We must now examine some of the specific rationales given in Orthodox communities for refusing to report suspected Jewish child abusers - or other criminals - to secular authorities. While these are matters of religious law, it will be seen that the interpretation of these concepts by contemporary rabbis is subject to, and an expression of, the underlying attitudes of the Orthodox community toward its surrounding communities and toward the issues posed by reporting one of "its own" to the representatives of non-Jewish institutions. Only when these attitudes, and their effects on members of the Orthodox Jewish community, are properly understood can we fathom the acts of institutions like Ohel.

2.4.1 *M'sirah*

Talmudic law contains a prohibition against *m'sirah*, or the "traducing" of one Jew by another to an extortionist (whether Jewish or non-Jewish) in order to cause the victim an injury. Although, strictly speaking, the law has nothing to do with reporting to law enforcement authorities - in fact, the Hebrew word *m'sirah* does not mean "informing," as often stated - the Talmud already cites a malicious report to a non-Jewish tax official as an example of such forbidden "traducing."[4] The reason for this, according to a typical explanation found in an influential nineteenth-century commentary, was entirely the result of the ugly experiences Diaspora Jewish communities had suffered at the hands of rapacious tax farmers and similar "officials," who were often hostile to the Jews and in general were little better than common criminals.[5] The consensus of contemporary Orthodox authority is that the principle of *m'sirah* does not prohibit reporting suspected criminal assaults

[4] Babylonian Talmud, *Baba Qamma* 116b-117a; *Gittin* 7a.

[5] *Arukh ha-Shulhan*, Hoshen ha-Mishpat 388:7.

(including sex abuse) by a Jew to secular law enforcement authorities, certainly not in a country with a functioning justice system (Dratch, 2009, p. 116).

That, however, does not prevent Orthodox Jews from condemning those who do report sex offenses to authorities as if they had, in fact, committed a cardinal sin. Nearly all of the Orthodox Jewish sex abuse victims who have spoken to the authors have described being sternly warned not to report what was done to them to police. Indeed, the authors have both been accused, by many Orthodox Jews, of committing *m'sirah* ourselves simply for publishing the facts of a few such cases. Clearly, the force of the principle has slipped its moorings in Jewish law and has taken on a life of its own. In fact, a declaration signed by fifty prominent rabbis appeared in a Yiddish-language Brooklyn newspaper in 2000, openly encouraging the murder of anyone who informed on a fellow Jew to secular authorities (Neustein & Lesher, 2009, p. 201).

Obviously, *m'sirah* is a handy club to swing at abuse victims who speak out. As a rationale for refusing to report crimes against children to police, however, it is does not pass muster with experts in rabbinic law.

2.4.2 *Lashon ha-ra*

M'sirah is probably the most frequently invoked rationalized invoked by Orthodox Jews for failing to report crimes against children, or for discouraging others from making such reports. However, apart from the question of "traducing" a fellow Jew, there are two separate but related issues that often appear in the discourse.

Jewish law contains a prohibition against slander, gossip and tale-bearing, collectively referred to in Jewish literature as "*lashon ha-ra*." Although it is commonplace for Orthodox community members to accuse abuse victims of violating this prohibition whenever they speak out about their experiences, this – like the invocation of *m'sirah* discussed above – quite plainly amounts to an abuse of Jewish law. As Rabbi Mark Dratch explains, using the prohibition to intimidate genuine victims from speaking out is itself *lashon ha-ra*:

> "*Lashon ha-ra* can be a tool of abuse, both when derogatory speech defames innocent people, destroying their reputations, and when warnings to refrain from derogatory speech are used to silence victims of abuse who cry out for help. . . . Victims of abuse need to speak out, for all kinds of personal reasons, in order to help themselves. . . . And the community needs to speak out in order to hold the perpetrators responsible and in order to protect other innocents from potential harm."

It is evident that the claim of "*lashon ha-ra*" will not take one any farther toward a "defense" of non-reporting of child abuse than the parallel issue of *m'sirah*. Still, members of the Orthodox community quite commonly invoke it to achieve exactly that result. Even Orthodox journalists are not immune. As the authors reported in 2002, an Orthodox news writer named Alan Borsuk has claimed publicly – and incorrectly, in our view – that being a religious Jew and being committed to publicizing the truth are, to some extent, inconsistent values because of the Jewish laws against *lashon ha-ra*:

> "The worlds of Orthodox Judaism and newspapering have some very different philosophic premises. Journalism's cardinal tenet of laying out the facts and letting the chips fall where they may is definitely in conflict with *Jewish tradition's strong emphasis on not saying things that unnecessarily harm others, even if they are true*. . . . The neutral or

accepting position that the news media take on a lot of social and lifestyle issues is very different from the strong stand Judaism takes . . ." (Borsuk, 1997).

Borsuk's assumption that truth-telling runs afoul of "Jewish tradition's strong emphasis on not saying things . . . even if they are true" was carried even further by an Orthodox Jewish anchorwoman for a local television news station whose viewing area included parts of New York, New Jersey and Connecticut. When one of the authors sought the station's news coverage of serious allegations of a sex abuse cover-up at Ohel in 1987, the Orthodox anchorwoman personally contacted her to urge her "not to publicize the alleged scandal," because "it was far better to have a rabbi settle the matter than to air it in the press." As we have previously reported, "The station never aired the story until the anchorwoman left the station several years later; thereafter, its feature length piece covering the story won an Emmy Award" (Neustein & Lesher, 2002: p. 83). Once again, Jewish law - as understood by experts - cuts one way, but cultural attitudes, fears and prejudices cut another.

2.4.3 *Hillul ha-shem*

A final rationalization used within Orthodox Jewish communities to silence victims of abuse is the prohibition against *hillul ha-shem*, which means "a desecration of God's name." The phrase itself requires some explanation. "Traditional Jewish law," writes Rabbi Dratch,

> "deems an act committed by a religious Jew that arouses public disgust (particularly on the part of non-Jewish observers) a 'desecration,' in effect of God Himself, since in the eyes of the Talmud Jews are identified with God through the responsibility of observing His law" (Dratch, 2009, pp. 116-117).

It is not difficult to see why the principle of *hillul ha-shem* is improperly applied to a truthful report of a violent crime. It is not the *report* of the act that constitutes the offense, but the act itself. To quote Rabbi Dratch:

> "First, it is the unethical behavior in and of itself - not merely discussing it - that constitutes a desecration of God's name. The abuser, not the abused, has committed *hillul Hashem*. . . .
>
> "Second, when efforts to deny or suppress the truth about a crime are exposed, the scandal is much greater than the exposure of the crime alone. And Jewish tradition insists that scandalous behavior will always come to light despite efforts to keep it hidden" (*Id.*, p. 117).

In a word, not only is reporting child abuse to authorities not an example of *hillul ha-shem*, a failure to report it actually amounts to a massive violation of precisely the same principle. Certainly, this element of religious law cannot be invoked to justify refusal to report such crimes.

It is fair to say that not one of the appeals to elements of Jewish law commonly deployed within Orthodox communities to defend a policy of suppressing abuse reports can withstand scrutiny. Yet the practice continues, for reasons we have already attempted to explore. Let us now turn to some of the typical results.

3. Some relevant histories

In 1990, on Yom Kippur - the most solemn day of the Jewish year - eight-year-old Yaakov Riegler was stabbed to death by his mother with a kitchen fork. The case attracted considerable public attention because, it turned out, Ohel - which was responsible for the boy's care at the time - had been clearly warned that the boy's mother was dangerously violent. Still, rabbis working with Ohel and the Jewish community overrode the admonitions of the city's child welfare administration to keep the child away from his abusive mother. Although this was not a case of child sexual abuse, it illustrates - as far too many sex abuse cases do - the power of rabbis working in concert with Ohel to override secular agency's authority to protect children.

In the wake of the boy's brutal killing, child welfare experts did not mince words in their criticism of Ohel. Clara Hemphill, writing for *New York Newsday*, reported that just weeks before the stabbing, Ohel had learned alarming facts about the boy's condition. However, "rather than call the State Central Registry in Albany - as required by law - officials said they called a Child Welfare Administration office in Manhattan which had nothing to do with the case. Ohel officials," according to Hemphill, "could not offer an explanation why they called the unit [in Manhattan] rather than the state hotline. Child welfare experts were astonished by the blunder"(Hemphill, 1990, p. 23).

Brenda McGowan, a professor at Columbia University's School of Social Work and an expert in foster care, commented to *Newsday* that Ohel's decision to call the unrelated Manhattan office, rather than the State Central Registry, was "insane" (Hemphill, 1990, p. 23). McGowan's was not a lone voice. Many child advocates and experts on foster care were just as astonished. What must not be forgotten is that Ohel is not an obscure institution working far from state authorities. Rather, it is a state licensed foster care agency with a multimillion dollar annual budget, much of which comes from New York and federal money. (In fact, Ohel pulls in even more government money than its budget reveals. For example, in fiscal year 2010 alone Ohel was awarded $900,000 in federal "earmarks" - that is, extra disbursements approved by individual Congressmen - approved by the later-disgraced Congressman Anthony Weiner, who in turn had received a substantial campaign contribution from Ohel's Executive Director, David Mandel.)

Yet the non-reporting in the Riegler was far from anomalous. Health care professionals connected with Ohel have stated openly that notwithstanding state law which mandates abuse reports to state authorities by such professionals, they - as observant Orthodox Jews - will not make such reports without first consulting a rabbi. For example, Dr. Susan Schulman, a Brooklyn pediatrician and a member of Ohel's Advisory Board, openly declared - in a recorded lecture she herself circulated - that she always asked a rabbi before making a legally mandated report, even knowing that by doing this she risked prosecution (Fifield & Lesher, 1996). (Although Dr. Schulman's astounding statement has been publicized in print at least since 1996, Ohel chose to feature Dr. Schulman on a video it produced, ostensibly to promote "awareness" of child sexual abuse, as recently as 2009.)

Similar evidence of Ohel's position on child abuse reporting can be gleaned from the example of Rosalie Harman. Ms. Harman, a former senior-level supervisor for New York City's Child Welfare Administration (CWA), testified at a New York State legislative hearing chaired by Senator David A Paterson (who later became Governor of New York) that she knew of a CWA employee whose responsibilities included overseeing Ohel. According to Ms. Harman, once the CWA employee began to express her "suspicion of fiscal irregularities with that agency . . . and asked for someone from the state to come and review the practices of Ohel she was . . . stopped in her tracks" and "taken away from that team" that oversaw Ohel (Harman, 1993, pp. 34-35).

The authors' years of investigation into abuses at Ohel confirm that the examples cited above define patterns that continue to inform Ohel's handling of child abuse allegations. The following three cases - all of which involve non-reporting of suspected child sexual abuse by the agency - typify the sort of problems our research has repeatedly uncovered.

3.1 Stefan Colmer

The outrage of the Stefan Colmer case is that it might never have happened. Before Colmer was ever criminally charged with sexually abusing two boys - for which he ultimately served a jail sentence - he participated in an "offender's program" run by Ohel, a program supposedly intended to help protect the Orthodox community from further abuse from "offenders" like Colmer. Yet he abandoned the program prematurely in 2002, without having been successfully treated, simply because he had decided to get married and didn't want to inform his new wife that he was a pedophile. During the following years, he sexually abused at least two thirteen-year-old boys.

The astonishing thing was that, from the time Colmer dropped out of its offenders' program until his arrest (in Israel) in 2007, Ohel did - nothing. It made no attempt to find out where Colmer was, or what he was doing, or whether he was spending any time alone with young boys. It never attempted to communicate with the Brooklyn religious school near which Colmer settled and from which, according to police sources, he lured potential victims to his house. In light of these facts, the *Jewish Week* reported,

> "Colmer's case raises several thorny questions: Should Ohel have agreed to treat Colmer, knowing that he had never been reported to the police? Is there a will on the part of the community and its institutions to reform reporting policies and practices to plug what appears to be a gaping hole in the reporting system, one that leaves children unprotected from men like Colmer? And, most pressing of all, who, in the end, should bear responsibility for what happened to the two innocent 13-year-old alleged victims of Colmer, whose lives will likely never be the same?" (Winston, 2009b).

In our view, other questions might have been added: Why didn't Ohel have a fixed policy that would have triggered some sort of action in the event Colmer refused to complete an agreed-upon therapy program as an offender? How many other dropouts were there from Ohel's offenders' program, and what did the agency do about those? Couldn't a program whose ostensible purpose was to protect the community have included a provision, agreed to in advance by the offender, that violation of Ohel's rules would result in, say, a report to the police or (assuming no crime had yet been committed) appropriate notification to protect potentialvictims? The fact that Ohel has offered no answers to any of these questions suggests that the Colmer case, unfortunately, does not stand alone.

3.2 Avrohom Mondrowitz

Avrohom Mondrowitz fled Brooklyn for Israel in late 1984, just as police were closing in for an arrest in what may be New York's worst-ever case of serial child sex abuse. Authorities believe that Mondrowitz - who was an administrator of a school for troubled youth, and a "child psychologist" (with a fake diploma) who "treated" children - sexually abused well over a hundred young boys, nearly all of them Orthodox Jews. He fled to Israel, which refused to extradite him. Justice continues to elude his victims, despite extraordinary efforts to renew the case against him, in which one of the authors has figured centrally (Lesher, 2009).

For our present purposes, the most important point is the fact that Mondrowitz obtained several of his victims from Ohel - and that the agency did nothing in response to their pleas for help (Lesher, 2009, p. 157). This allegation was made in print as long ago as 1999, when one of the police detectives who investigated the Mondrowitz case "told The [New York] Post that his 1984 investigation," while leading him to the conclusion that Mondrowitz had molested "hundreds of children - including some Ohel orphans," was stymied "when cops tried to question the agency." According to the detective, "They weren't cooperating. . . . 'Kids . . . had complained to Ohel and it was swept under the rug . . . [and] never reported.'"

Ohel officials have denied the detective's allegations. But one of the authors has personally interviewed one of Mondrowitz's other victims, who clearly remembers speaking, years ago, to an Ohel foster child who told him - and his parents - that he had reported Mondrowitz's abuse to Ohel officials, who had ignored him (Montero, 1999). The credibility of Ohel's denials in the Mondrowitz case may be gauged from the following case history.

3.3 Simcha Adler

Two typical themes dominate the case of Simcha Adler, a camp counselor employed by Ohel who, according to his victims, repeatedly raped them at knifepoint. First, Ohel seems to have made every possible effort to minimize the offender's punishment and to silence the victims. Second, Ohel claimed not to know of any danger posed by the abuser when, in fact, evidence suggests it did know.

According to press reports, Adler repeatedly and violently abused his eleven-year-old victims at a summer camp where he was their counselor, and then continued to molest and rape them at Ohel, where both were foster children. Yet the boys' complaints to Ohel officials were ignored - for more than a year - "until a worker caught [Adler] straddling Michael," as Douglas Montero reported in the *New York Post*.

Amazingly, although Ohel officials knew the abuse had been severe and chronic, it stood by silently as Adler plea-bargained for a sentence that did not involve even a single day of jail time. Still more amazingly, the plea bargain was concluded less than two months after his arrest.

Despite charges of sodomy and sexual abuse that could have resulted in a sentence of more than twenty years in prison, court records reveal that Adler's punishment was minimal: five years' probation and psychological counseling. His victims only learned of Adler's plea deal years later, and were outraged, as Montero reported:

> "'It's a crime that he could walk away . . . and have a normal life,' said Michael, now a mailroom worker in Midtown. 'This man ruined my life.' . . . . 'I was [angry], but I couldn't do anything - I wasn't smart enough to do anything,' said Robert, now a City College freshman who wants to be an optometrist" (Montero, 1999).

Here, in a nutshell, is a vivid illustration of Ohel's priorities. Ohel took no action when the boys complained of heinous abuse for over a year; Ohel never accepted any responsibility for what was done to them; Ohel never talked to the boys about the status of the criminal case. (One of the victims remembered "vaguely" that an Ohel officer told him, after the fact, that Adler was getting "probation; other than that, there does not appear to have been any communication between Ohel and the victims about the prosecution of their assailant.)

Ohel's only clear priority was self-protection: both victims charged that "Ohel swept the abuse 'under the rug' to avoid a legal battle that might ruin its reputation."

This confirms the first theme mentioned above: Ohel acted to minimize the consequences suffered by the abuser (and thus, by the agency itself), while doing nothing to aid the victims. This would be bad enough; but in fact, it goes hand in hand with the second theme - that Ohel knew far more all along than it admitted - as duly reported by Montero:

> "A former Ohel employee told The Post the boys' allegations were not taken seriously or investigated by Ohel because Michael was thought to be a 'liar.' . . .
>
> "The owner of a Borough Park building where Adler, until recently, had been living told The Post that the former counselor - who married in December and moved to Jerusalem - admitted to her several years ago that he was a pedophile. She said his confession came after Ohel officials knocked on her door and told her to keep an eye on her children" (*Id.*)

This is a singularly damning juxtaposition of facts. On the one hand, Ohel would do nothing for the victims because it assumed - why, we are not told - that the eleven-year-old accuser was a "liar." On the other hand, at the same time Ohel allegedly allowed young boys in its care to be raped at knifepoint, Ohel officials quietly warned the abuser's Orthodox Jewish landlord "to keep an eye on her children," which was all it took to elicit a "confession" from the abuser - though the Orthodox landlord, like the Ohel officials, apparently had no qualms about keeping the confession a secret.

This illustrates a kind of doublethink at work in Ohel that can only be explained as an intellectual method of protecting a culturally-ingrained set of priorities. Ohel's position cannot be described simply as refusing to believe young boys who reported abuse. In fact, the agency *did* believe them, or believed them at least enough of what they said to try to protect someone else's children. But the agency did this only when it could act without *publicly* acknowledging the reality of the victims' abuse and without forcing it to confront the abuser. What is at stake here is not simply ignorance. It is a systematic arranging of priorities so as to preserve the community homeostasis described above. Unfortunately, this approach has the effect of further victimizing children entrusted to its care.

4. Solutions

While the sort of fundamental rethinking of abuse issues that must take place if institutions like Ohel are to be truly reformed is likely years away, practical short-term strategies may still be suggested. This is particularly true because Ohel receives government money, which makes it accountable to state child welfare authorities, as well as to the federal government, as discussed below. The first major steps toward reforming the agency require little more than the political will to exert power already inherent in government authorities.

4.1 Federal mandate

Some years ago, Congress passed the Child Abuse Prevention and Treatment Act (CAPTA) for the purpose of helping the states create and maintain more effective child welfare systems.[6] The authors believe that this federal statute has the potential - so far,

[6] 42 U.S.C. § 5101 *et seq.*; 42 U.S.C. § 5116 *et seq.*

unfortunately, unused - to support a detailed federal inquiry into the child welfare system of any state that accepts federal money under this statute, as New York certainly does (Neustein & Lesher, 1999). Such an inquiry could, and should, include an examination into the proper oversight of agencies like Ohel. Has the agency complied with state reporting laws? Has it met government standards for maintaining the safety of foster children in its care? If not - and our research suggests it has not - federal funding should be terminated, a penalty that would almost certainly spur reform.

There are also federal civil rights statutes that Ohel's officials may be found to have violated if they have knowingly suppressed the reporting of child sex abuse. For example, Section 241 of Title 18 of the U.S. Code, provides that a conspiracy of two or more people "to . . . threaten, or intimidate any person in any State . . . in the free exercise or enjoyment of any right or privilege secured to him by the Constitution or laws of the United States" is a federal crime. Since access to the court system is just such a "right or privilege," this means a concerted effort by Ohel officials to prevent a child abuse victim from pursuing a criminal charge may justify federal prosecution. This point should be borne firmly in mind where Ohel's acts are at issue.

4.2 Investigation

Because of Ohel's close relationship with secular authorities, it necessarily falls under additional regulatory authority. To some extent, therefore, the nature of Ohel's apparent wrongs suggests its own remedy.

The first logical step would be a thorough investigation by the governments that have funded Ohel - those of New York City, New York State and the United States - to ensure that those funds have not been misappropriated. We have already discussed additional authority for such a probe under CAPTA. In any event, the misappropriation of government funds for an improper purpose (for example, the personal enrichment of an officer) would probably involve a violation of law.

Ohel's role in the non-reporting of suspected abuse to authorities might also implicate federal civil rights statutes, as discussed above. Even where there is no criminal violation, the facts unearthed by a federal investigation might support civil litigation by victims who were wrongfully intimidated or pressured not to approach police for protection.

5. Conclusion

This chapter aims at offering some guidance to scholars, advocates and policy makers who grapple with problems similar to those posed by Ohel. Ohel does not stand alone. It is quite possible that other institutions serving other insular, fundamentalist religious sects also act in violation of secular law and in violation of the public trust.

Analysis of Ohel is important for another reason. Given Ohel's central role in a closely knit and family-oriented Orthodox community, we must now consider and observe what happens when such an iconic institution comes under scrutiny for possibly violating mandates related to child welfare and safety (not to mention confidentiality).

Finally, we have attempted this exploration of Ohel because we believe that what has happened at Ohel, under the auspices of religious authority ostensibly designed to protect and nurture children, demands serious scrutiny from anyone concerned with the future of child welfare in today's religious communities. Many such communities enjoy unprecedented political power and opportunities in the United States. These opportunities can be used for good - as when community members use religious values to impress the importance of compassion and human dignity on political institutions - or they can lead to abuses. The authors hope to see the sort of abuses we have observed at Ohel quickly curbed so that both religious and government values may be better served in the future.

6. References

Barrett, W., & Bowles, J. (1994). Unorthodox Politics: Did Joe Hynes' Jewish Communityh Ties Influence Four Cases? *The Village Voice*, (September 6, 1994), pp. (13-18)

Borsuk, A. (1997). Old fashioned Jew, Old Fashioned Reporter. *Neiman Reports*, Vol. 51, (Fall 1997), pp. (15-18)

Brown, E. (2009). Straying the Course: Can Jewish and Secular Leadership Archetypes Rein in Religious Leaders? In: *Tempest in the Temple: Jewish Communities & Child Sex Scandals*, Amy Neustein, (Ed.), pp. (60-73), Brandeis University Press, ISBN 978-1-58465-671-5, Waltham, MA

Butler S. (1999). Because I Remember Terror, Father, I Remember You, by Sue Silverman: Reviewed by Sandra Butler. *Journal of Religion and Abuse*, Vol. 1, No.1, (1999), pp. (103-108), ISSN 1521-1037

Chayil, E. (2011). Orthodox Jewish Child Abuse: Shattering a Traumatic Silence, *One Voice* JFCAdvocacy@yahoogroups.com, (August 1, 2011)

Dratch, M. (2009). A Community of Co-enablers: Why Are Jews Ignoring Traditional Jewish Law by Protecting the Abuser? In: *Tempest in the Temple: Jewish Communities & Child Sex Scandals*, Amy Neustein, (Ed.), pp. (105-125), Brandeis University Press, ISBN 978-1-58465-671-5, Waltham, MA

Dorff, E.N. (2009). Foreword, In: *Tempest in the Temple: Jewish Communities & Child Sex Scandals*, Amy Neustein, (Ed.), pp. (ix-xiii), Brandeis University Press, ISBN 978-1-58465-671-5, Waltham, MA

Fifield, A. & Lesher, M. (1996). A Child's at Stake: A Custody Fight Becomes a Political Nightmare. *Village Voice*, (October 1, 1996), pp. (10, 12-13)

Featherman, J. (1995). Jews and Sexual Abuse, In: *Sexual Abuse in Nine North American Cultures: Treatment and Prevention*, Lisa Aronson Fontes (Ed.), pp. (128-155), Sage Publications, ISBN 0-8039-5435-2, Thousand Oaks, California

Glick, M. (2000). Dealing With "Orthodox" Child Molesters: A Response to the Community's Response. *Jewish Press*, (February 4, 2000), pp. (87-88)

Greenberg, I. (1990). Abuse in Jewish Families: Rabbis Can Help by Speaking Out. *Moment*, Vol. 15, No. 2, (April 1990), p. (49)

Harman, R. (1993). Public Hearing on Family Court System. *New York State Legislative Hearing Record*, (May 14, 1993), pp. (32-44)

Hemphill, C. (1990). The Agony of Yacov Riegler: Bureaucracy Fails to Save Brooklyn Boy. *New York Newsday*, (December 16, 1990), pp. (6, 22-23)

Lesher, M. (2009). The Fugitive and the Forgotten: Cracking the Cold Case of Rabbi Avrohom Mondrowitz, In: *Tempest in the Temple: Jewish Communities & Child Sex Scandals*, Amy Neustein, (Ed.), pp. (126-162), Brandeis University Press, ISBN 978-1-58465-671-5, Waltham, MA

Lesher, M. (2011). Their Brothers' Keepers : New York Should Stop Funding Separate, Private Police Forces for Orthodox Jews. *New York Post*, (July 31, 2011), pp. (21-22)

Mendelsohn, A. (2011). Wall of Silence: Sex Scandals in Religion, *Cogent/Benger Productions, Inc.* (May 16, 2011)

Montero, D. (1999). Victims Learn Kid-Sex Fiend Served No Time; Nightmare Lingers for Kid-Sex Victims, *New York Post,* (September 21, 1999), p. (3)

Neustein, A. & Lesher, M. (1999). Legislative Solutions to the Protective Parent Backlash. Family Violence and Sexual Assault Bulletin, Vol. 25, Nos. 2-3, pp. (19-26)

Neustein, A & Lesher, M. (2002a). Does the Jewish Community Sacrifice Victims of Sexual Abuse? *Jewish Exponent,* Vol. 211, No. 22 (May 30, 2002), p. (37)

Neustein, A & Lesher, M. (2002b). The Silence of the Jewish Media on Sexual Abuse in the Orthodox Jewish Community, In: *Sex, Religion, Media,* Dane S. Claussen, (Ed.), pp. (79-87), Rowman & Littlefield Publishers, Inc., ISBN 0-7425-1557-5, Lanham, MD

Neustein, A. & Lesher, M. (2008). A Single Case Study of Rabbinic Sexual Abuse in the Orthodox Jewish Community. *Journal of Child Sexual Abuse,* Vol. 17, Nos. 3-4, (September/October 2008), pp. (70-89), 1053-8712

Neustein, A. & Lesher, M. (2009). Justice Interrupted: How Rabbis Can Interfere with the Prosecution of Sex Offenders - And Strategies for How to Stop Them, In: *Tempest in the Temple: Jewish Communities & Child Sex Scandals,* Amy Neustein, (Ed.), pp. (197-229), Brandeis University Press, ISBN 978-1-58465-671-5, Waltham, MA

Shafran, A. A Matter of Orthodox Abuse. *Jewish Week,* (June 23, 2006)

Silberg, J & Dallam, S. (2009). Out of the Jewish Closet: Facing the Hidden Secrets of Child Sexual Abuse - And the Damage Done to Victims, In: *Tempest in the Temple: Jewish Communities & Child Sex Scandals,* Amy Neustein, (Ed.), pp. (77-104), Brandeis University Press, ISBN 978-1-58465-671-5, Waltham, MA

Staff Reporter (1991). Family of Sex Abuse Victim Driven From Home by Mob. *Guardian,* (August 2, 1991), p. 11

Staff Reporter (2009). Ohel's Halachic Advisor: OK To Cheat on Taxes? *Jewish Week,* (June 10, 2009)

Winston, H. (2009a). Brooklyn DA Announces New Plan To Urge Reporting of Abuse. *Jewish Week,* (April 2, 2009)

Winston, H. (2009b). A Suspected Pedophile Eludes the System. *Jewish Week,* (May 6, 2009)

Winston, H. (2011a). Abuse Case Tests Ohel's Adherence to Reporting Laws. *Jewish Week,* (February 23, 2011), pp. (1, 8)

Winston, H. (2011b). Ohel Campaign To Bolster Image Questioned: In wake of Jewish Week story, social service agency shared confidential files about abuse case with outsiders. *Jewish Week,* (May 31, 2011), pp. (1, 9)

13

Researching Sexual Abuse in Societies in Which Sexuality Is Regarded as Taboo: Difficulties and Proposed Solutions

Murat Topbaş and Gamze Çan
Karadeniz Technical University Faculty of Medicine, Department of Public Health, Trabzon Turkey

1. Introduction

Sexual violence is defined as any sexual act, attempt to obtain a sexual act, unwanted sexual comments or advances, or acts to traffic, or otherwise directed, against a person's sexuality using coercion, by any person regardless of their relationship to the victim, in any setting, including but not limited to home and work (1). In many countries a substantial proportion of women experiencing physical violence also experience sexual abuse. The term intimate partner abuse refers to the physical, sexual, and/or psychologial abuse of an individual perpetrated by a current or former intimate partner. While this term is gender-neutral, women are more likely to experience physical injuries and incur psychological concequences of intimate partner abuse (2).

Sexual abuse of women is commonly recognized as an important public health problem because of its attendant morbidity, mortality, and long-term impact on women's health (3-8).

2. Social and women associated characteristics

The features of societies determine women's responsibilities within those societies and represent the key to attitudes toward them. For example, the image of the child as representing the future of the community developed very early in Turkish society. Understanding of and sympathy towards motherhood and children are therefore among the factors that shaped Turkish traditions and customs (9). The elevated position ascribed to motherhood is even more apparent in the saying "*Paradise lies under [one's] mothers' feet.*" However, there are other perspectives that also judge a woman's position in society. For instance, the traditional Turkish saying "you must always keep a rod to a woman's back and a child in her belly" expresses a way of thinking that regards physical or sexual abuse of women as something quite natural.

Ninety-nine percent of the population of Turkey is Muslim. Islam recognizes that both men and women have sexual drives and rights to sexual fulfillment and affirms heterosexual relations within marriage and lawful relationships. But explicit discussion of sexuality is taboo in Turkey (10). Severe restrictions are imposed on sexuality under Islam, however. It is sometimes believed that if unsatisfied or uncontrolled, female sexuality might lead to social chaos (*fitna*), and that social order thus necessitates male control of women's bodies (9). Extramarital relations are forbidden in Islam. The woman has a duty to meet the sexual needs of the man to whom she is married. Although monogamy is common in Turkey in the strictly legal sense, the fact that society regards it as normal for a man to have extramarital relations outside religious laws, and that it is the man's wishes that play the determining role in the quantity, time, quality and form of sexual relations in marriage, makes the perception of the concept of sexual abuse difficult, for which reason it becomes a supposedly natural state of affairs for a woman to be exposed to sexual abuse.

The concept of approach to risk in terms of public health entails the principle of some service provision for all, but more for those at risk. In that light, all women may be at risk of sexual abuse, but some are at greater risk than others. These factors increase women's vulnerability. One of the most common forms of sexual violence around the world is that which is perpetrated by an intimate partner, suggesting that one of the most important risk factors for women - in terms of vulnerability to sexual assault - is being married or cohabiting with a partner. Other factors influencing the risk of sexual violence include:

- being young,
- consuming alcohol or drugs,
- having previously being raped or sexually abused,
- having many sexual partners,
- involvement in the sex trade,
- becoming more educated or economically empowered, at least where sexual violence perpetrated by an intimate partner is concerned and
- poverty.

Identification of women meeting these criteria will constitute the main objective for both research and for solving the problem.

3. Sources of data

The main sources of data for sexual abuse are police records, medical records, nongovernmental organization activities and survey research. The relationship between these sources and the global magnitude of the problem of sexual violence may be compared to an iceberg floating in water (11). The small visible tip represents cases reported to the police. A large part may be elucidated through survey research and the work of nongovernmental organizations. But beneath the surface remains a substantial although unquantified component of the problem.

Generally, sexual abuse has been a neglected area of research. The available data are scanty and fragmented. For example, police data are often incomplate and limited. Many women do not report sexual violence to the police because of shame, or from a fear of being blamed, not believed or otherwise mistreated. Data from medicolegal clinics may be biased towards the more violent incidents of sexual abuse. The proportion of women who seek medical services for immediate problems associated with sexual violence is also relatively small (1).

In addition to research aimed at determining the scale of the phenomenon in different societies, studies by nongovernmental organizations represent a further source of information. There is no screening program for abuse or violence towards women in Turkey. All that exists are the refuges or shelters known as "Purple Roofs," intended for women, or men, who seek their help and which provide judicial, social and psychological support for women exposed to violence.

4. Characteristics of existing studies

This section is intended to elicit conclusions by examining research on sexual abuse in terms of

- Method
- Aim and
- Study groups.

In terms of methodology, existing studies are mainly cross-sectional surveys based on an observational approach, while there may be a few case studies performed from patient presentations and fewer still of the quantitative focus group and in-depth interview type.

A simple description of the health status of a community, based on routinely available data or on data obtained in special surveys, is often the first step in an epidemiological investigation. In many countries this type of study is undertaken by a national centre for health statistics. Pure descriptive studies make no attempt to analyze the links between exposure and effect. They are usually based on mortality statistics and may examine patterns of death by age, sex or ethnicity during specified time periods or in various countries.

Cross-sectional studies measure the prevalence of disease and thus are often called prevalence studies. In a cross-sectional study the measurements of exposure and effect are made at the same time. It is not easy to assess the reasons for associations shown in cross-sectional studies. The key question to be asked is whether the exposure precedes or follows the effect. If the exposure data are known to represent exposure before any effect occurred, the data from a cross-sectional study can be treated like data generated from a cohort study.

Cross-sectional studies are relatively easy and inexpensive to conduct and are useful for investigating exposures that are fixed characteristics of individuals, such as ethnicity or blood group. In sudden outbreaks of disease, a cross-sectional study to measure several exposures can be the most convenient first step in investigating the cause.

Data from cross-sectional studies are helpful in assessing the health care needs of populations. Data from repeated cross-sectional surveys using independent random samples with standardized definitions and survey methods provide useful indications of trends. Each survey should have a clear purpose. Valid surveys need well-designed questionnaires, an appropriate sample of sufficient size, and a good response rate. Cross sectional studies are generally conducted "door to door" or "face to face" following appropriate sampling. The numerical data obtained are presented as prevalence and percentages.

Many countries conduct regular cross-sectional surveys on representative samples of their populations, focusing on personal and demographic characteristics, illnesses and health-related habits. Frequency of disease and risk factors can then be examined in relation to age, sex and ethnicity. Cross-sectional studies of risk factors for chronic diseases have been performed in a wide range of countries (12).

In these observational-type studies a "memory factor" problem, such as recalling or confusing past events, may arise when eliciting information from the interviewee. The memory factor does not represent a very significant drawback in terms of subject characteristics. But the characteristics of the person conducting the interview may affect study participation. The character of the interviewer is important in terms of subject confidentiality. Women may decline to participate in a study, for reasons such as the involvement of matters too private to be shared with someone encountered for the first time for the purpose of questionnaire administration or fear of her partner or partner's family, and this is important in terms of sources of error in observational-type studies.

One limitation of such studies is that only a small number of communities can be included, and random allocation of communities is usually not practicable; other methods are required to ensure that any differences found at the end of the study can be attributed to the intervention rather than to inherent differences between communities. Furthermore, it is difficult to isolate the communities where intervention is taking place from general social changes that may be occurring. Design limitations, especially in the face of unexpectedly large, favorable risk factor changes in control sites, are difficult to overcome. As a result, definitive conclusions about the overall effectiveness of community-wide efforts are not always possible.

Random and systematic errors are significant sources of error in epidemiological studies. There are three major sources of random error; individual biological variation, sampling error and measurement error. Systematic error (bias) comprises selection bias and measurement (or classification) bias. Selection bias occurs when there is a systematic difference between the characteristics of the people selected for a study and the characteristics of those who are not. Sample size and participation or refusal to take part represent a risk in terms of sources of error in studies of sexual abuse. While errors regarding sample size apply to all studies, an unwillingness to speak out because of the subject matter involved may hinder participation, and this may represent a more significant source of error.

Although there have been considerable advances over the past decade in measuring the phenomenon through survey research, the definition used have varied considerably across studies. There are also significant differences across cultures in the willingness to disclose sexual violence to researchers. Caution is therefore needed when making global comparisons of the prevalence of sexual violence (1).

With multi-factorial topics, the inability to control elements other than the factor investigated represents a significant limitation of cross-sectional studies. Because of the subject matter it is important for attention to be paid to this in cross-sectional surveys.

The number of studies regarding domestic violence and physical and sexual abuse is also limited. One of the main reasons for this is women's family loyalty and the fact that they ignore the physical and sexual abuse they suffer, a reluctance to apply to any legal or health institution, which stems from regarding such abuse as normal or at least putting up with it, and, in particular, the idea that even if they were to resort to such measures, abuse within the family is a purely domestic issue. This contradictory situation stems from changes in the nature of relations between men and women in Turkey in historical and social terms. However, its ancestral nature is particular to the Turks, and manifests deep psychological roots that need to be considered when evaluating Turkish group behavior (10).

Evaluated in terms of aims, existing research consists predominantly of prevalence studies aimed at determining the current situation. Studies provide analyses aimed at the scale of the subject representing narrow fields with small or large sample sizes. This approach is important as it will guide the subsequent cause, effect and intervention phases. Fewer case studies and qualitative studies are intended to provide information about causes.

In terms of study groups, cross-sectional survey studies are performed with married or pregnant women or with physicians. Participation levels for all groups constitute a significant problem. As explained above, this represents one of the sources of error in epidemiological studies. Eliciting information and discussing unmarried women's sex lives may be a problem, especially in societies in which sexuality is a taboo subject.

A participation level of 69% was reported in one cross-sectional study on the subject of sexual abuse with a study group made up of physicians. Physicians have also been shown to face severe problems in identifying relevant situations. Major barriers to physician identification of intimate partner abuse and referral of patients include patient-related barriers such as fear of retaliation, lack of disclosure, fear of police involvement and lack of follow up, mutual barriers such as cultural differences, lack of privacy and language differences, and provider-related barriers such as lack of training, lack of time, lack of resources/referrals and a sense of inefficacy (2).

When the study group is made up of physicians, the specialization of the group involved may also have an effect. Primary care physicians, internal disease specialists and obstetricians may produce different situation analyses. Obstetricians generally have a greater predisposition toward the subject, or may identify more cases. Generally speaking, primary care physicians tend not to add asking patients about sexual abuse to their routine procedures. Failure to identify patients at this stage represents a major missed opportunity. Standardization of protocols to be drawn up and procedures, as well as physician training, will increase interest and support on the subject (13,14).

5. Recommended solutions

Scientists with an interest in the subject in Turkey are aware that women are subjected to sexual abuse, but they face very great difficulties in conducting research intended to reveal the true position. The problems we envisaged prior to one study in which we investigated whether or not pregnancy had any effect on physical and sexual abuse, and the problems that arose during that research, are listed below. Our recommendations for Turkey and countries/societies resembling it in religious and social terms are also discussed:

1. Turkish society and Turkish women are unaware of and unable to fully comprehend the concept of sexual abuse. For that reason, awareness should be established before such studies, particularly using written and visual media, and research performed only afterward.

2. We observed in our research that even when women were forced to engage in sexual relations, or did so against their will, they put up with the situation, making no protest against it. Underlying this is the role of "satisfying the husband" that society imposes on women. However, this attitude changes as levels of education rise. This perspective declines if the woman is educated, is in paid employment and enjoys high status. Stratification should therefore be performed according to women's status when research is performed.
3. It is very difficult to perform screening / cross sectional studies / society-based research on the subject of sexual abuse. It is just about impossible to ask individuals or families identified for sampling in cross-sectional, cohort or descriptive studies questions about sexual abuse. In order to obtain more significant results from cross-sectional studies, given the difficulty in asking questions by way of questionnaires, research could be conducted on the basis of meetings with physicians at hospitals and clinics to which individuals apply and receive health services for any reason, with the security provided by the patient-doctor relationship.
4. Because of the difficulties involved in conducting descriptive, cross-sectional and cohort studies, it might be of greater benefit to perform quantitative research, such as focus group encounters, to reveal women's exposure to sexual abuse.
5. People who participate as project directors or interviewers in future research into such a sensitive subject must instill a sense of security in those taking part. The study team, and particularly those who will be involved in speaking to women, must be very well trained. That training must stress verbal communication, body language and general communication.
6. It is just about impossible to investigate extramarital sexual relations. For that reason, in planning research the study population should consist of women of reproductive age, 15-49, and married women only should be used, if possible.
7. It is effectively impossible in societies such as Turkey to ask about even a married woman's relations with different partners. The scale and nature of abuse in these relationships cannot therefore be established.
8. In Turkey, a woman's most important role in marriage is child-bearing. There is a strong preference for the child to be born to be male. Exposure to sexual abuse is therefore generally hidden because of that pressure. For that reason, questions should be asked investigating men and women's birth preferences and the results analyzed.
9. Sexual abuse is generally correlated with exposure to physical violence and emotional stress. Questions regarding physical and emotional abuse should therefore be asked before turning to sexual abuse. A second interview within the scope of the research should even be conducted if necessary because of the likelihood of sexual abuse in those responding positively to questions about those other forms of abuse.
10. It may be difficult to perform descriptive and/or cross-sectional studies in order to establish the nature, frequency and nature of and figures for sexual abuse. Studies should therefore be planned on the basis of more than one interview. This may help the woman taking part establish confidence in the study team and make it easier for her to provide more information about herself.
11. The person to conduct the interview coming from the local area may be either a positive or a negative factor. It may be positive in assisting women to establish a sense of trust, but negative in that women may be reluctant to share their secrets with a local.

12. Men should also perform studies. This will help educate men on an individual basis and also assist debate among men when the subject is raised, as well as establishing sensitivity/awareness.
13. Interview / questionnaire/data forms used must not be too long. Initial interview/scanning forms in particular must not be highly detailed for quantitative studies.

6. References

[1] WHO - Krug EG, Dahlberg LL, Mercy JA, Zwi AB, Lozano R, eds. World Report on Violence and Health. World Health Organization, Geneva 2002 pp: 149.

[2] Rodrigez MA, Bauer HM, McLoughlin E, Grumbach K. Screening and intervention for intimate partner abuse. JAMA 1999;281(5):468-474.

[3] Dunkle KL, Jewkes RK, Brown HC, Yoshihama M, Gray GE, McIntyre JA, Harlow SD. Prevalence and Patterns of Gender-based Violence and Revictimization among Women Attending Antenatal Clinics in Soweto, South Africa. American Journal of Epidemiology 2004; 160:230-9.

[4] Rodriguez AM, Bauer MH, McLoughlin E, Grumbach K. Screening and Intervention for Intimate Partner Abuse. JAMA 1999; 281(5): 468-474.

[5] Donohoe M. Violence and human rights abuses against women in the Developing World. Medscape Ob/Gyn & Women's Health 2003; 8(2). Available from: http://www.medscape.com/viewarticle/464255 (connecting date 23.04.2004).

[6] Martin SL, Mackie L, Kupper LL, Buescher PA, Moracco KE. Physical abuse of women before, during, and after pregnancy. JAMA 2001; 285:1581-1584.

[7] Velzeboer M, Ellsberg M, Arcas CC, Garcia-Moreno C. Violence against women: The Health Sector Responds. Pan American Health Organization, Silver Spring, Maryland, USA 2003. p. 4-7.

[8] Jewkes R, Sen P, Garcia-Moreno C. Sexual Violence. Chapter VI. World Report on Violence and Health. (Eds: Krug EG, Dahlberg LL, Mercy JA, Zwi AB, Lozano R) WHO, Switzerland; 2002. p149-81.

[9] Ornek SV. Geleneksel Kültürümüzde Çocuk (The Child in Our Traditional Culture). Türkiye İş Bankası Kültür Yayınları. Ankara, 1979. (in Turkish).

[10] Göka E. Kadın-erkek ilişkileri örneğinde "Türk Grup Davranışı" (In the relations between men and women: Turkish Group Behaviour). htpp://drerolgoka.20m.com/makale/015.htm (in Turkish)

[11] Jewkes R, Abrahams N. The epidemiology of rape and sexual coercion in South Africa: an overview. Social Science and Medicine 2002;55: 153 - 166.

[12] Bonita R, Beaglehole R, Kjellstörm T. Basic Epidemiology 2nd Edition. WHO 2006, Geneva.

[13] Freidman LS, Samet JH, Roberts MS, Hudlin M, Hans P. Inquiry about victimization experiences: a survey of patient preferences and physician practices. Arch Intern Med 1992; 152: 1186 - 1190.

[14] Parsons LH, Zaccaro D, Wells B, Stovall TG. Methods of and attitudes toward screening obstetrics and gynecology patients for domestic violence. Am J Obstet Gynecol. 1995; 173: 381-387.

14

Considering the Sexual Harassment as an Equivalent Incestuous

Claudio Cohen and Adriana Esturaro
University of São Paulo, São Paulo
Brazil

"Power is the great aphrodisiac"
Henry Kissinger
(The Nobel Peace Prize)

1. Introduction

Relationships formed in a professional setting may involve conflicts of interest arising from social functions determined by institutions, such as family, church, codes of ethics and labor laws. In these relationships, we can see emotions, characteristic of human beings, but which are limited by factors imposed by cultural identity. As every society develops its own culture, individuals acquire their values in relation to the social context in which they live. This cultural identity influences the creation of norms of conducts and the values linked to it.

An encounter with another person will always cause some sort of emotional disturbance, due to the adaptation to the presence of the other. This disturbance predominantly originates from our understanding of social structures and respect for the freedom of others, and can be perceived in different forms.

One of the forms of adaptation to the presence of the other emotional disturbance is sexual harassment, which is either an intimidation, bullying or coercion of a sexual nature, or an unwelcome or inappropriate promise of rewards in exchange of sexual favors (Paludi, 1991).

It includes a wide range of behaviors, from seemingly mild transgressions and annoyances, to actual sexual abuse or assault (Dziech, 1990).

It may also occur in a variety of different settings. For example, in education, many scholars point out that sexual harassment remains a "forgotten secret," with educators and administrators refusing to admit that the problem exists in their schools, or accepting their legal and ethical responsibilities to deal with it (Ibid).

Sexual abuse commonly occurs in workplaces, and can have several different forms, such as unwanted jokes, gestures, offensive words about clothing, unwelcome comments and wordplay, repeated requests for dates that are turned down, or unwanted flirting. It can be anything of sexual nature, from verbal to physical behavior (U.S. Equal Employment Opportunity Commission).

Polymorphous incest, according to Cohen (1992), "involves sexual relationships between people that take advantage of their positions or jobs to have sexual satisfaction with someone who has a subaltern position, and is considered an equivalent of incest". Professional relationships are vertically asymmetric, and may be equivalent to the parent-child relationship, that is, they have hierarchy of power and specific laws.

There is a relationship of power between bosses and their subordinates, between psychoanalysts and their patients, professors and students. This relationship of power is the central point of this discussion, because it has an element of social control in it (Foucault, 1993).

According to Foucault, sexuality and politics are the two most important taboos in society, with discourses filled with the search for desire and power, the struggle for control and the prohibitions related to them. (Foucault, 1993)

Our proposal is to demonstrate that sexual harassment in a professional environment is a type of incest and cannot be simply classified as sexual assault. In these cases, besides the abuse of power, violence towards the victim is frequent, and because of these factors, sexual harassment is called "polymorphous incest".

We will use Freud's psychoanalytical theory to explain the basis of sexual development, how sexuality develops normally, and what causes certain deviations in a way that a human being will show socially unacceptable sexual.

2. Definition of sexual harassment

According to the Universal Declaration of Human Rights, "all human beings are born free and equal in dignity and rights. They are endowed with reason and conscience and should act towards one another in a spirit of brotherhood". Sexual harassment is an offence to human rights.

Sexual harassment is a problem that afflicts the entire world. In the 1990s, the number of cases in United States increased, the profile of victims changed, and more laws were created in order to set new precedents.

People from different backgrounds, cultures and social positions have found themselves involved in sexual harassment cases, from presidents to church leaders.

Sexual harassment in the workplace is attracting increasing attention, nowadays, many countries have established laws forbidding this conduct in the workplace. This kind of offence is not only a problem of the Western world: the Egyptian Centre for Women's Rights (ECWR) describes the problem as a social cancer. A survey made by this organization showed that sexual harassment was experienced by 98% foreign women visitors, and by 83% Egyptian women.

The research team on sexual harassment at workplace of Women Watch-China showed that 23.9% of the interviewees reported having witnessed or heard about sexual harassment of other employees in the same company, 19.8% of the interviewees admitted having been sexually harassed, and 5.3% of interviewees admitted having sexually harassed others (Women Watch-China, 2010). This research team suggested helping companies to establish a mechanism to prevent sexual harassment at work, besides discussing and improving laws and regulations on the issue.

Sexual harassment is characterized by different actions, which may be comments of sexual nature such as jokes, insinuations or wordplay, or even verbal and physical abuse to obtain sexual favors. We have to emphasize here that sexual harassment is related with undesirable conducts that are not pleasurable for the receptor, that is, they are imposed, and uncorresponded. That is when we can see the difference with conducts in corresponded affective relationships.

However, sexual harassment has a component of the neurotic behavior in hysteria, observed by Freud when dealing with hysteria in three essays on sexuality. In hysteria, there is a contradiction: excessive sexual need on one side, and excessive sexual repression on the other. The person affected by this disorder likes to be harassed, and many times demonstrates interest in the proposal. However, he or she cannot act on it, and unconsciously uses this ambivalence, with a secondary benefit, playing the role of the victim.

Sexual harassment is one of the offenses to sexual freedom, and the perpetrator may be any person, men, women, and even the victim. However, what we would like to emphasize here is the contribution of the victim to the offense. As in the case of any crime, sexual harassment is also analyzed in criminology, the science that studies crime, criminality and their causes: the victim, social control of the criminal act, personality of the criminal and the way to insert him/her back into society.

Shecaria (2011) emphasizes that "victim studies are very important, because they enable the examination of the role of the victim as a trigger of the crime. Besides, they enable the study on judicial, moral, psychological and therapeutic assistance, especially in cases of violence or severe threat to the person, crimes that leave marks or traumas, making it possible to determine adequate measures, and enabling the indemnification of the victims by state programs, as occurs in several countries..."

Elias Neuman (1984), an Argentinean criminologist, emphasized that the victim may be the triggering factor in the etiology of crime and, in certain cases and circumstances, may assume a posture that contributes to the offense. In some cases, the notion of the victim's innocence should be set aside.

The worldwide trend is to relate sexual harassment to the work environment. In some countries, sexual harassment at work is considered a crime, whereas in other countries in the Middle East, there are no regulations on the subject.

The workplace is where several people have their jobs and, generally, have an intimate relationship for long periods. This environment creates an opportunity for people to get close to each other. This intense relationship between work colleagues may give rise to intimate relationships that may even lead to marriage, and it is an absolutely normal fact of life that people meet each other, feel attracted and decide to consolidate affective relationships.

However, there are situations in which affection is not corresponded. In these cases, sexual coercion may be practiced by people in superior hierarchic position, constituting sexual harassment. The behavior of the harasser may be beyond reasonable standards, and may involve exchanging sexual favors for permanence on the job; inadequate invitations involving promotions, and other situations.

Studies carried out in Brazil (Cohen et al.), and in other parts of the world (China and Egypt) demonstrated that women are more harassed than men. However, we should consider that, even if less frequent, men are also harassed. There is, though, a dark figure, because men do not report the crime because of fear of prejudice. Fazary (2004) states that "The 'dark figure' of crime is not some sinister character but a theory that postulates that we do not know how much crime is out there, and that with current methods of studying of crime we have no way of knowing the truth".

Failure to report an offense is very common, especially in cases of sexual abuse. There is a certain embarrassment on the part of victims to make the event public. In 1994, the matter was dealt with by the American film industry in the film "Disclosure", directed by Barry Levinson, a film on sexual harassment in which the man who is harassed by his new female boss.

The United States were the first country to make sexual harassment a crime, on the second half of the 1970s. From this moment on, other countries considered sexual harassment a crime. Among them, Spain, Portugal, France and Italy. In Brazil, it was introduced as a sex offense in the penal code only in 2001.

Although Brazilian regulations have make sexual harassment in the workplace a crime, we emphasize that the problem is much wider, as we will show in this discussion. Although there is a law that criminalizes sexual harassment, seldom do harassed people seek legal compensation for the problem. In most of the cases, the final legal decisions are do not favor those who appeal.

According to Pamplona Filho (2001), sexual harassment is any unwanted conduct of sexual nature which, although turned down, is continuously repeated, restricting the sexual freedom of the victim. This conduct is a violation of the free use of one's own body, and is deeply embarrassing. When occurs at the workplace, consequences are even more devastating.

However, this author, when dealing with the free use of the body, show us that sexual harassment may occur in other places and other social relationships, such as the academic world (professors, students, education workers); in hospitals (among doctors, aides and patients); in the religious world (among clergy and churchgoers).

These relationships, and even those between a boss and an employee, have an ethical-institutional structuring function that is called polymorphous incest or equivalent of incest. Institutions and relationships established between peers are moralistic and paternalistic, a reflection of the parent-child relationship (incest itself) and of its endogamy prohibition (Cohen, 1999).

In this context, Brazilian laws also consider it a crime, because it is another type of sex offense, such as rape. Penalties are greater when the offense is practiced by someone who has authority over the victim, such as a step father or mother, uncle or aunt, sibling, spouse, tutor, guardian, preceptor or boss.

3. Institutions: Ethical and moral aspects

It is important to demonstrate that laws are created based on a set of social factors. The most important of these factors are the institutions. Bleger (2001) defines institution as a set of norms that generate social values. Their essential function is to create rules for groups of individuals. The function of the Institution is to create values that transcend and characterized the individual. The institution comes before the professional relationship.

Social institutions are some of the ways that society uses to achieve satisfaction. In order to do that, regulatory tools are created and imposed to those who they aim at regulating. In Brazil and other countries, there are class entities that create norms of conduct for their members. Social acceptance of a given ideology, such as health, justice, or disease, is carried out by these entities. Institutes are moral representatives of the Institution. They are professional boards, courts, family, and others.

Conduct norms are filled with values that are linked to the interests of the institutions. What is expected from one professional is not always applicable to the other: expectations on the conduct of a teacher are different from those of a doctor, and so on. Institutions function as defense mechanisms against the most primitive anguishes of humans, strengthen the ego of their members, and make it possible for them to carry out their jobs (Jaques, 1969).

According to Cromberg's understanding "... when thinking that humans should be analyzed by their conscious acts and by social codes, I do not consider these codes all-embracing, once sexual and aggressive pulsions resist being domesticated by social codes, and make the psychological reality of humans highly complex. Besides, there is more to reality than that. There are intersubjective relationships that are not moderated only by social codes or necessity. These relationships produce imaginary effects that are privileged members of our psychological reality" (Cromberg, 2004).

Society establishes social codes based on cultural parameters, and does not accept sexual abuse. It will punish the aggressor once he/she is considered guilty. Different from the legal system, the activity of psychoanalysis is not limited to the identification of the aggressor, and to holding him/her accountable for what he/she did. It does not place the victim in a passive position, either. Human nature is more complex and mysterious than we can imagine.

Cromberg (2004), when talking about aggressive pulsions, does not refer to innate human nature, but to natural inclination towards aggressiveness.

When conduct norms are created, there are moral and ethical issues, with which we deal differently. Moral encompasses three characteristics: the values determined by it, which are not questioned; the fact that these values are imposed to everybody, and the punishment, when rules are disobeyed (Cohen and Segre, 2008). The expression of the values of society is given by the laws. Laws are not warranties of human behavior, once respecting the law depends on ethics, which are experienced differently by each member of society. Some accept the limits better than others. Institutions, with their conduct norms, abhor the attitude of those who practice sexual harassment. However, the existence of the law is no warranty that sexual harassment will not be part of crime statistics. Laws, without ethics, are useless.

The pillar that supports ethics is the perception of conflicts of psychological life. It is expected that individuals have resources to deal with his/her emotions in relation to reason, and that he/she may solve these conflicts coherently and with autonomy (ibidem). Cohen and Segre (2008) show the huge difference between moral and ethics: while moral has to be imposed, ethics should be grasped by the individual, it has to come from the inside.

According to Guirado (2010), intra and interinstitutional power relationships involve both agent-agent and agent-client relations. The power struggle shows, on one side, the one who sets the conduct norms, and on the other, the one who has to abide by it. However, the one who sets the norm also has to abide by it, he or she is not superior to the norm. Relationships established among peers, in other social scenarios different from hierarchical relationships at the workplace, may also be sexual harassment because when there is a breach of trust and the abuse of power.

Sexual conduct is not determined by a universal standard. Something that is acceptable for some is not for others. In some societies, exposing the body is acceptable and natural, while other societies demand the use of garments that cover the body as much as possible. Sexual-related behaviors may change from time to time, as individuals live and feel things differently depending on their time and culture. Social practices are determined by society, and culture strongly influences the way people relate to each other.

Humans live their sexuality very differently from the other living beings. First, because sex is not limited to reproduction, and second, because there are some peculiarities, such as desire, passion, fantasies, sensations and guilt. However, we should not banalize sexuality and reject the possibility of reproduction, one of the objectives of couples at reproductive age. Those couples that having difficulties in conceiving may use the services offered by a countless number of assisted reproduction clinics.

4. Sexuality and abuse of power

The structure and organization of human sexuality, specially in terms of sex differentiation and their position in relation to castration anxiety, is caused by the Oedipus complex, which also enables experimenting the ambivalence of desire.

Laplanche and Pontalis (1974) define the Oedipus complex as "an organized set of loving and hostile desires that the child feels toward the parents". In its so-called positive form, the complex is presented as in the history of Oedipus the king, who wishes for the death the rival, the character of the same sex, and has sexual desire for the character of the opposite sex. In the negative form, it is the opposite: love for the parent of the same sex, and jealous hatred for the parent of the opposite sex. In real situations, these two forms are found in different levels in complete form of Oedipus complex.

According to Freud(2001), the peak of Oedipus complex occurs between three and five years of age, during the phallic stage; its decline marks the latency stage. It is revived in puberty, and overcome, with greater or lesser success, in a special type of object-choice. Oedipus complex has a fundamental role in structuring the personality and in directing human desire Oedipal feelings come and go throughout life. As castration does not take place, there is nothing to prevent both the desire and the action. In this case, the problem is that the person will be held socially or criminally accountable for his/her.

Cohen et al. analyzed sexuality from a bioethical viewpoint, and observed that it is impossible to ignore the evolution of sexual context and ethics throughout history (Cohen et al., 2009).

When analyzing the historical aspects of human sexuality, Foucault brings an important contribution: the human being, in all its dimensions - social, politic, mental, ideological, cultural – is the central factor. For him, "the great game in history will be won by those who take hold of the rules, who take power from the ones who use power; it will be won by those who, in disguise, pervert the rules; who use the rules upside down and inside out; who put the rules against those who had imposed them" (Foucault, 1990).

This fragment shows us who is behind the power relationships, that is, who has control and creates the rules that domesticate the bodies and mainly, who use these rules for personal interests. This way, we go back to the idea of institutions as the keepers of power, the ones who determine rules and punishments for breaking these rules.

Power relationships have, on one side, someone who is dominant, and on the other side, someone who is dominated. This kind of essence was used by the Church to impose its values. According to Foucault (1990) , in the 18th century, society lived under powerful sexual repression; sex was reduced to mere reproduction, and the couple became the social model. Everything that is different from this standard became amoral and was banned, denied and silenced (Ibidem).

In the same piece, Foucault (1990) says: "until the end of the 18th century, three great explicit codes - besides the regulations related to costumes and opinions - ruled sexual practices: canonical rights, Christian pastoral power and civil law." These codes were centered in matrimonial relationships and determined what was licit and illicit in conjugal duties. Sex of a married couple was oppressive, full of rules and recommendations. In confession, married couples had to tell the priests all details of their sexual intercourses. In the 18th century, a system of surveillance mechanisms was in place. These mechanisms were coercive and corrective, and had the power to repress and silence the bodies, and suppress latent desires. The Church aimed at domesticating sex and bodies, and invested in restrictions to words and everything that was connected to sexual issues, in a way that anything that dealt with the theme was denied and considered degenerated.

Foucault (1990) proposed the study of what was in the margins of society: child sexuality, madness, criminals, those who love the other sex, maniacs, that is, a set of illicit issues that were on the edges of the social system. Power relationships discussed by him aimed at showing the elements that were on the borders of central issues, that is, to show how the discourse of power is gagged by culture, how stereotypes are build and how they are outside the social order. At this moment, it is possible to see the real interest of those who have a reductionist discourse on conducts considered wrong.

Freud, on his turn, developed a theory to explain the development of sexuality from the generation of the psychological subject. The organization of sexuality allows the subject to choose the object, with fixation in stages of development that bring him/ her greater pleasure. This can occur naturally or become a perverted fixation on an object. To Freud, humans are born as a polymorphous, perverse beings, and culture represses some perverse aspects. Transformation of perverse desires is part of the development of sexuality, and psychosocial development will repress pulsions. Thus, different from other animals, human sexuality will become independent of the reproductive function.

The theory of sexual selection was proposed by the British naturalist Charles Darwin, in 1871, in his book "**The Descent of Man, and Selection in Relation to Sex".** In his theory, he called "sexual selection" the process of choosing morphological and behavioral characteristics that may lead to successful mating, a process responsible for the evolution of characteristics that determine reproductive advantages. Instinct is related to biological sex. The sexual function of humans is innate and responsible for the preservation of the species. It is biological sex, proposed by Darwin, the reproductive function of all animals.

On the other hand, the development of sexuality is a long and complex process that begins at birth, and matures at puberty, the phase when reproduction and pleasure are associated. Freud demonstrated, in his studies on sexuality, that during psychosexual development, there is a change in object that provides sexual gratification. This finding made Freud develop his theory on the stages of sexual development. However, Freud emphasized that even a newborn have a germ of sexual motions. But sex life of a child is expressed in an observable way only after three or four years of age (Freud, 2001).

Freud called "pregenital" the stages of sexual development that come before puberty. The oral stage is the first one; sexual activity is not separated from nutrition. The second pregenital phase is the anal-sadistic organization. In this stage, activity is produced by pulsion for domination using body muscles. At this moment, the individual already shows sexual polarity, and a partial object. However, organization and subordination to reproductive function are still lacking. After that, sexual organization will only be defined in puberty, and the outcome is normal adult sex life, with a solid organization towards an external sex object (Freud, 1905). The third phase, which Freud called genital stage, is characterized by a greater or lesser organization of libido under the preponderance of the erogenous zone and object relationship (Laplanche and Pontalis,).

According to psychoanalysis theory and practice, in the development of human sexuality, the individual is born as a polymorphous perverse being dominated by sexual pulsions and death. He/she has to go through several stages, as demonstrated above, for his/her development, which will organize the Oedipus complex, his/her first experience aiming at humanizing the individual (Cohen, 1999).

Based on this theoretical referential of psychoanalysis, we understand that human psychological structure is supported by a tripod: genetic (complementary series), social (Oedipus complex) and individual factors (mental structure: id, ego and superego). The World Health Organization shows that health is biopsychosocial wellbeing, an integration of biological, psychological and social aspects (Cohen, 1999).

Therefore, human sexuality is nothing more than the product of symbolic constructions of one subject with the other, permeated by moral and social laws (religious law, Civil and Penal Codes, Conduct Codes). Conduct codes are important for the organization of society. However, they are worth nothing if the individual is not able to interpret them and act accordingly, as we can see if we analyze the situation of priests that harass churchgoers.

Choosing celibacy is an autonomous decision. It is understood that the choice was not forced upon the individual. Once on this path, the dogmas are presented to this individual together with the code of principles he/she has to follow, at the risk of punishment. Autonomy may only be created based on a respectful relationship. It comes from the perception of conflict between coherent decision-making and the ethical principles inherent to each human being.

There are reports from different parts of the world about churchgoers that were sexually harassed by priests. One example involves Cardinal Bernard Law, the archbishop of Boston, who turned a blind eye to the knowledge of sexual abuse committed by priests from parishes under his supervision. Not all individuals in a society are able to be ethical. In the case mentioned above, we have a Cardinal that knew the problem and turned a blind eye to it; and we have the priest who was carried away by his pulsions and moved away from the ethical principals of his function, using the trust bond established by the institution to which he belongs.

When a priest abuses churchgoers, he breaks up with the moral code and becomes socially incompetent for his function. When using autonomy to choose the religious path, the Church, as an Institution, recognized the aptitude of the person and authorized him/her to follow his wills, according to a legitimate code. This priest was fully instructed and made oaths. When he chose the break up with these commitments, he has to be held accountable for his actions by canonical, civil and penal laws. He will be punished, if the reports are accepted and the process continues. However, the difficulty in judging peers was observed not only in the Church, but in other Institutions.

Situations related to covering illicit acts are found in other social relationships; for example, when soldiers rape war prisoners with the consent of their superiors. This is also common in tribal wars in Africa, as in the case of Angolans raping immigrants who work in the mines of Luanda (source: doctors without borders). These are typical examples that involve individual ethics in relation to human rights. An army has a mission of recovering an invaded territory, as it was the case in Angola or American soldiers in Iraq. These soldiers committed crimes that harm human dignity, something that involves ethics and moral.

More than once, we heard of powerful people involved in sexual scandals, such as Bill Clinton, Arnold Schwarzenegger, Berlusconi, and more recently, Dominique Strauss-Kahn. What these people have in common, besides their public positions, is the power that their position gives them. They all seem to be above the law, and consider that they can do anything, without being punished. It is a narcissistic experience, common to any child, and is characterized by the total lack of respect and acceptance of the other. A regression to pre-Oedipian stages, specially because the ego and the id were not differentiated. The way out of narcissism is the possibility of socialization. Narcissistic subjects live in a reality that is not able to support the demands of the others, that is, they are subjects who talk about themselves to themselves, and are fragile in building relationships and projects. They are destructive and do not add values. To Joel Birman (

2005), postmodern society may be considered a culture of narcissism. Narcissism was approached by Freud several times. His referential starts in listening to the suffering of the patient, walks the path of pathology and reaches the definition of narcissism as a stage of libido development, a stage when looking at oneself is considered the object of love.

Many years have passed between Bill Clinton and Dominique Strauss-Kahn. It seems that, nowadays, society does not tolerate sexual abuse. In the case of Mr. Clinton, in 1998, he had the right to defend himself and kept his public position until the end of the case. Dominique Strauss-Kahn, on the other hand, was sent to prison and resigned from his public position.

A study carried out by Cohen et al. analyzed patients who reported doctor sexual abuses to the Sao Paulo Board of Medicine (CREMESP - Conselho Regional de Medicina do Estado de São Paulo). There were 150 reports of doctor sexual abuse in five years. From these, 63.96% were dismissed for lack of proofs, which is concerning, and only 22.67% of the cases were submitted to ethics and disciplinary processes. The age of the doctors involved ranged, in 87% of the cases, from 36 to 75 years old, the same age range of the harassers mentioned above (CREMESP, 2009).

We have to emphasize that sexual harassment is not an exclusive masculine offense, in which only men abuse women. Besides the cases cited above, there are reports of female teachers who sexually abused their students, such as Christine Scarlett, who was condemned to 5 years in prison for having sexual intercourse with a 17-year-old student. She became pregnant and was accused of sexual aggression and dissemination of obscenity to youth. Allena Willians, a medium school teacher, was indicted for having sexual intercourse with five boys between 13 to 15 years old. Other cases such as these appear in the news from time to time.

In spite of all these considerations drawn on harassers, the real focus of our interest is the game of power and the fantasy of imagining being in the control of the situation. What is this control that goes through the false perception of "considering" the other so submissive, he/she would never make things public? The other is treated as an object, not as a subject who has wills and wishes and may accept the proposal or turn it down, and may set a limit to the relationship. That is when the problem arises: the all-powerful person sees himself/herself facing a scandal, and will have to be responsible for his/her acts and respond legally to them. In these cases, the harasser pulsions are transferred to the other, making the victim responsible for the offense, and be free of guilt. Psychological functioning is compromised: this person was commanded by pleasure, and his/her fantasy had to be lived, no matter the consequences.

According to Laplanche and Pontalis (1984), and based on Freud, two basic principles regulate mental functioning: the pleasure principle and the reality principle. The pleasure principle is related to psychological activity that has the objective of avoiding suffering and seeking pleasure.

The reality principle is paired with the pleasure principle, changing it. As reality is imposed as a regulating principle, the search for pleasure does not take the shortest path, but takes turns and is postponed, as a consequence of the conditions imposed by the exterior world. This principle characterizes the preconscious-conscious system; psychoanalysis sets an intervention with this principle, as a type of pulsional energy working for the ego (Laplanche and Pontalis, 1984)).

Freud (2001) considered that pulsions may be understood, initially, only as psychological representations of an endosomatic, continuous source of stimulation, differentiating them from isolated, exciting stimulations that come from the outside (Freud, 1905). Therefore, Pulsion is one of the concepts that helps us to delimit animic and physical reality. Pulsion distinguishes these two realities, and gives them specific properties, which is the relationship between somatic sources and their targets. Tension is relieved by the pulsion, in a way that the impulse to act to satisfy this pulsion is intrinsically connected to the psychic history of the individual.

5. Sexual harassment as an equivalent of incest

Sexual harassment is characterized by the use of the pleasure principle by means of the endosomatic power given by the professional function, without respecting the reality principle that the other imposes to the harasser. Sexual harassment committed by doctors is considered an abusive, unethical, and incestuous act, due to the asymmetric nature of the doctor-patient relationship. (Cohen et al. 2009). All situations presented in this discussion, such as teacher-student and priest-churchgoer relationships, and those with hierarchic superiors, fit in what is called polymorphous incest or equivalent of incest.

In order to understand polymorphous incest or the equivalent of incest, it is important to observe some particular aspects related to human relationships. Depending on the place that one occupies in a given context, peer relationship is different. To Cohen, these relationships may be symmetric or asymmetric.

Asymmetric relationships among relatives and members of a family determine the following functions: the father as the one who sets the laws; the mother as the holder of emotions; the children as the ones who will learn to deal with reality. The objective of the family, in a given cultural context, is preservation. Professional relationships also fit in this asymmetric classification. Vertically, they are equivalent to the parent-child relationship, because they build this hierarchic scenario, with power and specific laws (Cohen, 1999).

Social and erotic relationships are symmetric. Social relationships are those between friends and have as objectives protection of the individuals and preservation of the social group; the values of the individuals in the group are similar. Erotic relationships make people close when seeking sexual pleasure, and may also have the objective of preservation of the species (Cohen, 1999).

We demonstrated that the search for sex relationships with peers with whom there is trust bond or preexistence of a professional relationship end up on Oedipal fantasies. Not even the superego or social moral will function as repressors, in a way that desire goes beyond limits.

This is the problem. The law exists, it is the moral factor. However, respecting it or not depends on individual ethics, because moral is imposed, and ethics have to be lived and understood. Ethics are based on the perception of the conflicts of psychological life (emotion vs. reason), and in the condition - that can be acquired - that we take coherent positions when facing these conflicts.

Not everybody lives and solves conflicts in an ethical manner, because psychological structure is not always adjusted for good mental functioning. Under the psychoanalytical point of view, the Ego should deal with internal and external conflicts. The ego has the function of better understanding ethics, because it is the part of the psychological apparatus that deals with pulsions that come from the Id, and orders that come from the Superego. (Cohen and Segre, 2008)

People who sexually harass other have a huge difficulty in adapting to the reality principle. Their emotions do not respect reason, because they are not able to take coherent positions when facing the limits and social functions imposed to them. The equivalent of incest, that is, power over the others given by social power, is repeated in sexual harassment when a boss starts to feel like a father, who has power over all the other members of the family and consequently, may abuse them.

6. Conclusion

Sexual harassment is not a contemporaneous phenomenon, exclusive of a given society. It does not depend of social and moral order, or even gender-related issues. It is generally seen as a type of sex crime, and not as an incestuous relationship.

However, cultural understanding of the way we deal with the attitudes involving sexual harassment can be changed.

We emphasize that our understanding of sexual harassment encompasses all relationships that involve power. This power is linked to a function given by an institution, and the person that accepted to be harassed was under pressure. Therefore, his/ her acceptance cannot be considered valid.

Sex relationships may be considered a special type of social relationship, one that is marked by respect to the other, and not on acting on incestuous impulses or perverse, polymorphous fantasies (child sexuality). Society imposes rules related to these issues.

Sexual perversion consequent to the abuse of power (sexual relationships between doctors and patients, teachers and students, bosses and employees, priests and churchgoers) should be considered an equivalent of incest, which we call polymorphous incest. It is clearly sexual abuse, because consent is not valid, because the harasser is only acting on Oedipal or pre-Oedipal fantasies. It is a socially illicit act, because it perverts professional function. It is abuse of power in an asymmetric relationship. It is a violent act, from an institutional viewpoint, because the individual takes advantage of preexisting professional trust to transform the professional relationship in another type of relationship. It apparently is an erotic sign (EROS) but, in fact, it is a sign of discharge of anguish (TANATOS).

Class entities, represented by social institutions, should reflect upon polymorphous incest and its individual and social consequences, in order to approach the problem in an unprejudiced way.

7. References

Birman, J. (2009) Mal -estar na atualidade: a psicanálise e as novas formas de subjetivação Civilização Brasileira. ISBN-13: 9788520004920. Rio de Janeiro.

Bleger, J. (2001). Temas de Psicologia. São Paulo: Martins fontes. ISBN-13: 9788533608771 São Paulo - Brasil.

Cohen et al.(2009) Sexual Harassment in the physician-patient interaction: analysis of charges against doctors in the state of São Paulo. Clinical Science; 64 (11)

Cohen, C & Segre, M. (2008) Bioética Editora da Universidade de São Paulo. ISBN 978-85-314-0304-0. São Paulo - Brazil

Cohen, C. (1993) O incesto um desejo. Casa do Psicólogo, São Paulo. BRAZIL

Cohen, C. (1999) Bioética e sexualidade nas relações profissionais. Associação Paulista de Medicina. São Paulo. São Paulo. BRAZIL

Cromberg R. U. (2004) In Nos olhares: mulheres e relações de gênero do Brasil- Fundação Carlos Chagas. São Paulo. BRAZIL

Darwin, C. (2010).The Works of Charles Darwin, Volume 21: The Descent of Man, and Selection in Relation to Sex (Part One). ISBN-10: 0814720641. NYU Press. New York - USA.

Dziech, B. W. & Weiner, L. The Lecherous Professor: Sexual Harassment on Campus. Chicago Illinois: University of Illinois Press, 1990

Fazari, G. M. . Research Strategy for Bringing to Light the Dark Figure of Campus Crime. Campus Law Enforcement Journal Volume:34 Issue:6 , 2004 Pages:32-34, to 36 Editor(s): Karen E. Breseman National Institute of Justice/NCJRS. Publisher Url: http://www.iaclea.org

Foucault, M (1990)The History of Sexuality, Vol. 1: An Introduction. Randon House, Inc ISBN 0-679-72469-9 . New York USA

Freud, S. (2001) The Complete Psychological Works of Sigmund Freud: "A Case of Hysteria" "Three Essays on Sexuality " and Other Works v. 7. Vintage. ISBN-13: 978-0099426585 New York - USA

Guirado, M. (2010) A análise institucional do discurso como analítica da subjetividade Annablume. ISBN 978-85-391-0127-6 São Paulo - Brazil.

http//www.womenwatch-china.org

Jaques, E. (1969) Os sistemas sociais como defesa contra a ansiedade persecutória e depressiva. Temas de Psicanálise aplicada. Zahar Editores. Rio de Janeiro - Brazil.

Laplanche & Pontalis. (1974) The Language of Psycho-Analysis W. W. Norton. ISBN-13: 978-0393011050. New York- USA

Neuman , E. (1984) Victimología - El rol de la víctima en los delitos convencionales y no convencionales. Editorial Universidad. ISBN-10: 9509072753 Buenos Aires.

Paludi, M. A. & Barickman, (1991) *Academic and Workplace Sexual Harassment*. SUNY Press.

Pamplona Filho, R. (2001) O assédio sexual na relação de emprego. LTR. ISBN-13: 9788536116891. São Paulo- Brazil

Shecaria, S.S (2011)- Criminologia- Editora Revista dos Tribunais. ISBN-13: 9788520339695 São Paulo-Brazil.

15

Sexual Abuse of Live-In Care Workers in Taiwan

Shu-Man Pan[1] and Jung-Tsung Yang[2]
[1]*Graduate Institute of Social Work, National Taiwan Normal University,*
[2]*Department of Sociology, National Taipei University,*
Taiwan

1. Introduction

Since 1993 Taiwan has become an ageing society. The growing number of old people increases the demands of long-term care. However, this trend has been ignored by the government. With little support from the government and decline of family size, middle-class families are likely to depend on paid employment for caring the family elderly. Every year thousands of migrant women from Southeast Asia enter Taiwan to work in private households as care workers providing care for the frail elderly or persons with severe disabilities.

Due to the lack of workplace protection and the live-in close relationship between employee and employer, these migrant women workers are vulnerable to exploitation and abuse in the workplace. However, the problem of abuse of live-in care workers have been largely ignored by Taiwanese feminist scholars of domestic violence and scholars of migration studies. This ignorance is also manifested in the policy of the government. Even though some studies of migration in Taiwan have recently revealed the disadvantages faced by live-in care workers in their employment (Lin, 1999; Lan, 2000 & 2006; Cheng, 2004; Loveband, 2004; Liang, 2011), few investigate the problem of sexual violence against migrant women workers in private households (Pan and Yang, 2012).

Accordingly, by analyzing the internal dynamics of Taiwanese households employing female migrant workers, this chapter aims to explore a topic ignored by the research on global migration and domestic violence. Drawing data from interviews and documents, this chapter illustrates how the cultural norms and family ideologies behind the foreign labor system reinforce the exploitation and abusive relationship. This chapter is divided into four sections following this introduction. First, this chapter analyzes the changes of population and family structure in Taiwan. Second, this chapter presents policies and regulations regarding live-in care workers. Third, this chapter illustrates the cases of live-in care workers who are sexually abused. Finally, this chapter investigates the internal dynamics of Taiwanese household employing live-in care workers.

2. Changes of population and family structure

2.1 Changes of population

The population structure of Taiwan has transformed over the past fifteen years. In 2010, the total population was approximately 23 millions. Persons aged over 65 constitute 10.7% of the total population (Council for Economic Planning and Development, 2008). This number is expected to increase up to 20% in 2025 and 38% in 2056 respectively (see Figure 1). The growing number of old people implies an increasing demand for care for the elderly. In 2009, the number of old people who need long-term care was 362,584 which constituted 1.55% of the total population. Two-thirds (245,551) are the frail elderly and one-third (117,033) are persons with severe disabilities. Most of the elderly live in the community and are cared by female family members (e.g., wife, daughter- in-law, and daughter), while about 15% are cared by live-in care workers at private homes (Ministry of Health, 2009).

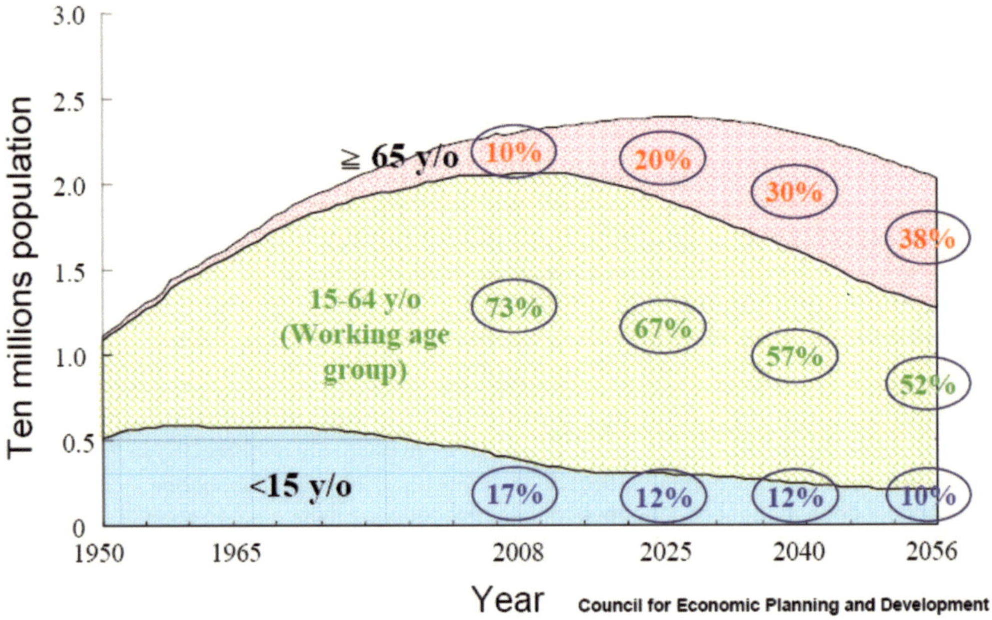

Fig. 1. Population structure of Taiwan in the next 50 years[11]

2.2 Decline of family size

Over the past fifteen years, the family structure of Taiwan has been shaped by a number of social forces. Firstly, a growing number of women received a high education. Women and men are almost equal in college and university education. This change has led to Taiwanese women's increasing involvement in labor force participation. In 2009, the women's labor force participation rate was 49.62% that improved 3.59% compared to 1999. The increase of women in labor force participation reduces the availability of women in providing unpaid care and domestic work.

Secondly, the decline of birth rate and family size are predicted to result in the shortage of younger people available to care for the elderly. In 2009, the birth rate of Taiwan was1.03 ‰

[1] The power point file entitled "Female labor force participation in Taiwan" has been presented by Taiwan Research Team at FLOWS Kick-off meeting, February 7th-9th 2011, in Aalborg University, Aalborg, Demark.

that decreased from 1.68 ‰ in 2000 (Ministry of the Interior, 2010). This implies that each family has less available manpower to care for the family elderly. Although the government has recently provided incentives to encourage young families to give birth of next generations, the birth rate continues to decline. This trend puts care for the elderly in urgency.

Thirdly, the family structure of Taiwan has also been shaped by the trends of modernization and urbanization. Currently, a growing proportion of the younger generation prefers to live without their parents in urban areas. In Taiwanese culture, however, filial piety is the fundamental principle governing family relations and this principle implies that the next generation, particularly sons, must take responsibility for caring the family elderly. Those who fail to care for their parents face severe criticism (Cheng, 2003; Lan, 2000; Pan and Yang, 2008).

Together, these factors make the elderly become a major concern for Taiwanese families. With little support from the government, however, Taiwan middle-class families are likely to depend on paid employment for providing care for the family elderly. In her studies on live-in care workers, Lan (2003b) names the trend of employing migrant women workers for providing care for the family elderly as 'outsourcing of filial piety' which in turn brings a significant influence on the family dynamics of Taiwanese household in everyday relation.

3. Policies and regulations regarding migrant live-in worker

The increasing number of migrant care worker in Taiwan has demonstrated how population changes affect the internal dynamics of family everyday life. In Taiwan, the term of "migrant care workers" usually refers to women from Southeast Asia providing care for the frail elderly or people with severe disabilities either in institutions or in private households. Currently, there are 190,000 live-in care workers from Indonesia, Vietnam, and the Philippines, constituting about 1% of the total population of Taiwan and representing 48 % of all migrant workers in Taiwan (see Figure 2).

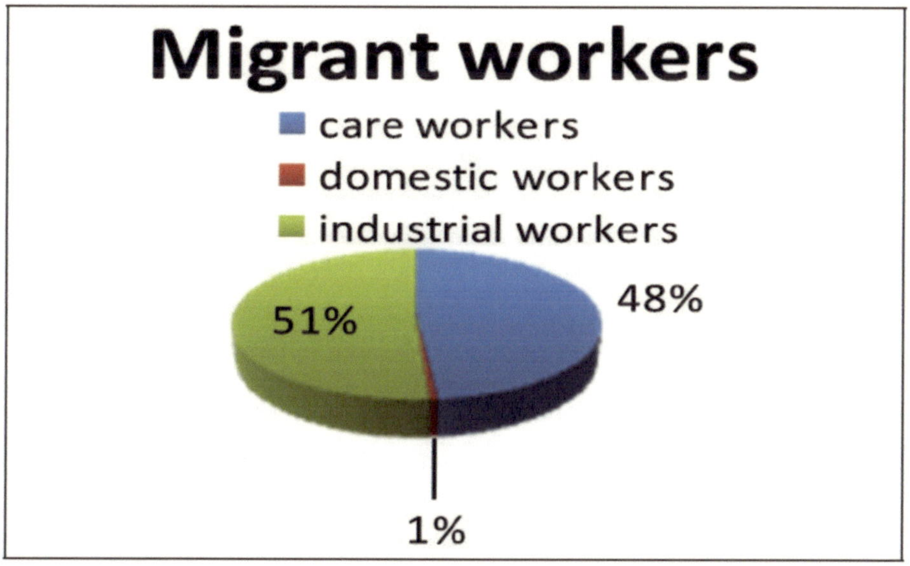

Fig. 2. Migrant workers in Taiwan - Source: Council of Labor Affairs (2011.3)

In 1989, Taiwan opened its gate to migrant workers. In 1992, foreign women can legally enter Taiwan as domestic workers and caregivers for the chronically ill, the elderly and the very young. Family could apply for live-in care workers based on the scores of the Activities of Daily Living (ADL) since then. Each year thousands of females from Southeast Asia enter Taiwan to work as care and domestic workers. Most migrant women workers work long hours up to 14-18 hours daily, without regular days off, for minimum wage (NT$ 17,942, approximately US$ 600). Migrant live-in workers are rarely allowed outside and are often prohibited from speaking with neighbors and outsiders. Even worse, this live-in working situation sometimes becomes a situation of abuse at the hands of their employers (Pan and Yang 2011).

Migrant women workers come to Taiwan to materially improve the lives of their families. However, to work in Taiwan these migrant women workers must ask the bank for a high interest loan. Repaying this money can cost over two-thirds of their salaries during their first year of work, and leave very little money to support their families. Most live-in care workers therefore hope to stay in the same household throughout their three-year working contract without being transferred to another employer. Immigration policy and labor law originally limited female migrant workers in Taiwan to a stay of just three years and this stay was extended to six years in 2007. This stay was extended to nine years in late 2008, and the requirement that they must work for the same employer throughout this period was removed.

According to Taiwan labor law, all migrant workers must be paid at least with the minimum wage. It is not uncommon to hear reports of live-in care workers being paid less than the minimum wage. Many live-in care workers find themselves working nearly around the clock, seven days a week. Some live-in workers are subjected to physical battery and sexual assault, but rarely reported to the police office because of the language barrier and their isolated living and working conditions. In the absence of hard evidence, accusations of sexual assault by their employers are more likely to lead to deportation than the redressing of their grievances.

4. Literature review

4.1 Sexual violence against migrant women workers

Since the early 1970s, sexual violence against women has become a central topic for women's liberation movement. Many researches, interventions and strategies have emerged to deal with many forms of sexual violence. However, only few researches have investigated this issue based on the perspective of the victim or in relation to migrant women workers.

Over the past ten years, there has been an extensive literature on the topic of global migration, particularly on the political economy of maid trade (Gibson, Law and McKay, 2001; Cheng, 2003; Lyons, 2007). Some feminist researches focused on the links between intrahousehold dynamics and migration (Chang, 2000;Yeoh and Huang, 1998 &2000; Lan, 2003a). Others explored the situation faced by migrant women workers (Abu-Habib, 1998; Huang and Yeoh, 2003; Loveband, 2004; Mantouvalou, 2006). But only few researches examined sexual violence against female migrant workers in their employments (Huang and Yeoh, 2007). Indeed, the empirical research on sexual abuse against female migrant workers is scant (Bach, 2003). Many studies only mention such sexual abuse but usually do not further analyze it. Even on those rare occasions when analysis is conducted, it tends to focus on general working conditions.

Recently, discussion on sexual abuse against migrant women workers has been from ILO (2003) and Human Rights Watch (2005). According to Human Rights Watch (2005), sexual abuse is likely to be underreported owing to the isolation of live-in care workers in the workplace and the deep social stigma attached to sexual assault. Huang and Yeoh (2007) investigated maid abuse in Singapore by using data from court transcripts and press reports and noted that most cases of physical abuse are perpetrated by women while most cases of sexual abuse are perpetrated by men.

Aihwa Ong (1991) argued that violence against live-in domestic workers in Asian families cannot ignore how the family and cultural norms shape family dynamics and relations in everyday life. In Taiwan, gender orders are deeply rooted in the traditional culture which is characterized by patriarchal family structure and the maintenance of traditional gender roles. This patriarchal culture encourages women to internalize values involving endurance and submission to maintain family harmony and moreover expects women to identify with family, by acting as self-sacrificing mothers, wives, and daughters. The influences of patriarchal gender orders on gender relations in everyday life maintain male dominance and female subordination within the family.

In Taiwan, many studies of migrant women workers have identified the power disparities between migrant women workers and their employers. But the power between employers and migrant workers is not monolithic and static. In her study on the dynamics involved in the relationships between Filipina domestics and their Taiwanese female employers, Cheng (2004) observed that globalization has introduced different relations and power dynamics within the private sphere. Taiwanese female employers redefine their domestic roles as household managers but struggle with deep anxieties associated with their womanhood and motherhood. Lan (2000, 2003b) also supported this argument by indicating that both live-in care workers and their employers negotiate their boundaries in the domestic politics of food, space, and privacy from one another on a daily basis.

Although replacing female family roles through their work, live-in care workers did not enjoy the same power as true female family members. Under the logic of kinship, which emphasizes blood and marital relations, live-in care workers are excluded and even seen as strangers. This position renders them powerless within the household. For instance, migrant women workers must obey all members of the family, even including young children. No regulations specify what work live-in domestic workers should or should not perform, and thus they are forced to provide twenty-four-hour care and perform endless household duties. If the families of their employers are dissatisfied with their work, migrant women workers are blamed or even beaten by their employers.

The working conditions of live-in care workers can be exacerbated by family kinship relationships. Unlike the West, in Taiwan, 'the family' signifies not a household but rather a network of family relationships that can include multiple households. In Taiwan, close relatives typically maintain close relationships by living either together or in close proximity to one another. However, while the provision of mutual support has many benefits, excessive emphasis on kinship ties can create problems for outsiders.

In sum, patrilineal kinship reinforces the power disparities between migrant women workers and their employers. However, the institutions of both immigration and labor system support this exploitation by patriarchal culture. Global migration can transform the traditional patriarchy faced by live-in care workers in their natal families, but the living and working conditions they face during their employment tie them to a multifaceted oppression.

One might expect that globalization lead to global migration, which would then attract the attention of scholars in different academic disciplines to study the different aspects of the global migration. There are indeed many such studies but very few of them are related to sexual abuse against migrant care workers. Furthermore, due to feminist advocacy, research on sexual violence against women has become important. Yet the sexual violence against migrant women is still ignored. So this chapter uses data drawn from in-depth interviews and documents from newspaper reports to examine the situations faced by live-in care workers in Taiwanese households within the context of transnational migration.

5. Research methods

5.1 Fieldwork

In Taiwan, live-in care workers suffering abuse from employers cannot seek help via existing channels designed to prevent domestic violence. Help mostly comes from church-affiliated NGOs providing shelter for battered migrant women workers. Most of these battered migrant women living in shelters submit arbitrations and wait to be transferred to other employers. Few file to sue for physical harm, sexual assault, or rape committed by their previous employers. Therefore, it was impossible for researchers to reach sexually abused migrant women workers directly, and all study participants were referred by church-affiliated NGO personnel throughout Taiwan.

5.2 Data collection

This study conducted fieldworks, including participant observation and in-depth interviews, between Sept. 2006 and Nov. 2007. Initially, this study performed participant observation at St. Christopher Catholic Church in Taipei as well as shelters for migrant workers organized by church-affiliated NGOs. Subsequently, this study performed in-depth interviews with 16 migrant women workers. Five of the 16 migrant women workers interviewed had experienced sexual abuse at the hands of their employers or their families, and three had experienced both sexual and physical abuse. The discussion in the following section is thus derived mainly from these five sexually abused migrant women workers.

Each interview lasted approximately 1.5—3.5 hours, and were mostly conducted either in English, in Chinese, or in the native language of the interviewees (with the assistance of translator). All participants were asked questions regarding their employers, their reasons for working in Taiwan, their living and working conditions, the process and pattern of abuse, and their efforts to seek help. All participants were fully informed of the study objectives, and in-depth interviews were conducted after obtaining written or verbal informed consent. Each study participant was provided with a US$ 20~$25 gift. All interviews were audio-recorded and transcripts are analyzed.

5.3 Participants

Table 1 lists the characteristics of the five migrant domestic workers who experienced sexual abuse by their employers (all identified by pseudonyms). Three of the five are from Vietnam, and two are from Indonesia and they are in their thirties and early forties. All but one was married and had children. All had experienced overwork, and some also had experienced inadequate rest and food. Additionally, they were frequently prevented from contacting friends, threatened with deportation, and subject to withholding of salary and documentation.

Name	Portraits
Beauty	A 39 year old married Vietnamese woman who was sexually assaulted by the brother of her employer.
Omar	A 36 year old married Indonesian woman who suffered physical abuse at the hands of the mother of her employer and sexual abuse at the hands of the father of her employer.
Snow	A 48 year old married Vietnamese woman who suffered severe physical abuse at the hand of the wife of her employer and sexual abuse at the hands of her employer.
Kim	A 44 year old single Vietnamese woman who suffered sexual assaults at the hands of her employer and his father.
Lisa	A 30 year old married Indonesian woman who suffered physical abuse at the hands of the mother of her employer and sexual assault at the hands of the father of her employer.

Table 1. Portraits of Sexual Violence against Migrant Women Workers

5.4 Data analysis

All of the interviews were audio recorded and transcribed. Each transcript was checked and read by two persons, the researcher and research assistant, to maximize familiarity with the phenomenon of abuse and ensure consistent interpretation. Thematic analysis was adopted for the data analysis. Data were interpreted based on categories related to socio-cultural contexts, family care and housework arrangements in everyday situations, and the concept of micro disciplinary technology was adopted to describe physical and sexual abuse. This study also probed scenarios and activities that can be identified and assigned to thematic interpretations of the problems of sexual abuse faced by these five migrant domestic workers in the Taiwanese households in which they worked.

5.5 Documentary analysis

This study conducted a documentary analysis of the newspaper reports and court transcripts to understand the situation faced by sexually abused migrant women workers. Since 1992, there were approximately 104 cases of sexual violence against live-in care workers reported by the newspapers. Perpetrators of fifty-five cases (approximately 53%) reported by the newspapers were sentenced while 49 cases were not guilty.

Furthermore, this study also used data from court transcripts. Between 2001 and 2010, there were nine cases from judicial court. Seven perpetrators of nine cases were sentenced while two perpetrators were not guilty. Six victims of nine cases are Indonesian and the other three victims are from Filipina, Vietnam, and China. Eight victims of nine cases were sexually abused by their employers and relatives. One victim was sexually abused by her agent. The incident of sexual abuse occurred mainly in the household of their employer while one incident occurred in outside of the employer's household.

The numerical discrepancy between cases reported by newspapers and cases reported by judicial courts is primarily due to the lengthy nature of Criminal Law procedures. Almost no employers are willing to hire abused migrant care workers, and particularly when they are involved in lawsuits. Consequently, most sexually abused migrant care workers choose not to press charges. The cases of some sexually abused migrant care workers are simply not represented in the court records owing to no sentence being handed down.

6. The family secret of multiple abuse

Taiwan currently hosts an estimated 190,000 live-in care workers, mainly from Indonesia and Vietnam. Restricted by onerous regulations associated with the foreign labor system, migrant women workers often experience workplace exploitation and abuse. Despite the high risk of sexual abuse at the hands of employers, few official complaints are made and few stories of abuse become public. Such incidents of sexual abuse frequently remain secret because of the isolated nature of workplaces and the deep social stigma associated with sexual assault.

As Radford & Tsutsumi (2004) observed, globalization increased opportunities for violence by men in rich countries against poor women from the Third World. However, the abusers include both female and male employers. According to the fieldwork of Pan and Yang (2011), physical abuse against live-in care workers tends to occur following sexual abuse within individual households. Domestic workers suffering sexual abuse at the hands of family members not living in the same household as their employer do not generally also suffer physical abuse. In the case of sexual assaults of domestic workers by perpetrators living in the same household as the employer, victims are frequently also suffering physical abuse at the hands of the wife.

The following cases illustrate the circumstances of three of five study participants who endured sexual abuse during their employment as domestic workers in Taiwan.

6.1 Case 1

Beauty is a 39 year old married Vietnamese woman and a mother of three children. To improve the living conditions of her family, Beauty decided to work in Taiwan as live-in care worker. The broker told Beauty that she would only be responsible for caring for the brother of her employer, who was suffering from a mental illness. However, after her arrival Beauty was instead sent to care for the father of her employer, who was staying in a hospital. The father died after two months, and Beauty was then sent back to the home of her employer to care for the mother of her employer and his newborn daughter.

Beauty was employed by a typical Taiwanese family composed of multiple households and enormous numbers of relatives. Beauty had to do housework for these family relatives everyday. Rising at 4:30 am, Beauty began cleaning and washing up, then took 'A-Ma' (the mother of her employer) to the nearby park to exercise. Beauty then had to return home sufficiently early to prepare breakfasts for the family. In the daytime, all family members went to school or work. Alone with only 'A-Ma' and a young baby girl, Beauty was responsible for taking care of them. While the baby was sleeping after lunch, she had to do housework for nearby relatives and then returned to prepare dinner. By the time she had completed all of her work, it was typically almost 11 pm. Usually Beauty took her meals only after everyone else had finished, but she said that since the family gave her enough to eat she felt it was okay.

An incident occurred when Beauty was cleaning the house of the older brother of her employer. Beauty and the older brother of her employer were the only persons at home, and the brother, lying on the bed dressed only in his underpants, asked her for a massage. As Beauty later said, 'that was really embarrassing'. Beauty gently refused and complained to 'A-Ma' when she returned home. Unfortunately, the situation did not improve, and on a subsequent occasion the older brother touched her inappropriately while she was working at his home. She ran back home and complained to 'A-Ma' again, and in response was dismissed without reason.

During the interview, Beauty had already spent several months living in a shelter operated by the church-affiliated NOG, and was waiting for a new assignment to another household. After suffering an incident of sexual harassment, Beauty preferred not to complain because, in her words: "every member of this family was good to me".

6.2 Case 2

Omar is a 36 year old Indonesian woman who is married and a mother of two sons. Omar was working in Taiwan for the first time, after having previously worked for six years in Malaysia and Brunei. The household of her employer comprised eight family members, including the couple employing her, their parents, their three young children, and one adult brother. Besides caring for this large household, Omar also had to do housework for another brother of her employer, who was married and lived nearby.

Omar had to get up at 6 am every day and begin the daily work of cleaning the five-story house, washing clothes, and preparing breakfast for the parents of the employer, 'A-Ma' and 'A-koun.' She also prepared lunch and dinner for the whole family.

Omar suffered sexual harassment from 'A-koun', the 77 year old father of her employer, who had limited mental function. Despite working in a big house, Omar had no private space of her own, instead sharing a room with the parents of her employer where she slept on the floor beside their bed. At night, 'A-koun' frequently touched her. She complained about this situation to 'A-Ma' (his wife) who did nothing to help but did become jealous.

One afternoon when Omar was bathing 'A'Koun', he asked her for sexual services. Subsequently, 'A-koun' played with himself in front of Omar, and continued to do this regularly. When Omar complained to her broker, the employer, and 'A-Ma', their response was simply 'it is okay, he is just an old man. It doesn't matter'. Omar felt sad and angry that nobody cared about what she was going through. Omar eventually decided not to tolerate her situation any longer and phoned the Department of Labor, which gave her the telephone number of a church-affiliated NGO. She then ran away.

6.3 Case 3

Snow is a 48 year old married Vietnamese woman and a mother of two sons. To support her poor family, Snow came to Taiwan two years ago to work as a live-in care worker. While she knew that she would have to work for a family with multiple households, she had no idea how harsh the work would turn out to be. Following sexual and physical abuse at the hands of her employers, she eventually underwent psychotherapy at a shelter established by a Vietnamese pastor. The father described his impression of Snow as follows: 'as a human being her dignity was totally destroyed by this family. Recently her smile has returned and she has also gained some weight.'

For the past two years, Snow worked for a middle-aged couple. Her employer was a busy businessman, with a wife who stayed at home. The wife demanded Snow cover her mouth with a surgical mask while in the house. Failure to comply was punished with a US$3.5 deduction from her salary. Every day Snow had to perform housework for three relatives, including two sisters of her employer, in addition to preparing dinner for the employer and his wife. Consequently, Snow only had time for one meal per day herself. Whether Snow ate lunch depended on her employer's wife. If the wife ate lunch, she might give the leftover rice or noodles to Snow. But if the wife did not eat lunch, Snow also went without lunch. Sometimes Snow was allowed to cook, but only plain noodle soup, without even salt or oil. Consequently Snow was perpetually starving. Facing food deprivation and an excessive burden of housework, Snow lost significant body weight. Snow's employer and his sisters all knew what Snow was experiencing, but nobody was willing to intervene against the wife. The sisters of Snow's employer secretly fed Snow when she worked at their houses.

Snow did not have a room of her own despite the house having numerous empty rooms. Instead, Snow was forced to sleep outside on the balcony. Snow used to put an umbrella up if it was raining, and paid a heavy price if the umbrella did not work. Snow's telephone card was held by her employer's wife, who prevented her from making phone calls. One day when Snow forgot to put her mouth mask on, her employer's wife cursed her hysterically and hit her around the head. Snow was beaten by the wife almost daily, depending on her mood swings.

One day, when her employer was not at home, his wife hit Snow's head against the wall. Snow pleaded for the beating to stop, but the wife continued. Snow eventually fainted and the wife dashed water on her face. Snow asked her broker to come and arrange a change of employer but her broker refused to get involved. The sisters of her employer then cared for Snow and asked her to see the doctor, but Snow was unwilling.

Snow suffered abuse not only from the wife of her employer but also from the employer himself. She recounted that her employer had asked her to have sexual relations with him when his wife was not at home on three or four occasions. When Snow refused, her employer threatened to send her back to Vietnam, and so Snow consented under duress. One day Snow told her employer's wife about this situation, and the wife responded by beating her more frequently than ever. Snow could not talk to anyone outside the family except when disposing of the garbage in the evening. One day while Snow was waiting for the garbage car, a fellow Vietnamese female worker asked why she had bruises. Snow told this woman her horrible situation and the woman gave her the Vietnamese pastor's cellular phone number. Snow phoned the pastor, and then fled the house by taxi.

Taiwanese society has low tolerance for sexual violence against women, but migrant women workers are often an exception. The exploitation of migrant women workers as sexual objects is sometimes taken as a way of protecting marital relations by reducing the probability of affairs involving male family members. Consequently, families typically prefer to treat this issue as a family secret, creating a conspiracy of silence. The story of Beauty, described above, reflects this family conspiracy to hide sexual violence against migrant women workers. When Beauty refused to have sex with her employer's brother, her employer immediately sent her to the office of the Department of Labor. In the stories of Omar and Snow, the wives of the perpetrators avoided dealing with the behavior of their husbands, and instead expressed their negative emotions such as anger and jealousy through physically abusing the victims of that behavior.

The most common threat made to migrant women workers was being sent back to their home countries. This threat was frequently made by employers subjecting workers to unreasonable work expectations, including working for multiple employers and providing sexual services. For example, Snow was forced to have sexual relations with her employer under threat of being sent back to Vietnam. Her employer's wife knew of this incident but offered no sympathy, instead yelling: 'why don't you leave my house?' contradicting this on other occasions by saying 'If you dare to leave, I would not let you back again.'

The reasons behind the prevalence of sexual harassment and assault of migrant women workers in households are unclear. Some attribute the phenomena to a lack of personal space, as occurs in the cases of Omar and Snow, while others attribute it to the patriarchal culture of Taiwan. This study has demonstrated that employers frequently utilize strategies such as threats of dismissal and being sent back to their home countries, as well as coarse language, to discipline female migrant workers and ensure their compliance, obedience and subordination. However, the PGFDW reinforced exploitation in everyday household relationships.

7. The media, the law and abused live-in care workers

The informal and personalized nature of domestic work increases the risk of live-in domestic workers being abused, yet such abuse is rarely reported to the authorities. The results of this study have also revealed the discrepancies of number between abused and reported. For example, since 2001 there were approximately 100 newspaper reports on sexual assaults against migrant women workers in Taiwan, but there were only nine cases presented in Court Proceedings. Besides, according to one advocator of a famous NGO for migrant workers in North Taiwan, the organization provided helps for 400 abused migrant women workers every year, but she believed that the number of being abused migrant women workers should be higher than 400 hundred cases (The United Daily News, Oct. 17,2007, C2).

Reasons for not reporting to the authorities or not escaping from the workplace are threats by perpetrators to 'terminate the contract' (Min Sheng Daily News, Dec. 3, 2004, A4) and 'send you back to home country' (The United Daily News, Dec. 29, 2007, C2). In 2005, the newspaper revealed that more than fifty Vietnamese women workers were raped by a broker and his son (The United Daily News, May 27, 2005, C4). One Catholic father from a NGO for Vietnamese workers pointed out that the tragedy of these abused Vietnamese women workers is caused by the regulations governing foreign labor worker in which migrant workers are not allowed to change their employers and switch employment categories. The father called this 'the murder by the system' (The Min Sheng Daily News, May, 19, 2005, A2).

According to the Court Proceedings and newspaper reports, most perpetrators of sexual assault against migrant women workers are their employers, their employer's relatives and brokers. Few incidents are caused by the strangers. Most abused migrant women workers endured sexual abuse in their employment for a long period of time (The United Evening News, Dec. 16, 2000, No.5) and suffered from physical harms and psychological trauma (The United Evening News, Jan. 2, 2004, No. 6; The Liberty Times, Sept. 17, 2008, B2). Some even attempted to commit suicide (The United Evening News, Dec. 16, 2000, No. 5).

According to Pan and Yang's study (2012), the abuse against live-in care workers is prevalent in Taiwan, because families tend to treat this issue as a family secret. But a case drew much national attention. Rose, a Filipina live-in care worker, was raped by her employer who is a famous legislator in Taiwan. After the incident, Rose escaped from the workplace and seeked helps from the Manila Economic and Cultural Office (MECO) in Taipei. The MECO reported to the Taipei City Center for Prevention of Domestic Violence and Sexual Assault (TCCPDVSA). One NGO for migrant worker rights in Taipei tried to help Rose. Rose was sent back to the Philippines a week later. This legislator claimed that he is innocent while his wife made a compromise with Rose via the MECO. Rose was paid for US $ 28,000 but she had to go back to her home country and never tells the truth of this incident again (The United Daily News, Feb. 16, 2004, A3). The week before Rose left Taiwan, there was nobody who could contact with her even the workers of this NGO. Rose told her friends that she was confined by the MECO and forced by administers of the MECO to sign a compromised contract with her employer's wife (The United Daily News, Feb. 17, 2004, A3).

According to Ong (1991), Asian families typically regard workers as children who should obey their 'parents' (i.e. supervisors). Taiwanese family dynamics and relations in everyday life are significantly influenced by the patriarchal family value and cultural norms, which maintain male dominance and female subordination within the family. This patrilineal culture and gender norm may put live-in care workers at a double disadvantage within Taiwanese household. Migrant women workers are expected to act as a daughter of this family but they do not have the same right as daughters.

Taiwanese often perceive migrant women workers as the property of the family. Some employers may assume that live-in care workers would like to do anything even sexual trade for money since they mostly come from poor families. Consequently, the employers who raped the live-in care workers did not feel guilty for their behaviors because they thought they paid for the trade. One guy raped the migrant women worker who takes care of his grandmother when his grandfather was not at home. He said, 'it's a loss not to do this when my grandfather was not at home' (The United Daily News, March 22, 2008, A19). Many perpetrators of sexual assault against live-in care workers have argued that the incident is a kind of 'sexual trade.' For example, as the Court Proceedings of N1 and N2 show, the live-in care workers were forced to have sex with their employers, but their employers claimed that the migrant women worker agreed to have sex with him because he gave money to her (see Table 2).

No.	Nationality	Perpetrators	Place of incident	Help-seeking	Sentence
G1	Indonesia	Employer's relative	Perpetrator's home	Report to the Police office	Yes
G2	Indonesia	Employer	Employer's home	Report to the Police office	Yes
G3	Vietnam	Employer's Son	Employer's home	Report to her broker and the authority	Yes
G4	Indonesia	Broker	Motel	Run away	Yes
G5	China	Employer	Employer's home	Call her friend	Yes
G6	Indonesia	Employer	Employer's home	Report to her broker	Yes
G7	Indonesia	Employer	Employer's home	Call 113 (hotline for prevention of domestic violence and sexual abuse)	Yes
N1	Filipinos	Employer	Employer's home	Escape from the workplace	No
N2	Indonesia	Employer	Employer's home	Cal 113	No

Table 2. Bio-data of Victims from Court Proceedings (2001~2010)

The above discussions revealed that most perpetrators of sexual assaults against migrant women workers are neither recidivists nor persons with criminal records. Many of them are from middle class with highly educated background (The United Daily News, Aug. 20, 2003, A8). Why did they dare to do this and did not care about how the family would react to this incident? It is not easy to explain this. It seems that this is related to many factors. Pan and Yang (2012) called this prevailing phenomenon of sexual violence against migrant women workers in Taiwan 'conspiracy of silence.' And, Anderson (2001) attributed this phenomenon to the multifaceted oppression embedded in the dynamics of race, gender, and class. Feminist scholars such as Mantouvalou (2006) and Pyle (2006) characterized the living circumstances faced by migrant domestic workers in industrial countries as 'domestic slavery' or 'modern-day slavery.'

8. Conclusion

No matter what globalization means this term gains its tremendous popularity even outside the academic. Sometimes it means global migration, which brings up the optimistic argument but the pessimistic argument also play its role to show the old dark side recurrent in the new context of global migration. Yet by repeating old argument, many studies indicate the old but still important issues such as the exploitation of migrant care workers. This study demonstrates how the aging population and the low birth rate in Taiwan intersect with the trend of global migration and bring in migrant care workers and analyzes the exploitation of these worker such as overwork even work for multiple households which is against the law.

But this study also argues that exploitation cannot fully explain the whole situation of migrant care workers by showing the sexual abuse against these workers, which is ignored by studies of migration and sexual violence against women. Although this study does not present the specific characteristics of this sexual abuse compared to other sexual violence, it seem that most migrant women care worker are sexually abused by the employers and their relatives and these workers suffered from long-term and continuous sexual abuse. It is very difficult for these workers to file a suit, because they face the employers who have tremendous power over them and the labor regulations and the policy by the government. This study has investigated the social-cultural context in Taiwan, which leads to the sexual abuse by the employer and his relatives. This study also reveals prejudice/stereotype/ideology, which operates in this context to justify or cover up the sexual abuse. For example, why the sexual abuse against care workers tends to be covered up by the family is this not related to race, class, and indifference to the outsider/foreigner status or xenophobia and micro-power politics. The male employers justify their abusive behavior by claiming that this is a trade and they had already paid the money. Is this justification not related to gender discrimination or the kind of stereotype that if the migrant women worker is willing to sell her labor, she is willing to have sex with the employer for money?

9. Acknowledgments

The authors would like to thank the National Science Council of the Republic of China, Taiwan for financially supporting this research under Contract No. NSC 95-2412-H-003-MY2. The authors are grateful to all those who assisted with or participated in this study. The authors would like to thank research assistants, Kai-Chi Chuang and Pei-Fang Hsieh, for their assistance in putting this study together, and Ted Knoy is appreciated for his editorial assistance.

10. References

Abu-Habib, Lina (1998), "The Use and Abuse of Female Domestic Workers from Sri Lanka in Lebanon," Gender and Development, 6(1): 52-56.

Anderson, Bridget (2001), "Why Madam has so Many Bathrobes: Demand for Migrant Domestic Workers in the EU," Tijdschrift voor Economische en Sociale Geografie, 92(1): 18-26.

Bach, Stephen (2003), Selectoral Activities Progrmme: Working Paper— International Migration of Health Workers: Labour and Social Issues, International Labour Office, Geneva.

Chang, Grace (2000), Disposable Domestics: Immigrant Women Workers in the Global Econnomy, New York: Routledge.

Cheng, Shu-Ju Ada (2003), "Rethinking the Globalization of Domestic Service: Foreign Domestics, State Control, and the Politics of Identity in Taiwan", Gender & Society, 17(2), 166-186.

Cheng, Shu-Ju Ada (2004), "When the Personal Meets the Global at Home: Filipina Domestics and Their Female Employers in Taiwan," Frontiers, 25(2): 31-52.

Council for Economic Planning and Development (2008), "Population estimation from 2008 to 2056 in Taiwan," Council of Economic Planning and Development, Republic of China, Taiwan.

Gibson, Katherine, Lisa Law & Deirdre McKay (2001), "Beyond Heroes and Victims", International Feminist Journal of Politics, 3(3): 365-386.

Huang, Shirlena & Brenda S. A. Yeoh (2007), "Emotional Labour and Transnational Domestic Work: The Moving Geographies of 'Maid Abuse' in Singapore," Mobilities, 2(2): 195-217.

Huang, Shirlena & Brenda S. A. Yeoh (2003), "The difference gender makes: State policy and contract migrant workers in Singapore," Asian and Pacific Migration Journal, 12 (1-2): 75-97.

Human Rights Watch (2005), Maid to Order: Ending Abuses against Migrant Domestic Workers in Singapore, Human Rights Watch.

International Labour Office (2003), Preventing Discrimination, Exploitation and Abuse of Women Migrant Workers: An Information Guide, Geneva: Gender Promotion Programme, International Labour Office.

Lan, Pei-Chia (2000), Global Divisions, Local Identities: Filipian Migrant Domestic Workers and Taiwanese Employers, Ph.D. Dissertation, Department of Sociology, NorthwesternUniversity Press.

Lan, Pei-Chia (2003a), "Maid or Madam? Filipina Migrant Workers and the Continuity of Domestic Labor," Gender & Society, 17(2): 187-208.

Lan, Pei-Chia (2003b), "Negotiating Social Boundaries and Private Zones: The Micropolitics of Empoying Migrant Domestic Workers," Social Problems, 50(4):525-549.

Lan, Pei-Chia (2006), Global Cinderellas: Mirgrant Domestic and Newly Rich Employers in Taiwan, London: Duke University Press.

Liang, Li-Fang (2011), "The Making of an 'Ideal' Live-in Migrant Care Worker: Recruiting, Training, Matching and Disciplining", Ethnic and Racial Studies, (forthcoming Article).

Lin, Chin-Ju (1999), "Filipina Domestic Workers in Taiwan: Structural Constraints and Personal Resistance," Taipei: Taiwan Grassroots Women Workers' Centre.

Loveband, Anne (2004), "Positioning the Product: Indonesian Migrant Women Workers in Taiwan." Journal of Contemporary Asia, 34(3): 336-348.

Lyons, Lenore (2007), "Dignity Overdue: Women's Rights Activism in Support of Foreign Domestic Workers in Singapore", Women's Studies Quarterly, 35(3&4): 106-122.

Mantouvalou, Virginia (2006), "Servitude and Forced Labour in the 21st Century: The Human Rights of Domestic Workers," Industrial Law Journal, 35(4): 395-415.

Ministry of Health (2009), "National Citizen Health Survey," Ministry of Health, Republic of China, Taiwan.

Ministry of the Interior (2010), "Population Statistics," Ministry of Interior, Republic of China, Taiwan.

Ong, Aihwa (1991), "The Gender and Labor Politics of Postmodernity," Annual Review of Anthropology, 20: 279-309.

Pan, Shu-Man and Jung-Tsung Yang (2008), "Cultural constructions of female homelessness in Taiwan", Journal of Social Distress and the Homeless,17 (3), 53-71.

Pan, Shu-Man and Jung-Tsung Yang (2012), "Strangers in the Family: Abuse of Migrant Domestic Workers in Taiwan", Asian Journal of Women's Studies, (forthcoming).

Pyle, Jean L. (2006), "Globalization and the Increase in Transnational Care Work: The Flip Side," Globalizations, 3(3): 297-315.

Radford, Lorraine, & Kaname Tsutsumi (2004), "Globalization and Violence against Women—Inequalities in Risks, Responsibilities and Blame in the UK and Japan," Women's Studies International Forum, 27(1): 1-12.

Yeoh, Brenda S.A. & Shirlena Huang (1998), "Negotiating Public Space: Strategies and Styles of Migrant Female Domestic Workers in Singapore," Urban Studies, 35(3): 583-602.

Yeoh, Brenda S.A., & Shirlena Huang (2000), "Home" and "Away": Foreign Domestic Workers and Negotiations of Diasporic identity in Singapore", Women's Studies International Forum, 23(4): 413-429.